D1756997

Molecular Biology of Lung Disease

Molecular Biology of Lung Disease

EDITED BY

PETER J. BARNES

MA, DM, DSc, FRCP
Professor of Thoracic Medicine
National Heart and Lung Institute
and Honorary Consultant Physician
The Royal Brompton Hospital, London

AND

ROBERT A. STOCKLEY

MD, DSc, FRCP
Consultant Physician
Birmingham General Hospital

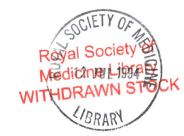

OXFORD

Blackwell Scientific Publications

LONDON EDINBURGH BOSTON

MELBOURNE PARIS BERLIN VIENNA

1994

© 1994 by
Blackwell Scientific Publications
Editorial Offices:
Osney Mead, Oxford OX2 0EL
25 John Street, London WC1N 2BL
23 Ainslie Place, Edinburgh EH3 6AJ
238 Main Street, Cambridge
   Massachusetts 02142, USA
54 University Street, Carlton
   Victoria 3053, Australia

Other Editorial Offices:
Librairie Arnette SA
1, rue de Lille
75007 Paris
France

Blackwell Wissenschafts-Verlag GmbH
Düsseldorfer Str. 38
D-10707 Berlin
Germany

Blackwell MZV
Feldgasse 13
A-1238 Wien
Austria

First published 1994

Set by Setrite Typesetters, Hong Kong
Printed and bound in Great Britain
by Hartnolls Ltd, Bodmin, Cornwall

DISTRIBUTORS

Marston Book Services Ltd
PO Box 87
Oxford OX2 0DT
(*Orders*: Tel: 0865 791155
          Fax: 0865 791927
          Telex: 837515)

USA
Blackwell Scientific Publications, Inc.
238 Main Street
Cambridge, MA 02142
(*Orders*: Tel: 800 759-6102
              617 876-7000)

Canada
Times Mirror Professional Publishing Ltd
130 Flaska Drive
Markham, Ontario L6G 1B8
(*Orders*: Tel: 800 268-4178
              416 470-6739)

Australia
Blackwell Scientific Publications Pty Ltd
54 University Street
Carlton, Victoria 3053
(*Orders*: Tel: 03 347-5552)

A catalogue record for this title
is available from the British Library

ISBN 0-632-03344-4

Library of Congress
Cataloging in Publication Data

Molecular biology of lung disease/edited
by Peter J. Barnes, Robert A. Stockley.
      p.   cm.
   Includes bibliographical references
   and index.
   ISBN 0-632-03344-4
   1. Lungs — Diseases — Molecular
aspects. I. Barnes, Peter J., 1946–
II. Stockley, Robert A.
   [DNLM: 1. Lung Diseases — genetics.
2. Lung Diseases — physiopathology.
3. Lung Diseases — immunology.
WF 600 M718 1994]
RC756.M65   1994
616.2'407 — dc20
DNLM/DLC for Library of Congress

Contents

Contributors

SIMON C. AFFORD PhD
Liver Research Laboratories, Clinical Research Block, Queen Elizabeth Hospital, Birmingham, B15 2TH, UK

PETER J. BARNES MA, DM, DSc, FRCP
Professor, Department of Thoracic Medicine, Cardiothoracic Institute, Dovehouse Street, London SW3 6LY, UK

MICHAEL J. BIRRER MD, PhD
National Institutes of Health, National Cancer Institute, Biomarkers and Prevention Research Branch, 9610 Medical Center Drive, Suite 300, Rockville, Maryland 20850, USA

DAVID BURNETT PhD, FRCPath
Lung Immunobiochemical Research Laboratory, The Clinical Teaching Block, The General Hospital, Steelhouse Lane, Birmingham B4 6NH, UK

ROBIN W. CARRELL PhD, FRCP, FRCPath
Professor, Department of Haematology, University of Cambridge, MRC Centre, Hills Road, Cambridge CB2 2QH, UK

JACK A. ELIAS MD
Pulmonary and Critical Care Section, School of Medicine, LCI 105, 333 Cedar Street, PO Box 333, New Haven, Connecticut 06510–8057, USA

VINCENT C. EMERY BSc, PhD
Department of Virology, Royal Free Hospital School of Medicine, University of London, Rowland Hill Street, London NW3 2PF, UK

GREGORY P. GEBA MD
Pulmonary and Critical Care Section, Department of Internal Medicine, School of Medicine, LCI 105, 333 Cedar Street, PO Box 333, New Haven, Connecticut 06510–8057, USA

BALARAM GHOSH PhD
Professor, Johns Hopkins Asthma and Allergy Center at the Francis Scott Key Medical Center, 5501 Hopkins Bayview Circle, Baltimore, Maryland 21224, USA

PAUL D. GRIFFITHS BSc, MD, MRCPath
Professor, Department of Virology, Royal Free Hospital School of Medicine, University of London, Rowland Hill Street, London NW3 2PF, UK

JAMES C. HOGG MD
Professor, Pulmonary Research Laboratory, McDonald Research Wing, Room 100, St Paul's Hospital, 1081 Burrard Street, Vancouver, BC V6Z 1Y6, Canada

MICHAEL C. IANNUZZI MD
Pulmonary and Critical Care Medicine, Henry Ford Hospital, 2799 West Grand Boulevard, Detroit, Michigan 48202–2689, USA

LAN JORNOT PhD
Respiratory Division, Hôpital Cantonal, Universitaire de Genève, 24 rue Micheli-du-Crest, 1211 Genève 14, Switzerland

ALAIN F. JUNOD MD
Respiratory Division, Hôpital Cantonal, Universitaire de Genève, 24 rue Micheli-du-Crest, 1211 Genève 14, Switzerland

NOOR A. KALSHEKER MSc, MD, FRCPath
Professor, Department of Clinical Chemistry, Queen's Medical Centre, University Hospital, Nottingham NG7 2UH, UK

GEOFFREY J. LAURENT PhD
Department of Thoracic Medicine, National Heart and Lung Institute, University of London, Emanuel Kaye Building, Manresa Road, London SW3 6LR, UK

DAVID A. LOMAS MRCP
Department of Haematology, University of Cambridge, MRC Centre, Hills Road, Cambridge CB2 2QH, UK

DAVID G. MARSH PhD
Professor, Johns Hopkins Asthma and Allergy Center at the Francis Scott Key Medical Center, 5501 Hopkins Bayview Circle, Baltimore, Maryland 21224, USA

PETER K. MAYS PhD
Department of Biochemistry and Molecular Biology, Jefferson Institute of Molecular Medicine, Jefferson Medical College, Thomas Jefferson University, Philadelphia PA 19107, USA

KEVIN MORGAN PhD
Department of Clinical Chemistry, Queen's Medical Centre, University Hospital, Nottingham NG7 2UH, UK

JULIA M. POLAK DSc, MD, FRCPath
Professor, Department of Histochemistry, Royal Postgraduate Medical School, Hammersmith Hospital, DuCane Road, London W12 0NN, UK

RORY J. SHAW BSc, MD, FRCP
Chest and Allergy Clinic, St Mary's Hospital, London W2 1NY, UK

S. BERTEL SQUIRE BSc, MRCP
Department of Virology, Royal Free Hospital School of Medicine, University of London, Rowland Hill Street, London NW3 2PF, UK

ROBERT A. STOCKLEY MD, DSc, FRCP
Professor, Lung Immunobiochemical Research Laboratory, The Clinical Teaching Block, The General Hospital, Steelhouse Lane, Birmingham B4 6NH, UK

EVA SZABO MD
National Institutes of Health, National Cancer Institute, Biomarkers and Prevention Research Branch, 9610 Medical Center Drive, Suite 300, Rockville, Maryland 20850, USA

ELIZABETH SZTUL PhD
Department of Molecular Biology, Princeton University, Lewis Thomas Laboratory, Princeton, New Jersey 08544, USA

GIORGIO TERENGHI PhD
Blond McIndoe Centre, Queen Victoria Hospital, East Grinstead, Sussex, RH19 3DZ, UK

RALPH J. ZITNIK MD
Pulmonary and Critical Care Section, School of Medicine, LC1 105, 333 Cedar Street, PO Box 333, New Haven, Connecticut 06510–8057, USA

Preface

The past 5–10 years have seen enormous advances in the development of techniques in molecular biology and their application to the pathogenesis and clinical management of respiratory disease. The identification of genetic risk factors may help respiratory physicians determine susceptibility to diseases of the lung and take preventative measures or design specific intervention therapies. Molecular biology also provides a means for speedier and more specific diagnosis of respiratory diseases. The application of molecular biology in research has already led to many new insights in respiratory disease. Gene therapy is already a reality with the treatment of adenosine deaminase deficiency and, more recently, the first human studies of delivery of the cystic fibrosis transmembrane regulator to the lungs of patients with cystic fibrosis.

However, all this is happening at a time when many physicians have not had the time or the inclination to learn the terminology used in molecular biology or the power and limitations of the methodology. This book aims to bridge this gap in their knowledge whilst making the understanding of molecular biology as user-friendly as possible. We approached authors with established reputations who were using the techniques in the respiratory field with a remit to make their impact comprehensible to the non-expert. We hope that we have succeeded. Any book on molecular biology is rapidly outdated but our aim is to demonstrate the broad principles and its scope, as applied to respiratory diseases. We hope that this book will be used as a springboard for further reading in this rapidly advancing field.

Peter J. Barnes
Robert A. Stockley

1 Molecular biology: principles and applications

ROBERT A. STOCKLEY

Introduction

Although the term molecular biology should be applied to the study of all molecules involved in cell structure and function, it has been utilized largely to encompass the events involved in gene structure, function and manipulation. The advances being made in this branch of science are so rapid that the mere act of putting pen to paper often outdates the article being written. However, molecular biological technology is being applied to the understanding of pathogenesis, susceptibility, diagnosis and, more recently, the treatment of diseases in all branches of medicine. Many of the techniques employed are now automated and available as pre-packaged kits with almost cookery-book application and are becoming widely used.

The purpose of this opening chapter is to lay the foundation that will enable the non-expert to negotiate the following chapters successfully. There will be some repetitions (where appropriate) throughout the other chapters, but it is hoped that this introduction to some of the terminology and basic principles will also provide the necessary background for more general reading. Keywords and phrases have been highlighted in **bold** type and a short glossary is provided at the end. Further, more comprehensive texts are available from an array of standard textbooks and manuals.

The building blocks

Genes are functional units of DNA located on the chromosomes and the complete gene collection of the organism is referred to as the **genome**. Structural genes contain the information that determines the amino acid sequence of proteins whereas regulatory genes do not produce proteins but regulate the transcription of structural genes. Only about 1% of the DNA in human cells is involved in protein synthesis.

The genes of nucleated cells (**eukaryotes**) are composed of double-stranded DNA with each strand wound around each other in a double helix. The DNA is then compressed by three further levels of coiling. First, the double helix is coiled around spherical histone beads (which are DNA-binding proteins) to form a **nucleosome**. The nucleosomes are then coiled to form a cylinder and these are finally coiled as loops.

Each strand of DNA is made up of varying combinations of four similar but distinct **nucleotides**. These have a common deoxyribose sugar linked at the 5′ end to a phosphate group and at the 1′ end to one of four bases: adenine (A), thymine (T), cytosine (C) or guanine (G). The nucleotides are linked by a 3′–5′ phosphodiester bond as indicated in Fig. 1.1 resulting in a backbone consisting of alternating deoxyribose and phosphate groups with a free 5′ phosphate at one end (5′ end) and a free 3′ hydroxyl group at the other (3′ end). This is shown diagrammatically in Fig. 1.1. The bases project at right angles from the backbone and the double helix is stabilized by hydrogen bonds between bases on opposite strands. Base pairing is fixed and can only occur between A and T (two hydrogen bonds) and C and G (three hydrogen bonds).

Thus the nucleotide sequence of one strand determines the other and both strands are referred to as **complementary**. This specific pairing is utilized to identify specific DNA sequences using known complementary DNA (cDNA) sequences as probes (see below).

One strand of DNA is known as the **coding** strand and its complementary strand is the **template**. During gene transcription the template is used to make a complementary RNA (cRNA) strand that becomes the messenger RNA (mRNA). The mRNA is similar to the coding strand of the DNA with two exceptions.

1 The sugar backbone is ribose (gain of O at the 2′ position [Fig. 1.1] to make a hydroxyl group).

2 The base thymine is always replaced by uracil which now pairs with adenine. mRNA is always described as the **sense** strand and hence the

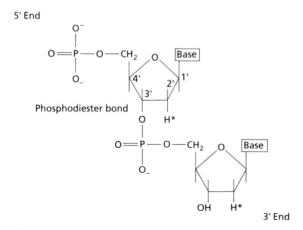

Fig. 1.1 Basic structure of DNA strand showing two deoxyribose sugars joined by a phosphodiester bond (3′–5′). The sugars are connected to the bases (A, T, C or G) as shown. The asterisk at the 2′ H atom represents the site of hydroxylation, which is a feature of ribose sugars incorporated into RNA.

template is an **antisense** sequence and its cDNA sequence (the coding strand) is a *sense* sequence (Fig. 1.2).

The order of nucleotides in a gene determines the signals that bind and activate the gene, where transcription starts, which sequences are transcribed into mRNA and which amino acids are assembled to make the protein. By convention the initial letters of the bases of the nucleotides are used in writing DNA sequences and only that of the coding strand 5′ to the left is given. Sequences to the left are said to be 5′ or *upstream* and those to the right, 3′ or *downstream*.

Genes vary in length from a few hundred to several thousand base pairs. The protein coding sequences are divided into blocks (**exons**) which are interspersed with non-coding regions (**introns**). The function of introns is largely unknown but they may contain some regions which enhance gene transcription. At the 5′ end of the gene, upstream from the coding sequences, are special sequences which control gene expression. Some of these are common for all genes whereas others may be specific only for certain genes. This area of the gene can contain few or multiple binding sites for promoting and enhancing the transcription. Figure 1.3 shows a simplified diagram of an idealized gene. The **promoter** region (up to 100 base pairs) always contains two recognized elements, the CAAT box (usually GGTCAATCT) and TATA box (usually TATAAA). The latter sequence binds a TATA box binding factor to form a stable transcription complex which is required before the promoter region can be recognized by an **RNA polymerase** which is required to generate RNA. The promoter region may also contain specific binding regions for other proteins including the products of proto-oncogenes which can influence transcription both positively and negatively. Further upstream are **enhancer** regions which include sequences that bind glucocorticoids. These enhancers are thought to be activated by such binding and the DNA loops around to bring the bound element in contact with the promoter region. When both promoter and enhancer regions are activated, gene transcription is enhanced (Fig. 1.4). Enhancer

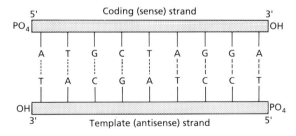

Fig. 1.2 Diagrammatic representation of DNA duplex showing base pairing. Shaded areas show deoxyribose−phosphate backbone. **Nucleotide** bases are shown as per convention: A, adenine; C, cytosine; G, guanine; T, thymine. Adapted from Owen CA, Stockley RA. *Thorax* 1990; 45: 52−6.

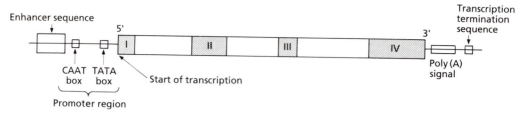

Fig. 1.3 Diagrammatic representation of a typical gene. Shaded areas show exons; white areas show introns. From Owen CA, Stockley RA. *Thorax* 1990; 45: 52−6.

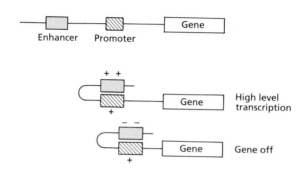

Fig. 1.4 Relationship of enhancer and promoter elements to gene transcription.

regions can be at some distance and even 3′ to the gene they activate and are usually tissue specific. Theoretically, the function of these regulatory nucleotide elements is determined partly by their sequence but also by experimentally introducing them into a **reporter** gene used in a variety of transcription/translation assays [1, 2].

Transcription

An outline of the process of gene **transcription** is shown in Fig. 1.5. Once RNA polymerase has bound and become activated on the template, transcription starts and runs 5′−3′ producing a **primary** RNA **transcript** with ACG and U paired with TGC and A, respectively, on the template. This process continues until a termination sequence on the template (ATT, ACT or ATC) is reached, resulting in UAA, UGA and UAG, respectively, in the RNA transcript. Before this termination sequence but 3′ to the end of the gene, a sequence of thymine (50−200 bases) results in a similar sequence of adenine in the RNA [poly(A) tail] which stabilizes the RNA transcript. In addition, the primary transcript becomes modified at the 5′ end by the addition of a 7-methylguanosine residue (**capping**) which is essential for protein synthesis.

The final modification within the nucleus involves the removal of the introns (**splicing**). At the end of each exon is a 5′ splice site (donor site) and at the start of the next exon is a 3′ splice site (acceptor site):

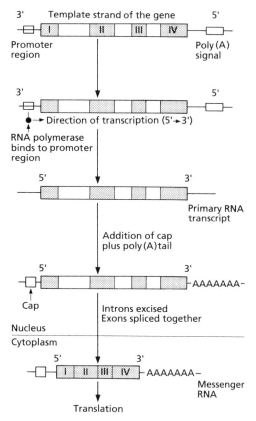

Fig. 1.5 The process of gene transcription to mRNA. Shaded areas show exons, white areas show introns. Adapted from Owen CA, Stockley RA. *Thorax* 1990; 45: 52–6.

```
          C          A
5' _____ or AG--|--GU or    AGU
          A        |  G

              Splice site

          C        | G
   or AG--|--or _____ 3'
          U        | A
```

the two ends then join.

This process can be further complicated by the process of alternative splicing where combinations of exons can be joined or omitted to generate different mRNA species and hence different protein products with different functions (e.g. calcitonin and the calcitonin gene-related peptide).

Following this final processing step the mRNA is exported from the nucleus where it becomes attached to the ribosome on the endoplasmic reticulum and is **translated** into protein.

Translation

This is the process whereby mRNA is used to generate a linear sequence of amino acids. In order to execute this process the nucleotide sequence of the mRNA is 'read' in sequential groups of three. Each triplet is referred to as a **codon**. There are 64 potential codon combinations of the four nucleotides, A U C G, but only 20 amino acids, thus several codons encode for the same amino acid. For instance, UCC, UCU, UCA and UCG all code for serine and hence the genetic code is said to be *redundant* or *degenerate*. The exceptions are AUG and UGG, which are the only codons that generate methionine and tryptophan, respectively, and the stop codons UAA, UAG and UGA that act as termination signals to end translation.

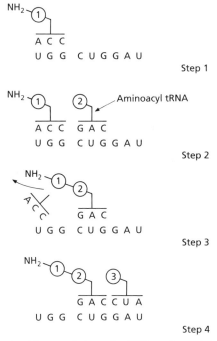

Fig. 1.6 Steps involved in translation of mRNA to its protein product. Complementary tRNA to consecutive codons binds to the mRNA bringing a single respective amino acid, which is passed on to the lengthening chain as the tRNA disengages (steps 1−4).

The process of translation commences with the first codon AUG, although in this instance it does not code for methionine. The reason is largely unknown but may relate to the 5′ CAP. Thereafter codons are read in sequence. This involves a further molecule, the **transfer RNA (tRNA)**. This molecule consists of an anticodon at its 5′ end with complementary triplets to the mRNA codon and a CCA sequence at its

3' end which is attached covalently to a specific amino acid. A second tRNA molecule then attaches to the next codon downstream and the amino acid attached to the first tRNA molecule is transferred to the end of the second and so on (Fig. 1.6). Eventually, a termination signal is reached which binds a release factor. At this point the ribosome dissociates and the polypeptide chain is released.

In practice, the matching of the tRNA codons does not have to be perfect for *every* codon as long as the first two nucleotides match. This means that a mismatch or **wobble** can, in some instances, be tolerated for the third nucleotide and explains why only 31 different tRNA molecules are required for the 64 codons.

This whole process is one of biochemical matching and is subject to manipulation. Indeed, recent research [3] has enabled a new codon to be devised together with a new tRNA that carries a new amino acid (iodotyrosine). This potentially opens up the genetic code and can enable new proteins to be constructed.

Once the polypeptide chain is released it undergoes protein folding (based on the amino acid sequence), post-translational modifications and cellular sorting.

The tools of molecular biology

The applications of molecular biology are dependent upon four simple principles:

1   The specific base pairing of DNA and RNA sequences.
2   The specificity of restriction enzymes (**nucleases**) for known sequences on double-stranded DNA.
3   The ability of DNA to replicate itself and make RNA.
4   The ability of RNA to generate its respective DNA.

Hybridization

Probes are known nucleotide sequences that can be radiolabelled or attached to another potential marker, such as fluorescein, digoxygenin or biotin, thereby enabling them to seek out and identify their natural matched partner.

Double-stranded DNA can be dissociated (denatured) by heating or treatment with alkali. If the temperature is then lowered or the solution neutralized, the two strands will eventually reassociate (**anneal**). The better the match, the earlier this will occur (conditions of higher stringency). If probes are introduced into the system, base pairing will take place only between complementary sequences to form a duplex (**hybridization**). If the conditions for hybridization are of high stringency probes can be used to identify DNA sequences that differ by as little as one nucleotide (Fig. 1.7). This approach can be used to identify DNA from the Z variant of α_1-antitrypsin, where a single nucleotide change at codon 342 alters the amino acid from glutamic acid to lysine [4].

If uncertainty remains about the specificity of the probes and their binding this can be confirmed by a series of *protection assays*. These depend on the ability of the enzymes, S1 nuclease and RNAse, to digest single-stranded DNA and RNA, respectively. If probe binding mismatches

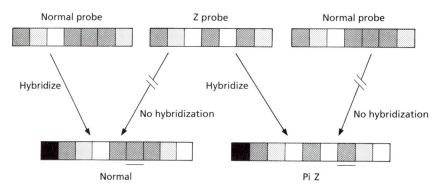

Fig. 1.7 Use of specific oligonucleotide probes to detect DNA sequences. Note hybridization only occurs under stringent conditions when the match is perfect.

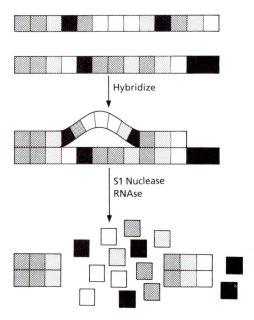

Fig. 1.8 Principle of enzyme protection assays. Hybridization of complementary sequences to form the relevant duplex results in protection of the single strand from enzyme digestion. Any unprotected areas are cleaved into their respective nucleotides.

by as little as a single nucleotide the separation of the two strands at this point is seen by the respective enzyme as a single strand and hence digested. The partially complementary strands therefore break at these points (Fig. 1.8). It is then a simple matter to determine whether the remaining strands are the exact length of the probe that has been used or whether significant mismatch has occurred, resulting in shorter segments. Indeed this ability of the enzymes and chemicals to cleave minor mismatches has been used as a rapid screening method to detect mutations in genes such as the tumour suppressor gene p53 in lung cancer [5].

Restriction enzymes

Restriction endonucleases are bacterial enzymes that cleave specific base sequences of double-stranded DNA. More than 300 enzymes have been isolated, recognizing in excess of 85 distinct DNA sequences. The predictability of these enzymes allows DNA to be cleaved and joined with known specificity at known sites and is critical for the generation of probes, the cleaving of DNA into manageable fragments and restriction fragment length analysis (see below).

The enzymes are divided into two classes. Class 1 enzymes recognize a specific nucleotide sequence and then cleave the DNA at a fixed distance away, whatever the actual sequence at that site. Class 2 enzymes, however, only cleave DNA at recognized sites and always in a specific manner. For this reason class 2 enzymes are more useful in recombinant DNA technology. The class 2 enzymes are 'sequence specific' recognizing sequences that are 3−6 base pairs in length and possess a twofold rotational symmetry (palindrome). The number of cuts made by each enzyme in a length of DNA is solely dependent upon the number of recognition sequences present in the DNA. The enzymes can cut both strands of DNA between base pairs resulting in 'blunt' ends. For example, the enzyme Sma1 cuts the sequence:

5'-CCC GGG-3'   5'-CCC + GGG-3'
                    to produce two fragments
3'-GGG CCC-5'   3'-GGG + CCC-5'

Alternatively, the enzyme may make a staggered cut, resulting in 'sticky' ends:

EcoR1 cuts 5'-G AATTC-3'   5'-G   +   AATTC-3'
                         to produce
            3'-CTTAA G-5'   3'-CTTAA   +   G-5'

This latter effect is useful in joining DNA sequences derived from two different sources if both have been cut with the same enzyme. Overlapping sequences will join spontaneously by hydrogen bonding. Indeed, if enzymes have produced blunt ends, annealing can only be achieved if the ends are lengthened asymmetrically to produce complementary 'sticky ends'.

Replicating enzymes

DNA polymerases are enzymes which possess the ability to duplicate and repair DNA. As DNA replicates the two strands open up to form a replication fork. In the presence of new nucleotides, pairing takes place in the fork and the enzyme DNA polymerase joins these together in a 5'–3' direction to make new double strands. The replication fork then moves on in a process described as 'unzipping' until two complete new double strands have been made (Fig. 1.9).

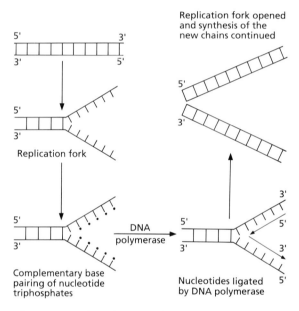

Fig. 1.9 Schematic representation of DNA replication. From Owen CA, Stockley RA. *Thorax* 1990; 45: 52–6.

This process of replication forms the basis of the **polymerase chain reaction** (PCR), which is shown diagrammatically in Fig. 1.10. This technique is used to amplify as little as one sequence of DNA or RNA (after it has been made into DNA) into quantities large enough to measure, manipulate or use to probe new sources. The sequence can be amplified more than a million times in a few hours. In essence the sequence of the DNA to be amplified has to be known. **Primers** complementary to alternate sides and opposite ends of the putative DNA duplex are mixed with the heat-denatured DNA. The primers anneal to their respective strands and in the presence of DNA polymerase and an

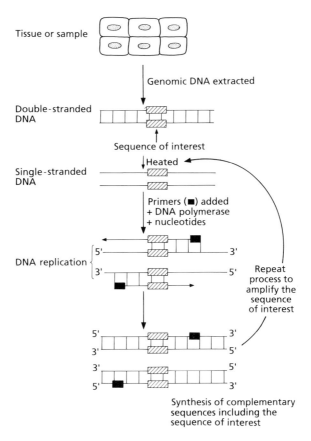

Fig. 1.10 Representation of the polymerase chain reaction. From Owen CA, Stockley RA. *Thorax* 1990; 45: 52−6.

excess of deoxyribonucleotide triphosphates they generate new double strands. The mixture is then heat denatured to generate four single strands (two new and the two original strands) and the cycle is repeated. The technique has been used to identify low copies of *Pneumocystis* sequences [6] and the human immunodeficiency virus [7] and recently mycobacterial DNA in sarcoid tissue [8]. Other illustrations of its use are described in subsequent chapters. However, it is critical to check the specificity of the amplified product by assessing the DNA between the known primers. This can be done by sequencing or the use of a specific probe to the desired intervening sequences.

RNA polymerase

RNA polymerases are enzymes which initiate the transcription of DNA to RNA as described above. These enzymes, with the appropriate promoter, are critical in the generation of RNA probes (see below).

Reverse transcriptase

This is an enzyme made by retroviruses as a means of incorporating their RNA into the genome of the host for the purpose of self-replication. The enzyme reverses the normal transcription process by making copies of DNA from RNA. The DNA is then incorporated into the host DNA and replicates making new copies of the RNA virus. The enzyme has also been of major use in DNA cloning and with the PCR to detect low copies of tissue RNA by first changing them to DNA (see below).

Probes

If specific DNA or RNA sequences are being sought in a mixture there has to be a complementary probe developed and labelled so that hybridization can be achieved and visualized. The nature of the probe depends upon its purpose and specificity. For instance, the genome is large and nucleotide combinations are likely to be repeated. This is particularly true in genes which code for proteins with similar function where sequence homology can be 50% or more. The longer the probe the less the importance of sequence homology. In addition, longer probes can be labelled more extensively, if required, to ensure a greater signal.

Nucleotides can be linked biochemically and short chains produced as required. This results in **oligonucleotides**, which can be designed to hybridize with specific DNA or RNA sequences. The ideal size is 20–30 nucleotides in length, which increases specificity while reducing cost and risk of error. Such probes are usually used for PCR, RNA recognition, site-directed mutagenesis and the identification of specific minor genetic defects (see below).

Genomic probes are complementary to DNA sequences that include exons and introns and are usually derived from a source of whole DNA. This has conventionally been obtained from liver tissue, divided into small fragments by restriction enzymes and cloned into an appropriate vector resulting in a multitude of different clones (*liver library*). When a specific probe is sought the whole library has to be screened to identify the small number of clones bearing the sequence of interest. This has conventionally been achieved by identifying the product of the DNA sequence from the appropriate *vector* (usually grown in bacteria), either immunologically or enzymatically as the cloned DNA is transcribed and translated. Of course the cloned DNA may only produce a fragment of the product since only a fragment of the gene may have been cloned and this may provide some difficulty in their identification.

An alternative approach is to make an *expression library*. This facilitates the process of obtaining a probe as it depends upon the fact that not all genes are expressed in all tissues. If it is known that a gene of interest is expressed by a certain cell type, this can be harvested, the mRNA isolated, exposed to reverse transcriptase to make the corresponding DNA, cloned into a vector and then grown in the appropriate bacteria. Again the probe can be identified by the appearance of the protein product. In this instance the whole of the protein is made. The probe (cDNA) will only hybridize with the coding regions (exons) of the gene.

RNA probes can be made from the corresponding cDNA. In this instance the vector containing the cDNA is 'designed' so that the site of insertion of the cDNA contains different transcriptional promoters at either end that can be activated to transcribe either the template DNA or the coding sequence. The importance of transcribing both strands is to develop an internal control. Normally the **template** is transcribed to form RNA which is designated the sense orientation.

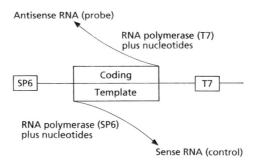

Fig. 1.11 Generation of sense and antisense RNA probes using 'specific' RNA polymerase promoter regions at either end.

In order to develop an RNA probe it is necessary to make RNA that is complementary, i.e. antisense and thus has to be transcribed from the **coding** sequence of DNA. This can be achieved by having a promoter at the 'wrong' end of the DNA insert and in the reverse orientation so that it transcribes the 'wrong' DNA sequence. The promoter at the 'right' end makes the 'right' RNA in a sense orientation (Fig. 1.11). Once an insert has been placed between the promoters in a suitable plasmid vector, it is grown in the appropriate bacterium and harvested. The plasmid is then linearized by cleaving one side and can be mixed with promoter DNA-specific RNA polymerase (in this case SP6 or T7). In the presence of radiolabelled nucleotides the respective sense and antisense probes can be generated and harvested by size separation from the plasmid enzymes and free nucleotides. When used as probes only the antisense RNA probe should bind to tissue RNA and the sense probe should not bind (negative control).

Cloning

Cloning is the mechanism whereby multiple identical fragments of DNA are generated, usually in bacteria. Since the bacteria do not take up foreign DNA very efficiently the fragments are inserted into special forms of DNA (vectors) that can enter and replicate in the bacteria. The choice of vector depends primarily on the size of DNA to be cloned. **Plasmids** are used for up to 10 kilobase pairs, **bacteriophages** for 5–20 kilobase pairs and **cosmids** (a hybrid of plasmid and bacteriophage DNA) for large sequences of 40–50 kilobase pairs.

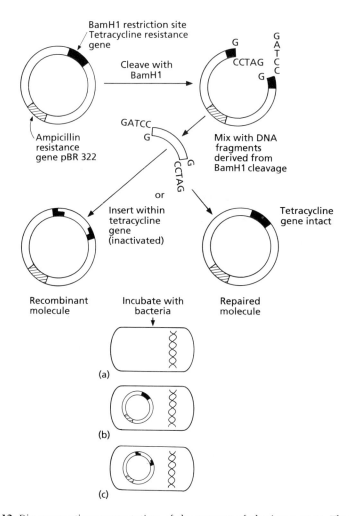

Fig. 1.12 Diagrammatic representation of the process of cloning a gene. The DNA sequence is cloned into a plasmid and then inserted into a bacterium. The successful recombinant plasmid is identified by its ability to alter the antibiotic sensitivity of the bacterium. (a) No plasmid: sensitive to ampicillin and tetracycline. (b) Repaired plasmid: resistant to ampicillin and tetracycline. (c) Recombinant plasmid: resistant to ampicillin and sensitive to tetracycline. From Owen CA, Stockley RA. *Thorax* 1990; 45: 147–53.

Plasmids are used where possible and consist of a circular duplex of DNA. Many are now custom designed to include an array of restriction sites (usually one for each enzyme) as well as genes coding for a marker such as antibiotic resistance which allows the successfully transfected bacteria to be identified. For example, the plasmid pBR 322 carries the ampicillin- and tetracycline-resistant genes and a restriction site for the enzyme BamH1 (see Fig. 1.12). Incubation of the plasmid with BamH1 cleaves the tetracycline-resistant gene and leaves 'sticky' ends. If the DNA to be cloned is cut with the same enzyme and mixed with the plasmid some will insert itself into the plasmid in the presence of the enzyme DNA ligase, interrupting the tetracycline-resistant gene. The plasmids are then incubated with bacteria and some enter, resulting in **transformation**. The few bacteria that have been transformed by the recombinant plasmid are identified by their antibiotic resistance profile. These are then grown in bulk culture, lysed and the plasmids obtained by centrifugation. The plasmids are then treated again with BamH1 and the insert (cloned DNA) is released. This is separated from the remaining plasmid by gel electrophoresis, identified by size and harvested by cutting the appropriate band out of the gel (see Fig. 1.13).

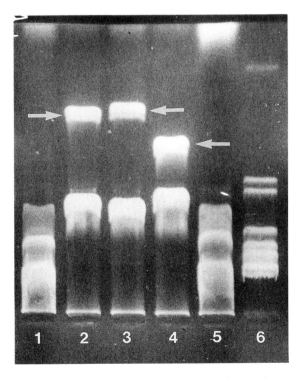

Fig. 1.13 Electrophoretic gel of plasmid preparation. Tracks 1 and 5 are plasmid plus restriction enzyme. Tracks 2–4 are plasmids that contained various DNA inserts that have been separated (arrowed) by the restriction enzymes. Track 6 contains DNA size markers.

Applications

The ability to cleave, mend and duplicate DNA in a controlled manner enables many strategic methodologies to be employed in biological sciences. The potential, and hence application, of these techniques is advancing rapidly and our knowledge of disease susceptibility, diagnosis and therapy has already been greatly advanced. In this section examples are given to illustrate how these techniques have been applied or are being considered in clinical science and medicine.

Genetic studies

Early genetic studies were driven by clinical observation of a recognized abnormality of protein defects (haemoglobinopathies, α_1-antitrypsin deficiency). In such an example, identification of the gene follows a logical though often tedious pathway. Cloned sequences of DNA were screened in an **expression** vector (see below) to identify those associated with the protein (usually detected immunologically). Once the respective DNA sequences were identified they could be harvested and used as probes for further studies.

The labelled probe could be used to identify the chromosomal location of the gene by *in situ* **hybridization** in healthy subjects. Following this or often before chromosomal localization the same probe could be used to study the gene. Sequences of the gene could be identified in genomic DNA and partial characterization obtained by simple dot-/slot-blotting and **Southern** blotting. In the former, denatured DNA (single stranded) is dotted on to a nitrocellulose membrane and the remainder of the membrane is coated with non-human DNA to block all other potential binding sites. The membrane is then incubated with the labelled probe, washed thoroughly, developed and the presence and quantity of the signal assessed. This provides evidence for the presence of the DNA and a semiquantitative measure of its amount. If the gene has been deleted, as with a section (see below) of the short arm of chromosome 3 in small cell lung cancer, no signal will be obtained with a probe to the aminoacylase-1 gene [9].

Further information can be obtained by the process of Southern blotting. The principles of this technique are outlined in Fig. 1.14. This method, devised by E.M. Southern, is probably one of the most quoted methodologies in molecular biology. Briefly, genomic DNA is extracted and exposed to digestion by one or more restriction endonucleases to generate multiple fragments of varying sizes dependent upon the frequency and distribution of the relevant restriction sites. The sample is then electrophoresed in a size separation gel. The gel is then blotted on to nitrocellulose which gives an imprint of single-stranded DNA fragments. All non-specific binding sites are blocked with non-human DNA

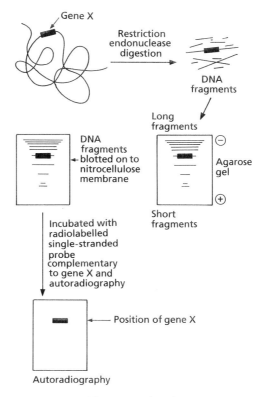

Fig. 1.14 Principles of Southern blotting to identify a DNA sequence in the genome. From Owen CA, Stockley RA. *Thorax* 1990; 45: 147–53.

and then the membrane is mixed with the labelled probe, which is identified by an appropriate label. It only hybridizes with its cDNA fragment and the number and size of the bands depend upon the probe and where the DNA has been cut by the restriction enzymes. By using different enzymes and probing each digest separately, it is possible to derive a **restriction map** (i.e. a plan of the number, nature and position of the restriction sites) of the gene. This principle of Southern blotting is often used for **restriction fragment length analysis** (see below).

Once the gene has been located it can be analysed further to determine whether it is 'normal'. Part of this process will involve the assessment of the fragments produced by restriction endonucleases. Genetic abnormalities may delete or introduce restriction sites that differ from normal. For instance in sickle cell anaemia a single base substitution (GAG → GTG) results in the loss of a restriction site for the enzyme, M*ST*II [10]. Digestion with this enzyme produces larger fragments than expected in DNA from such patients using a β-globin DNA probe. However, the most complete method is to determine the actual nucleotide sequence as this will also detect changes that do not involve restriction sites.

DNA sequencing

The ability to sequence genes has provided the knowledge of basic gene structure and function. In addition, it enables minor gene defects to be identified that may or may not affect gene function. Furthermore, gene sequencing has facilitated the development and confirmation of genetic manipulation. The technology has now been refined to the extent of the development of automatic gene sequencing.

The most commonly used method for DNA sequencing was described by Sanger *et al.* [11] and uses an enzymatic dideoxynucleotide technique. Incorporation of a dideoxynucleotide into gene elongation terminates the process and can be used to determine the sequence of the four nucleotides.

In brief, the DNA molecule to be sequenced is first cloned in a bacteriophage. A synthetic oligonucleotide, with a sequence complementary to about 15 bases of the phage sequence 3′ to the DNA insert, acts as a primer for DNA synthesis. The **Klenow fragment** of DNA polymerase is then used to synthesize DNA complementary to the DNA being sequenced in the presence of free nucleotides. Unlike the whole DNA polymerase the Klenow fragment lacks 5′−3′ exonuclease activity and can thus assemble dideoxynucleotide triphosphates. Since these nucleotides lack the 3′ OH group (see Fig. 1.1), they can no longer act as recipients of chain elongation so the chain becomes terminated. Four reaction mixtures are set up, each containing all four nucleotides, one of which is labelled with ^{32}P, and a low concentration of the dideoxynucleotide triphosphates (one in each tube). The net result is a series of partially synthesized radioactive DNA molecules with a common 5′ end and varying lengths to a base specific 3′ end as one of the dideoxynucleotides becomes incorporated. The use of four mixtures means that a dideoxynucleotide should be incorporated into every nucleotide in at least one of the lengthening sequences in one of the tubes, thereby stopping the process.

The DNA of each of the reaction mixtures is then denatured and electrophoresed to separate them by size in adjacent lanes. The radioactive bands of DNA are detected by autoradiography and the sequence can be read directly from the autoradiograph as the chain sequence is stopped (Fig. 1.15). The sequence data can be used to determine whether the correct piece of DNA has been amplified by PCR; whether a predetermined mutation has been introduced as in site-directed mutagenesis (see below); where the introns and exons are (in genomic cloning); what the amino acid sequence of the gene product is (reverse genetics, see below); and the size of the putative mRNA. In addition, once the normal gene has been sequenced this technique enables a variety of gene defects to be identified.

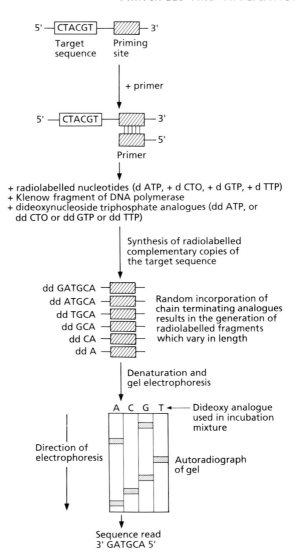

Fig. 1.15 DNA sequencing by the Sanger technique. The order on the sequence gel is complementary to the gene being sequenced. From Owen CA, Stockley RA. *Thorax* 1990; 45: 147−53.

Gene defects

A **gene mutation** is a change in the base sequence from normal. These may arise spontaneously or be the result of DNA damage due to ultra-violet light, γ-irradiation or chemicals such as nitrous acid or acridines. The consequences of such mutations depend upon their extent, nature and site. For instance, minor mutations in the controlling sequences are more likely to alter gene function than major defects in the intervening (non-coding) sequences.

A **point mutation** is an alteration in a single base resulting in a substitution. This does not affect the reading frame of the gene as the number of bases remains unaltered. The new base is 'read' with its two partners in the respective codon. The mutation may be silent if the substitution results in an alternative codon with the same function (for example CTT→CTC which both code for lysine). Alternatively, the 'message' relayed by the codon may change producing a new amino acid in the protein chain (for example GAG→AAG will replace glutamic acid with lysine). In this instance the effect will depend upon the importance of the amino acid to protein structure and function. The change may have no apparent effect or may grossly alter protein function. For instance, the change of the amino acid at position 342 on the α_1-antitrypsin molecule has a major effect on protein secretion due to polymerization in the endoplasmic reticulum [12], resulting in marked serum deficiency. Another example is the substitution of arginine for methionine at the active site (amino acid — 358) of the same protein which results in a change of function from an elastase inhibitor to antithrombin-III-like function [13]. Finally, the point mutation may result in a termination codon. For instance, GAG (glutamic acid)→TAG (stop) in codon 279 of the glucokinase gene leading to diabetes [14].

A mutation which results in the insertion or deletion of one or two bases will alter the reading frame from that point onwards (a **frameshift mutation**). If bases are deleted the reading frame moves forwards towards the 3' end (3' frameshift), whereas insertions retard reading (5' frameshift). These frameshifts result in the generation of a new amino acid sequence and commonly result in the appearance of premature stop codons. This gives rise to an absence of mRNA [15] or a truncated protein which is highly unstable [16].

Sometimes defects can be greater, ranging from deletions of a single codon, thereby missing a single amino acid but producing the remainder of the protein [deletion of phenylalanine at position 508 on the cystic fibrosis (CF) transmembrane receptor] [17], to intron exon deletions (exon 19 in the dystrophic gene in Duchenne muscular dystrophy Kobe) [18].

Genetic counselling

Although the identification of these defects explains the disease, current technology does not enable them to be repaired *in vivo*. Nevertheless, knowledge of the defects has had a major effect on diagnosis, prognosis and genetic counselling. For instance, identification of the point mutation in the Z variant of α_1-antitrypsin enables it to be identified with the use of specific oligonucleotide probes [4] as outlined in Fig. 1.7. It could be argued that this approach is inappropriate since plasma sampling already identifies the significant deficiency associated with disease. However, it is not possible to obtain plasma samples *in utero* and yet the defect can still be identified by chorionic villus sampling and examination of DNA [19]. The need for such an approach is clearly dependent upon the need or desirability of early termination. Superficially this does not appear to be the case in α_1-antitrypsin deficiency since most subjects live until their fourth and fifth decades, even if they smoke in later life [20]. However, severe neonatal jaundice also occurs in α_1-antitrypsin deficiency and may cause death. Studies have shown that such an occurrence is associated with a high incidence of similar problems in a subsequent affected child. In this instance prenatal diagnosis and consideration of termination may be indicated.

The case for such studies in CF may at first glance appear stronger. The common codon deletion (F508) is associated with worse prognosis due to severe pancreatic disease but variable pulmonary disease [21]. However, many such individuals are now surviving well into adult life and their long-term outlook may improve with new approaches to therapy (see below). Nevertheless, genetic studies can prove informative since many defects have been identified on the CF gene and some are associated with much milder lung disease [22]. The identification of such defects and their implications make genetic counselling much clearer.

Finally genetic studies probably become most useful when the phenotypic appearance of the disease is delayed into late adulthood. By this time families have been formed and the genetic defect passed on inadvertently. Huntington's chorea is the best known and most well characterized of these diseases. It is now possible to identify the predisposition to this autosomal dominant disease well in advance of presentation [23]. The knowledge and its implications for future generations can therefore be imparted with greater degrees of certainty.

Restriction fragment length polymorphism

When the gene or gene defect is not known an alternative and often preliminary approach is that of restriction fragment length polymorphism (RFLP). This depends upon the fact that the human genome is very polymorphic. On average 1 in 250 bases is polymorphic and one in six of these result in the loss or gain of a recognition site for a restriction enzyme. Most of the polymorphisms are situated in the 95% of the genome that is not transcribed and therefore do not affect the phenotype of the individual. The polymorphisms are, however, identified as changes in the length of DNA fragments produced by the relevant restriction enzyme on Southern blotting. This principle is illustrated in Fig. 1.16 with reference to a polymorphism of the 3' flanking region of the α_1-antitrypsin gene that eliminates a restriction site for the enzyme Taq1.

To be useful clinically the polymorphism should be rare in a healthy

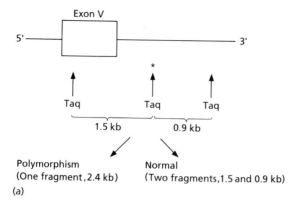

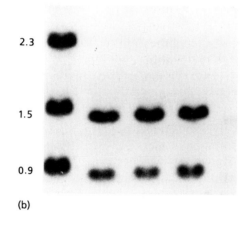

Fig. 1.16 Polymorphism of the α_1-antitrypsin (AAT) gene. Three restriction sites to the enzyme Taq1 are normally present in this region but in some individuals the middle site is absent. DNA cleavage of this area of the gene results in two fragments (normal) or one (polymorphism). Electrophoresis of the fragments and identification with a cDNA probe to this region produces two bands (normal), one band (homozygote with the polymorphism) or three bands (shown here) for a heterozygote with one normal gene and one with the polymorphism. kb, kilobase. (Gel kindly supplied by Professor N. Kalsheker, Nottingham.)

population but common in the disease state. Thus, if the RFLP is closely and stably linked to the abnormal gene (linkage disequilibrium) it can be used as a genetic marker even if the true gene is unknown and can actually narrow down the search for the gene. This approach was in fact used in the search for the CF gene [24]. Unfortunately, the use of RFLP is limited because few diseases are the result of single mutations and even these may not alter a restriction site.

However, when such linkages exist their significance can be confirmed by the co-inheritance of the disease phenotype and the RFLP. This relationship is confirmed by the **LOD** score. In most instances the gene is unknown and the polymorphism (if present) could relate to any one of 350 or more restriction enzymes. The process is therefore usually very tedious and potentially requires the assessment of most of the genome and all restriction enzymes. Thus it is exceptionally fortunate when linkage is found relatively early during familial studies as recently seen with immunoglobulin E (IgE) responsiveness and chromosome 11 [25]. In this study linkage was found when only the 17th gene probe and one restriction enzyme were used.

The process of genetic linkage depends on the disease and an identified polymorphism cosegregating, i.e. the individuals with the disease show the polymorphism and those without do not. This is facilitated in large family studies where disease penetration is usually absolute (heterozygotes also manifest the disease phenotype). However, because genetic material may cross-over during meiosis, the polymorphism may become separated from the disease and this is more likely the further the polymorphism and defective gene are apart. Separation of the two is due to recombination, and the proportion of siblings in whom this occurs determines the **recombination fraction**.

For example, if five of 10 siblings have disease A and polymorphism B, but only one sibling without the disease has the polymorphism, the recombination fraction is probably one of 10 or 0.1. This value is used to describe how far apart the gene and polymorphism are on the genome. For this example the two loci are said to be 10 **map units** or **centimorgans** apart.

Having defined the incidence of polymorphism B and disease A the recombination fraction is calculated. This value depends on many other factors, including the number of siblings available for study and the penetration of the disease. The calculations are tedious and usually carried out with the aid of a computer program [26]. The likelihood (or odds) that this recombination fraction is correct, is conventionally expressed as its logarithm, the $\log_{10}$ of the odds or LOD score.

The process is repeated with several families and the LOD scores are added together and the sum is plotted for each recombination fraction. The maximum likely estimate of the recombination fraction is the value that corresponds to the peak of the summated LOD scores. Thus in the example given above, if the maximum LOD score at a recombination of 0.1 is 4.0 or above it means that the odds are more than 10 000 to 1 that a linkage occurs at this distance (10 centimorgans) between the gene and the polymorphic marker. In other words the RFLP is close (within 10 centimorgans) to the defective gene causing the disease.

Once the close association has been determined it is possible to move along the chromosomal DNA using overlapping probes until the gene is identified. At this point the gene sequence can be established and its protein product predicted — the method of **reverse genetics**.

This kind of approach was applied to the disease, CF. A useful RFLP was identified and the chromosomal localization of the CF gene found [27]. Subsequently, the gene itself was identified and its product predicted to be a transmembrane receptor [28]. Further studies confirmed that the gene product was associated with a chloride channel [29] and this was defective in CF [30].

Assessment of RNA

Once the gene is transcribed it is possible to assess the form and function of the transcript. The cellular RNA can be dotted or slotted on to nitrocellulose and assessed by hybridization with an appropriate probe as for DNA. The results are usually confirmed by size separation followed by absorption on to nitrocellulose as for Southern blotting and DNA (see Southern blotting above). When RNA is being probed the method is referred to as **Northern blotting**. Again semiquantitative data can be obtained by densitometry scanning.

Quantification of RNA can lead to an overestimation of the importance of the observation. There is a tendency to assume that a positive signal indicates RNA that is being transcribed and that the strength of the signal relates to the amount of protein that will be made. However, it must be emphasized that all RNA is not translated and it is often measured at a single time point, failing to take into account RNA half-life or translational efficiency. Further precautions or assessment of RNA can provide a more complete picture.

First, it is important to assess only the stable polyadenylated form of RNA. This can be achieved by prior purification of this type of RNA by binding it to a complementary column (oligo dT — a series of thymine nucleotides that bind the poly(A)tail of RNA). More recently this preparative step has been overcome by the use of a 'poly(U)' nitrocellulose, which again will bind the poly(A) form of RNA.

Second, increases in mRNA may be transient so it is important to study the time course as protein production will lag behind. Furthermore, over a prolonged period the protein can have accumulated long after the mRNA has been 'turned off' and catabolized. This is particularly true of mRNA to acute phase reactants which have multiple AU sequences and are thus rapidly catabolized [31]. This catabolism can be assessed by the measurement of mRNA half-life. At a known time point transcription is terminated by the use of an agent such as novabiocin and sequential RNA harvesting allows the subsequent catabolism of the preformed mRNA to be assessed.

When mRNA is assessed together with the protein product further information can be obtained. For instance, if steady state mRNA does not increase despite an increase in production of its product it will be clear that translational efficiency has been increased. Alternatively, an increase in mRNA production associated with no change or a decrease in its product suggests an unstable or rapidly catabolized transcript (confirmed by half-life studies).

Finally, mRNA can be identified within individual tissues and cells by *in situ* hybridization using specific antisense cRNA probes. This provides evidence that the tissue or cell in question has the capability to produce a given protein (confirmed by immunohistochemistry and tissue/cell culture).

Expression vectors and translation systems

Expression vectors are vehicles used to generate the products of the gene or its RNA. For gene expression the most commonly used technique is to insert the relevant cDNA into an appropriate plasmid with the necessary controlling sequences. The recombinants are then introduced into bacteria (often *Escherichia coli*) by the process of transformation, and the bacteria grown in bulk culture. These are then lysed and the product purified.

An alternative approach is to use an animal cell which can be an oocyte, fertilized egg or even an embryo. The most commonly used system is the *Xenopus* (toad) oocyte because they are easily obtained, large (0.8−1.2 mm) and with a large nucleus. Single-stranded DNA can be introduced into the nucleus by microinjection. It is then converted into double-stranded DNA and assembled into chromatin. The exogenous DNA can then be transcribed by RNA polymerases leading to the formation, transport and translation of RNA. The protein is then secreted by the oocyte into the culture medium.

The oocyte can also be used to study mRNA by injecting it into the cytoplasm. Alternatively, the process of translation and post-translational protein modification can be studied in a **cell-free** translation system. The mRNA is added to a lysate of rabbit reticulocytes or wheat germ, which contains all the necessary ingredients for translation.

The system used depends upon the desired result. For instance, if a large amount of the product is required it is important to have a robust self-replicating system. In this instance bacterial transformation is the most appropriate. This sort of technology has been used to generate the human hormones, insulin and growth hormone, as well as α_1-antitrypsin used in replacement therapy. In addition, it has been used to generate proteins that are difficult to harvest from other sources because of their low concentrations such as cytokines including interleukin-1 (IL-1) and the colony-stimulating factors. Although many of these products have been generated for patient treatment, these recombinant proteins are now the major source for biomedical experimentation. The only concern is that these proteins do not undergo many of the normal intracellular processing steps such as glycosylation. This has led to some concerns over antigenicity [32] and whether function is preserved correctly.

In addition to protein production these systems have been used to determine the mechanisms of disease processes. For instance, subjects with α_1-antitrypsin deficiency produce normal quantities of mRNA but only 10−15% of the normal plasma protein. Experiments have shown that the mRNA is translated normally in cell-free systems [33] but the protein is not secreted in the intact cell due to a defect in intracellular processing [34].

Site-directed mutagenesis

Oligonucleotide site-directed mutagenesis is a technique used to alter a gene in a specific way, either to improve its product or gain insight into protein function. The gene in its pure single-stranded form is cloned into an appropriate vector and a complementary oligonucleotide is synthesized, which contains the intended mutation. Under carefully controlled conditions this oligonucleotide will still hybridize with the DNA strand and can be used as a template for DNA extension to form a heteroduplex (see Fig. 1.17). This is then transformed into a bacterium and is 'repaired' by bacterial DNA polymerase to correct the mismatch. Since the bacterium does not know the correct sequence it will either produce the original or the mismatch sequence. A radiolabelled complementary mismatch oligonucleotide is used to probe the bacterial colonies under highly stringent conditions to find the 'new' sequence. The DNA is harvested and the mutation confirmed by conventional DNA sequencing.

This process has been used to determine the importance of cysteine residues on β-receptor ligand binding [35]. In addition, the active site of α_1-antitrypsin has been altered from methionine (358) to valine, which renders the protein resistant to oxidation, a process that inactivates it as an elastase inhibitor [36]. Oxidative inactivation of α_1-antitrypsin has been implicated in chronic lung diseases and an oxidation-resistant form may have therapeutic potential.

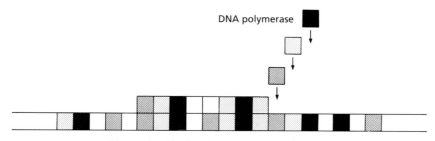

DNA polymerase

Oligonucleotide site-directed mutagenesis

Fig. 1.17 Site-directed mutagenesis. An oligonucleotide containing the desired mutation is hybridized with the normal gene and extension is carried out with DNA polymerase. This is introduced into a vector and then a relevant bacterium, which replicates and 'repairs' the mismatch. There is a 50% chance that the normal sequence will be repaired to match the mutation.

The techniques of mutagenesis can be taken further and new proteins can be designed. For instance, it is possible to combine portions of two or more proteins to make a **chimera** with functions of the original constituents. This approach has been taken with the receptor-binding domain of IL-2 and the active part of the diphtheria toxin [37]. This limits the cellular destruction of the functional part of the diphtheria toxin to cells with IL-2 receptors. Some haematological malignancies express large numbers of high affinity IL-2 receptors and this chimera has been used already with some success [37]. This opens new paths for therapeutic approaches to tumours previously unresponsive to conventional therapy.

Transgenic animals

The study of the pathogenesis of genetic diseases has and will be advanced by the study of animal models into which an abnormal gene has been introduced. These transgenic animals (usually mice) enable the effects of the gene to be observed. As such these animals are mainly a research tool providing basic information on the pathogenicity of the gene defect.

The relationship of α_1-antitrypsin deficiency to liver disease has been clarified by such studies. There has been debate concerning whether the liver disease in α_1-antitrypsin deficiency is due to the low plasma levels of the protein failing to protect the hepatocyte from proteinase-induced damage or whether the intracellular accumulation of protein itself is the cause. The introduction of the abnormal α_1-antitrypsin into mice resulted in liver damage and accumulation of the protein in hepatocytes [38]. Since the mouse has its own protective α_1-antitrypsin and since no such effects were seen when the normal α_1-antitrypsin gene was introduced, it can be concluded that hepatic damage is a result of intracellular α_1-antitrypsin accumulation.

Perhaps more exciting for the future is the potential to replace genes with faulty ones in animal models. Recent studies have shown that homologous gene targeting is possible [39]. The faulty gene is joined to a marker gene for drug resistance. This is then introduced into cells from a mouse embryo at the blastocyst stage of development. In some instances the construct will recombine with the natural copy of the gene and can be identified by the drug resistance. These are then reintroduced into a blastocyst resulting in mice with both the natural and artificial gene. Selective breeding then results in animals with only the new gene. This provides the opportunity to develop animal models of diseases such as CF by the introduction of the abnormal CF gene in the embryonic stem cell and indeed such studies are currently under way. Clearly the development of such an animal model will provide a major breakthrough in the understanding and management of CF.

Therapy

Understanding the genetic basis of disease opens up new concepts and potential for treatment by replacement or inactivation of defective genes. For example, most tumours are associated with overexpression of oncogenes or a loss of normal tumour suppressor genes. Experimentation has already shown that it is possible to suppress cell proliferation by two approaches:

First, expression of an abnormal oncogene (c-*myc*) can be prevented by the use of specific antisense oligonucleotides that inactivate the abnormal mRNA. This in turn leads to a reduction in cell replication [40]. Second, replacement of the wild-type (p53) tumour suppressor gene can suppress growth of a malignant sarcomatous cell line [41].

Molecular biology has already resulted in the production of a variety of proteins that can be used in replacement or supplementation therapy. The most advanced studies in respiratory disease are with α_1-antitrypsin which has been aerosolized and shown to be effective within the lung of patients with deficiency [42] or excess elastase activity [43].

Perhaps the most challenging, however, is the possibility of gene therapy itself. In principle this seems relatively straightforward, especially when a gene is absent or not transcribed, but may be less realistic when an abnormal gene is expressed and disease is a direct result of its product. Nevertheless, advances are being made both *in vitro* and *in vivo*. The α_1-antitrypsin gene has been introduced into airways epithelial cells *in vitro* [44] and this can also be achieved *in vivo* [45]. Similarly the CF gene can be introduced into epithelial cells and will correct the chloride channel defect in CF [46]. Thus in both of these diseases where manifestations occur within the lung it may be possible to transfer a normal gene to the human airways epithelium in the near future. Clearly the methodology works, although several problems still exist.

The transfer of the α_1-antitrypsin gene has been mediated by a non-replicating adenovirus [45]. This 'infects' the epithelial cell and inserts the new gene into the cellular DNA via reverse transcriptase. This process occurs at random and although most of the genome appears non-functional it could interrupt vital gene function (including oncogenes and tumour suppressor genes). In addition, the cellular target is non-replicating and thus therapy has to be repeated. Although this is a minor problem in practical terms, it may prove impractical if respiratory host defences become activated on repeated exposure preventing the viral vector from 'infecting' the epithelial cells. Other means of gene delivery are being explored including cell receptor-mediated endocytosis [47], which should not evoke a host immune response.

However, even if delivery, safety and successful expression are achieved, they may not alter the course of disease. The lung damage may be self-perpetuating and hence therapy may have to be started at birth. In addition, it has been suggested that replacement of the CF gene may not alter the disease if the abnormal gene is still expressed. This is based on the observation that subjects who do not express the CF gene have milder pulmonary disease [22]. The implications are that no gene is better than the abnormal gene and perhaps the abnormal gene in some way makes the disease worse. If so, replacement of gene function would only prove effective if the abnormal gene is also inactivated.

However, despite these potential difficulties, gene therapy can be effective [48]. As more is learnt about disease processes in general, the potential for intervention in new and meaningful ways increases.

As stated at the start of this chapter the purpose was to introduce the reader to the terminology, methods and concepts of molecular biology. With the increasing use of these techniques it becomes critical for both scientists and clinicians to understand the basic language of the science. It is hoped that this introductory chapter will enable the non-specialist reader to negotiate the remainder of the book and other general reading as painlessly as possible. In addition, it is hoped that the problems as well as potential of this branch of science have been placed in perspective.

Glossary of useful terms

anneal Joining of two complementary strands of DNA by hydrogen bonding between base pairs.

antisense Strand of DNA transcribed to make mRNA (template). A sequence complementary to mRNA.

bacteriophage Bacterial virus that can be used as a cloning vehicle.

capping Addition of methylate guanine residue to the 5′ end of the RNA transcript.

centimorgan (also called map unit) Unit of measurement for the distance between two loci on a gene.

chimera An artificial construct of part or all of two or more proteins.

cloning Introduction of fragments of DNA into bacteria in order to make millions of identical copies.

coding strand of DNA (sense) The strand that is not transcribed but which has the same sequence as mRNA (with T instead of U).

codon Three consecutive bases that code for an amino acid or function signal (start/ stop/splice).

complementary base pairing Hydrogen bonding between two bases of opposite strands of DNA.

cosmid Hybrid cloning vector composed of a plasmid and bacteriophage used to clone large pieces of DNA.

denaturation Separation of complementary strands of nucleic acid by heat or alkali.

DNA polymerase Enzyme that catalyses DNA synthesis.

enhancer DNA sequence that modifies gene transcription.

exon Sequence of DNA that codes for part of the amino acid sequence of a protein.

expression Translation of a gene sequence to make mRNA.

frameshift mutation Insertion or deletion of one or two nucleotides that disrupts the normal reading frame.

gene Functional unit of DNA that gives rise to a protein.

genome Total genetic material of a cell.

hybridization *(see also anneal)* Joining of complementary nucleotide sequences.

in situ **hybridization** The use of a labelled antisense probe to identify specific mRNA in tissues or probe to identify chromosomal location of a gene.

intron Sequence of a gene that does not code for a protein.

Klenow enzyme Fragment of DNA polymerase that catalyses DNA synthesis and can utilize dideoxynucleotides (used in sequencing).

LOD score Log_{10} of the likelihood that a given RFLP is close to a gene that influences the phenotypic appearance of a disease.

map unit See *centimorgan*.

messenger RNA (mRNA) (sense orientation) Modified gene transcript that is the template for protein production.

mutation Change in base sequence of DNA.

Northern blotting Size separation and identification of mRNA by probing.

nuclease Enzyme that catalyses the degradation of nucleic acids by breaking phosphodiester bonds.

nucleotide Single unit of nucleic acid.

oligonucleotide Short sequence of nucleotides.

oligonucleotide-directed mutagenesis Technique which mutates the nucleotide sequence of a gene to alter its product in a known way.

penetration The frequency with which a gene manifests itself.

plasmid Self-replicating circle of double-stranded DNA found in bacteria. The most commonly used cloning vehicle.

point mutation Substitution of a nucleotide in DNA sequence.

poly(A) tail Sequence of adenine nucleotides at the 3′ end, which stabilizes mRNA.

polymorphism One or more naturally occurring alternative nucleotide sequences at a recognized genetic location. Usually identified by the alteration of a restriction site.

primary transcript Initial RNA made from the DNA template which still contains the sequences complementary to the introns.

primer Short single-stranded DNA molecule complementary to flanking sequences of a DNA template and acts as a growing point during DNA synthesis.

probe Single-stranded DNA or RNA sequence used to identify its complementary partner.

promoter Regulatory sequence of DNA essential for gene transcription.

recombinant DNA New DNA molecule constructed *in vitro* from two or more different DNA sequences.

recombinant fraction A measurement of the separation of a gene marker from the disease gene due to DNA recombination.

restriction endonuclease Enzyme which recognizes short sequences on double-stranded DNA and cleaves it at this point or nearby.

restriction map Location of restriction enzyme cleavage sites on a sequence of DNA.

reverse transcriptase Enzyme which generates single-stranded DNA from mRNA.

RNA polymerase Enzyme which catalyses the synthesis of RNA from the DNA template.

sense Strand of DNA which gives the nucleotide sequence similar to mRNA (T instead of U) and provides information regarding the amino acid sequence of the gene product (coding strand).

Southern blotting Size separation and identification of DNA sequences using a specific probe.

splicing The process whereby the non-coding regions are excised from the primary mRNA transcript.

template DNA (antisense orientation) Sequence from which RNA is transcribed.
transcription Transfer of genetic information from DNA to RNA.
transfer RNA (tRNA) Triple nucleotides attached to specific amino acids that join to complementary codons on mRNA for protein synthesis.
transformation Process by which extraneous DNA is taken up by a cell.
transgenic Introduction of a foreign gene into the genome of an organism.
translation Process by which mRNA is made into protein.
wobble The ability (in some instances) for hybridization to occur and be effective with a degree of nucleotide mismatch.

References

1 Simone VD, Ciliberto G, Hardon E *et al. Cis* and *trans*-acting elements responsible for the cell-specific expression of the human α_1-antitrypsin gene. *EMBO J* 1987; 6: 2759−66.

2 Boam DSW, Clark AR, Docherty K. Positive and negative regulation of the human insulin gene by multiple transacting factors. *J Biol Chem* 1990; 265: 8285−96.

3 Bain JD, Switzer C, Chamberlin AR, Brenner SA. Ribosome-mediated incorporation of a non-standard amino acid into a peptide through expansion of the genetic code. *Nature* 1992; 356: 537−9.

4 Kidd VJ, Wallace RB, Itakura K *et al.* α-1-Antitrypsin deficiency detection by direct analysis of the mutation in the gene. *Nature* 1983; 304: 230−4.

5 Curiel DT, Buchhagen DL, Chiba I *et al.* A chemical mismatch cleavage method useful for the detection of point mutations in the p53 gene in lung cancer. *Am J Respir Cell Mol Biol* 1990; 3: 405−11.

6 Wakefield AE, Pixley FJ, Banerji S *et al.* Detection of *Pneumocystis carinii* with DNA amplification. *Lancet* 1990; 336: 451−3.

7 Ou CY, Mitchell SW, Krebbs J. DNA amplification for direct detection of human immunodeficiency virus-1 (HIV-1) in DNA of peripheral mononuclear cells. *Science* 1988; 239: 295−7.

8 Saboor SA, Johnson NMcI, McFadden J. Detection of mycobacterial DNA in sarcoidosis and tuberculosis with polymerase chain reaction. *Lancet* 1992; 339: 1012−15.

9 Miller YE, Minna JD, Gazdar AF. Lack of expression of aminoacylase-1 in small cell lung cancer. *J Clin Invest* 1989; 83: 2120−4.

10 Orkin SH, Little PFR, Kazazian HH *et al.* Improved detection of the sickle mutation by DNA analysis. *N Engl J Med* 1982; 307: 32−6.

11 Sanger F, Nicklen S, Coulsen AR. DNA sequencing with chain-terminating inhibitors. *Proc Natl Acad Sci USA* 1977; 74: 5463−7.

12 Lomas DA, Evans DLC, Finch JT, Carrell RW. The mechanism of Z α_1 antitrypsin accumulation in liver. *Nature* 1992; 357: 605−7.

13 Owen MC, Brennan SO, Lewis JH, Carrell RW. Mutation of antitrypsin to antithrombin. α_1-Antitrypsin Pittsburgh (358Met − Arg), a fatal bleeding disorder. *N Engl J Med* 1983; 309: 694−8.

14 Vionnet N, Stoffel M, Takeda J *et al.* Nonsense mutation in the glucokinase gene causes early-onset non-insulin-dependent diabetes mellitus. *Nature* 1992; 356: 721−2.

15 Nukiwa T, Takahashi H, Brantly M, Courtney M, Crystal RG. Alpha-1-antitrypsin null_Granite Falls, a non expressing alpha-1-antitrypsin gene associated with a frameshift to stop mutation in a coding exon. *J Biol Chem* 1987; 262: 11999−12004.

16 Sifers RN, Brashears-Macatee S, Kidd VJ, Muensch H, Woo SLC. A frameshift

mutation results in a truncated alpha-1-antitrypsin that is retained within the rough endoplasmic reticulum. *J Biol Chem* 1988; 263: 7330−5.

17 Kerem BS, Rommens JM, Buchanan JA *et al*. Identification of the cystic fibrosis gene: genetic analysis. *Science* 1989; 245: 1073−9.

18 Matsuo M, Masumura T, Nishio H *et al*. Exon skipping during splicing of dystrophin mRNA precursor due to an intraexon deletion in the dystrophin gene of Duchenne muscular dystrophy Kobe. *J Clin Invest* 1991; 87: 2127−31.

19 Kidd VJ, Globus MS, Wallace RB *et al*. Prenatal diagnosis of α_1 antitrypsin deficiency by direct analysis of the mutation site in the gene. *N Engl J Med* 1984; 310: 639−42.

20 Larsson C. Natural history of life expectancy in severe alpha-1-antitrypsin deficiency, PiZ. *Acta Med Scand* 1978; 204: 345−51.

21 Kierem E, Corey M, Kerem B-S *et al*. The relation between genotype and phenotype in cystic fibrosis − analysis of the most common mutation ($\triangle F_{508}$). *N Engl J Med* 1990; 323: 1517−22.

22 Cutting GR, Kasch LM, Rosenstein BJ *et al*. Two patients with cystic fibrosis nonsense mutations in each cystic fibrosis gene, and mild pulmonary disease. *N Engl J Med* 1990; 323: 1685−9.

23 Meissen GJ, Myers RH, Mastromauro CA *et al*. Predictive testing for Huntington's disease with use of a linked DNA marker. *N Engl J Med* 1988; 318: 535−42.

24 Wainwright BJ, Scambler PJ, Schmidtke J *et al*. Localisation of cystic fibrosis locus to human chromosome 7 cen-q22. *Nature* 1985; 318: 384−5.

25 Cookson WOCM, Sharp PA, Faux JA *et al*. Linkage between immunoglobulin E responses underlying asthma and rhinitis and chromosome 11q. *Lancet* 1989; i: 1292−4.

26 Lathrops GM, Lalouel JM. Easy calculations of LOD scores and genetic risks on small computers. *Am J Hum Genet* 1984; 36: 460−5.

27 Tsui L-C, Buchwald M, Barber D *et al*. Cystic fibrosis locus defined by a genetically linked polymorphic DNA marker. *Science* 1985; 230: 1054−7.

28 Riordan JR, Rommens JM, Kerem B-S *et al*. Identification of the cystic fibrosis gene: cloning and characterization of complementary DNA. *Science* 1989; 245: 1066−73.

29 Anderson MP, Rich DP, Gregory RJ, Smith AE, Welsh MJ. Generation of cAMP-activated chloride currents by expression of CFTR. *Science* 1991; 251: 679−82.

30 Frizzel RA, Rechkemmer G, Shoemaker RL. Altered regulation of airway epithelial cell chloride channels in cystic fibrosis. *Science* 1986; 233: 558−60.

31 Shaw G, Kamen R. A conserved AU sequence from the 3′ untranslated region of GM-CSF mRNA mediates selective mRNA degradation. *Cell* 1986; 46: 659−67.

32 Gribben JG, Devereux S, Thomas NSB *et al*. Development of antibodies to unprotected glycosylation sites on recombinant human GM-CSF. *Lancet* 1990; 335: 434−7.

33 Verbanac KM, Heath EC. Biosynthesis processing and secretion of M and Z variant human alpha-1-antitrypsin. *J Biol Chem* 1986; 261: 9979−89.

34 Bathhurst IC, Errington DM, Foreman RC, Judah JD, Carrell RW. Human Z alpha-1-antitrypsin accumulates intracellularly and stimulates lysosomal activity when synthesised in the *Xenopus* oocyte. *FEBS Lett* 1985; 183: 304−8.

35 Dixon RAF, Sigal IS, Candelor MR *et al*. Structures required for ligand binding to the beta adrenergic receptor. *EMBO J* 1987; 6: 3269−75.

36 Courtney M, Jallat S, Tessier LH *et al*. Synthesis in *E. coli* of α_1 antitrypsin variants of therapeutic potential for emphysema and thrombosis. *Nature* 1985; 313: 149−51.

37 Lemaistre CF, Rosenblum MG, Reuben JM *et al*. Therapeutic effects of genetically engineered toxin (DAB_{486} IL-2) in patients with chronic lymphatic leukaemia. *Lancet* 1991; 337: 1124−5.

38 Sifers RN, Finegold MJ, Woo SLC. Alpha-1-antitrypsin deficiency: accumulation or degradation of mutant variants within the hepatic endoplasmic reticulum. *Am J Respir Cell Mol Biol* 1989; 1: 341−5.

39 Riele H te, Maandag ER, Clarke A, Hooper M, Berns A. Consecutive inactivation of both alleles of the pim-1 proto-oncogene by homologous recombination in embryonic stem cells. *Nature* 1990; 348: 649−51.

40 McManaway ME, Neckers LM, Loke SL *et al.* Tumor-specific inhibition of lymphoma growth by an antisense oligodeoxy-nucleotide. *Lancet* 1990; 335: 808−11.

41 Chen P-L, Chen Y, Bookstein R, Lee W-H. Genetic mechanisms of tumour suppression by the human p53 gene. *Science* 1990; 250: 1576−80.

42 Hubbard RC, McElvaney NG, Sellers SE *et al.* Recombinant DNA-produced α_1-antitrypsin administered by aerosol augments lower respiratory tract anti-neutrophil elastase defenses in individuals with α_1-antitrypsin deficiency. *J Clin Invest* 1989; 84: 1349−54.

43 McElvaney NG, Hubbard RC, Birrer P *et al.* Aerosol α_1-antitrypsin treatment for cystic fibrosis. *Lancet* 1991; 337: 392−4.

44 Chytil A, Garver R, Crystal RG. Human α_1-antitrypsin production by human epithelial cells infected with a retroviral vector containing the human α_1-antitrypsin gene. *Am Rev Respir Dis* 1988; 137: A371.

45 Rosenfeld MA, Siegfried W, Yoshimura K *et al.* Adenovirus-mediated transfer of a recombinant α1-antitrypsin gene to the lung epithelium *in vivo*. *Science* 1991; 252: 431−4.

46 Rich DP, Anderson MP, Gregory RJ *et al.* Expression of cystic fibrosis transmembrane conductance regulator corrects defective chloride channel regulation in cystic fibrosis airway epithelial cells. *Nature* 1990; 347: 358−63.

47 Curiel DT, Agarwal S, Romer MU *et al.* Gene transfer to respiratory epithelial cells via the receptor-mediated endocytosis pathway. *Am J Respir Cell Mol Biol* 1992; 6: 247−52.

48 Culver KW, Osborne WR, Miller AD *et al.* Correction of ADA deficiency in human T lymphocytes using retroviral-mediated gene transfer. *Transplant Proc* 1991; 23: 170−1.

2 Analysis of protein synthesis

DAVID BURNETT AND SIMON C. AFFORD

Introduction

The purpose of this chapter is to discuss the methods for the analysis of specific protein synthesis by cells in the lung, although the principles clearly apply to all organ tissues. It is hoped that the information gathered here will be a guide to those planning an investigation or help those with an interest in molecular medicine, but limited experience, to make some sense of the literature. The significance of the effects of metabolic inhibitors such as α-amanitin or brefeldin might be obvious to some cell biologists, but not necessarily to a chest physician. The effects of the commonly used inhibitors of protein synthesis and processing will be explained in the text and are summarized for reference in Table 2.1 and Fig. 2.1. There are many stages in the cellular production of a mature protein, some of which are discussed in other chapters. The expression of proteins can be controlled at each of the stages from the initial transcription of the gene to the post-translational processing of the protein product.

The analytical techniques used to study the synthesis, processing and secretion of proteins are all essentially concerned with one of two approaches. The first is to detect and characterize the protein product itself. The second is to study the expression of the messenger RNA (mRNA), which codes for the protein of interest. The development of molecular genetics has seen the use of 'molecular biology' techniques become *de rigueur* and the demonstration of specific mRNA transcripts in a cell or tissue is, by many, considered synonymous with the translation and synthesis of the protein product. It will become evident that this assumption is not necessarily true and that methods employing 'molecular biology' and 'traditional' protein biochemistry are complementary and both approaches are necessary.

Detection of translated protein

The first step in an investigation is likely to be a 'broad approach'. It would be appropriate to determine first whether the protein is present in the tissues of interest. Frequently, a protein is detected in increased

Table 2.1 Inhibitors of protein synthesis and processing

Transcription inhibitors	*Translation inhibitors*
Actinomycin D	Anisomycin
α-Amanitin	Cycloheximide
Novabiocin	Puromycin
Inhibitors of secretion	*Glycosylation inhibitor*
Brefeldin	Tunicamycin
Monensin	

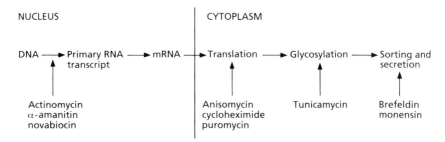

Fig. 2.1 A greatly simplified schema of the stages in protein synthesis showing the points at which metabolic inhibitors act.

concentrations in a biological fluid such as lung secretions [1] and this raises the question of which particular cell type is responsible for its synthesis.

An initial approach could be based on the analysis of whole, homogenized lung tissue using a variety of methods which rely on specific antibodies to the protein of interest. These include gel precipitation methods, radioimmunoassay and enzyme-linked immunosorbent assay (ELISA). Alternatively, if the protein has a functional activity, for instance that of an enzyme, this can also be used as the basis of an assay to detect or measure the protein in the sample. Clearly, this approach does have disadvantages. In particular, tissue homogenates represent the products of many cell types; they often include contaminating blood, and the results would therefore provide little information other than confirming the protein is present. Thus, more specific and accurate methods need to be considered.

Immunohistochemistry

The use of immunohistochemistry to detect the presence of proteins in cells has become a standard method in many laboratories. Immunohistochemical detection of surface markers, for instance, is used routinely for identifying different populations of leucocytes. The binding of the antibody to the target protein is visualized with either an enzyme- or fluorochrome-linked antibody (Fig. 2.2) [2]. The method has the advantage of not requiring the purification of cells; it can be used effectively on frozen or paraffin tissue sections as well as smears or cytocentrifuge preparations of cells. Despite the versatility of this technique, there are several potential problems in interpreting results:

1   It is important with all methods using antibodies as probes that the antibodies are specific. One potential problem is that an apparently specific antibody raised to a protein purified from one source, plasma for instance, may cross-react with another intracellular protein. Polyclonal antisera, which recognize several epitopes on an antigen, are regarded by some to be by definition less specific than monoclonal antibodies which react with a single epitope. Nevertheless, a cross-reaction by one species of antibody in a polyclonal antiserum may not be evident if it represents only a small proportion of the total spectrum of antigenic determinants (epitopes), whereas cross-reaction of a monoclonal antibody will be total if the antibody reacts with a shared epitope on two different proteins.

2   A protein identified within or on a cell might be present as a result of uptake from the surrounding environment, rather than the result of active synthesis.

3   The presence of a protein can represent material which was produced and stored previously by the cell but is no longer actively synthesized. For instance, blood and tissue neutrophils can be stained immunohisto-

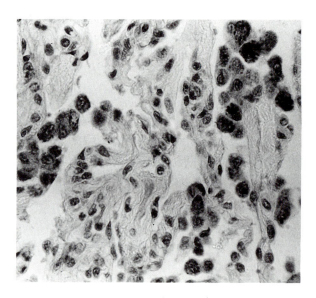

Fig. 2.2 Immunohistochemical localization of α_1-antichymotrypsin in alveolar macrophages. The formalin-fixed section of lung was incubated with a specific sheep antibody to α_1-antichymotrypsin and antibody binding was detected with a horseradish peroxidase-conjugated donkey antibody to sheep immunoglobulin G (IgG).

chemically for granule proteins, such as the enzymes elastase and cathepsin G [3, 4], demonstrating the presence of these proteins in the mature cells. The granules are formed, and their constituents synthesized, at the promyelocytic or myelocytic stages of differentiation in the bone marrow [5] and mature neutrophils cannot synthesize these proteins [6].

4 Cells can produce proteins that are not stored but are rapidly secreted and the intracellular levels are too low to detect. It is possible, by treating the cells with the ionophore monensin or with brefeldin A (Fig. 2.1), to prevent the transport of proteins from the endoplasmic reticulum or Golgi; these proteins therefore accumulate in sufficient quantity to be identified. This method has been used, for instance, to demonstrate the synthesis of the tissue inhibitor of metalloproteinases (TIMP) by a variety of cell types [7].

In association with immunohistochemistry, the localization of the cells responsible for the synthesis of a protein can be confirmed by the detection of specific mRNA transcripts (see below).

Immunochemical detection of synthesized protein

Once cells suspected of synthesizing a protein of interest have been identified it will be necessary to isolate them for more detailed study. Purified cells in primary culture, or suitable cell lines, can be analysed in a number of ways for evidence of the synthesis of a specific protein. Cell cultures can be subjected to immunohistochemistry, as indicated above, or cell lysates and conditioned medium can be analysed by a variety of immunological assays including gel immunodiffusion methods, radio-immunoassay or ELISA for the presence of protein. These results alone will not prove that active synthesis has occurred although the time course may provide strong evidence in the absence of added protein. *De novo* protein synthesis can be confirmed in two ways. First, cultures can be maintained in the presence of inhibitors of protein synthesis; if the cells are actively synthesizing the protein, quantitative immunoassays should detect decreasing or static amounts of the protein within the cells or secreted into the culture medium. Several inhibitors are available (Table 2.1; Fig. 2.1) to block synthesis at the level of transcription of mRNA from the gene (actinomycin; α-amanitin; novabiocin), at the level of translation of protein from mRNA (puromycin; anisomycin; cycloheximide), or to prevent transport of the synthesized protein from the endoplasmic reticulum (brefeldin A) or Golgi (monensin).

A second approach is to label newly synthesized protein with radio-labelled amino acids. The cells are cultured in the presence of the radiolabelled amino acids, usually ^{35}S-methionine or ^{35}S-cysteine, which will be incorporated into the polypeptide chains of proteins synthesized during the period of culture. The efficiency of incorporation is increased by using cell culture medium deficient in the chosen radiolabelled amino acid (methionine-free culture medium is commercially available for this purpose from suppliers of cell culture media). The conditioned medium and cell lysates can be harvested and subjected to immunochemical analysis, such as immunoelectrophoresis followed by autoradiography (Fig. 2.3). The immunoprecipitate obtained with a specific antibody will be visible on the autoradiograph if *de novo* synthesis of the protein has occurred. Further confirmation of the specific incorporation of the radio-labelled amino acid into synthesized protein can be obtained with control cultures containing the appropriate inhibitors mentioned above (Fig. 2.3). An alternative method of analysis is to isolate the protein of interest from the radiolabelled cell culture material and subject it to sodium dodecylsulphate—polyacrylamide gel electrophoresis (SDS—PAGE) followed by blotting on to a nitrocellulose membrane [8]. Autoradiography of the membrane will reveal specific incorporation of amino acid and give additional information regarding the molecular mass of the protein product. A refinement of radiolabelled amino acid incorporation is pulse—chase. The cells are incubated (pulsed) with the radiolabelled amino acid for a short period, after which the culture medium is replaced by one without a radiolabel. Subsequent recovery (chase) and analysis of cell lysates and conditioned medium reveal information about the time and location of each step of protein construction and secretion from the translation stage [9].

Detection of RNA transcripts

It follows from Watsons' dogma (DNA = RNA = protein) that the synthesis of a protein by a cell must be preceded by the transcription of mRNA from the gene. The detection of specific mRNA is therefore often a convenient and powerful approach if used in conjunction with analysis for the protein product. This is necessary because examples exist showing that mRNA does not always lead to the production of the protein product, especially if the mRNA is abnormal (see below).

Most of the basic methods for the analysis of DNA and RNA are described in detail by Sambrook *et al.* [10].

In situ hybridization

In situ hybridization is analogous to immunohistochemistry, utilizing complementary DNA (cDNA), RNA (cRNA) or oligonucleotide probes to detect mRNA rather than antibody to detect protein. As with immuno-histochemistry, the advantage of this method is that pure cell preparations are not essential; the method can be used satisfactorily on tissue sections prepared appropriately (Fig. 2.4). Nonetheless, as with antibodies, it is important that the specificity of the DNA or RNA probes is confirmed by

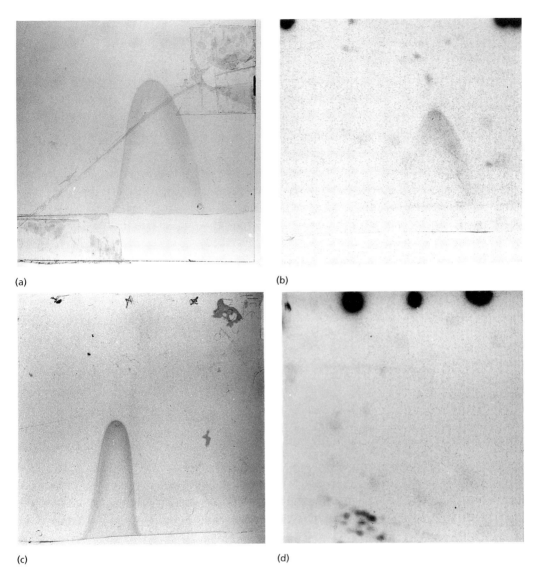

(a)   (b)

(c)   (d)

Fig. 2.3 Two-dimensional (crossed) immunoelectrophoresis of conditioned medium from cultures of alveolar macrophages in the presence of ^{35}S-methionine, demonstrating incorporation of the radiolabelled amino acid into *de novo* synthesized α_1-antichymotrypsin. The proteins in the medium, mixed with pure 'carrier' α_1-antichymotrypsin, were separated by electrophoresis in agarose gel (the first dimension, see a) and then electrophoresed, at right angles to the first dimension, into agarose containing a specific antibody to α_1-antichymotrypsin, which formed a visible immunoprecipitate in the gel following staining with Kenacid blue (a). The gel was washed to remove non-precipitated proteins and autoradiographed, revealing the immunoprecipitate to contain ^{35}S-methionine (b) and thus suggesting incorporation of the radiolabelled amino acid into newly synthesized α_1-antichymotrypsin. In order to confirm the specificity of incorporation, cell cultures were also incubated with cycloheximide. The stained gel from this control showed an immunoprecipitate due to the presence of carrier protein (c), but there was no incorporation of ^{35}S-methionine (d), demonstrating that cycloheximide had inhibited synthesis of α_1-antichymotrypsin by these cells. The dark spots on the upper edges of the autoradiographs (b) and (d) correspond to where ^{35}S had been dotted on to the gels (marked on (a) and (c)) for orientation purposes.

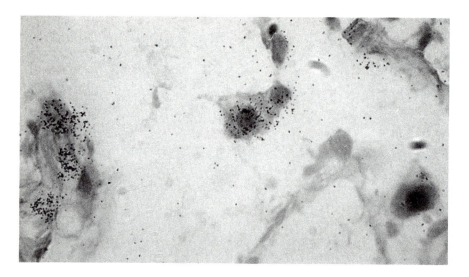

Fig. 2.4 *In situ* hybridization using a radiolabelled cRNA probe, demonstrating hepatocyte growth factor mRNA in a limited number of cells within a section of human lung tissue.

the size of the transcripts seen on Northern blotting. *In situ* hybridization is covered comprehensively in Chapter 3.

Blotting techniques

With a cDNA probe, whole lung tissue preparations (with the same reservations as for protein detection), or cell cultures, can be used to detect the presence of mRNA by means of blotting. Northern blotting involves the separation of the different mRNA species by size in agarose gel, followed by transfer to a membrane where they are probed with labelled (usually radiolabelled with ^{32}P-nucleotides) cDNA probes and autoradiographed to detect specific transcripts (see Chapter 1 and Fig. 2.5). This method is useful in a number of ways. First, the detection of a transcript of appropriate size confirms the specificity of the probe. The detection of multiple transcripts might indicate multiple genes encoding for closely related proteins or alternative splicing of transcripts from a single gene. Alternatively, it can indicate that the conditions of hybridization of the probe to the blotted RNA are not stringent enough and 'unrelated' RNA species, with areas of homology, are being detected (see Chapter 1). Given that the conditions of stringency are satisfactory, this method is a powerful and semiquantitative tool for detecting mRNA species. Northern blots can be scanned by densitometry and the results related to total RNA loaded on to the agarose gel, or to initial cell numbers, to indicate the amount of specific mRNA per cell. Once the specificity of a cDNA probe is established, dot- or slot-blotting (see

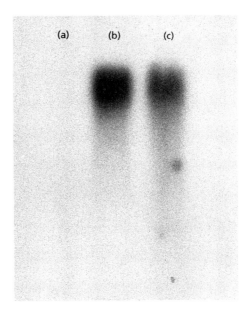

Fig. 2.5 Northern blotting of RNA using a radiolabelled cDNA probe for neutrophil elastase. The results show the absence of mRNA for elastase in mature neutrophils (a) but a 0.9 kilobase (kb) transcript in bone marrow (b) and U937 myelomonocytic cell line (c).

Chapter 1 and Fig. 2.6) can be used as a semiquantitative method to assay mRNA. These techniques, where RNA preparations are not electrophoresed but simply transferred to a suitable membrane, such as nitrocellulose, before probing with the labelled cDNA, are easier to perform than Northern blotting. The autoradiographs can be scanned by densitometry for quantification or the portions of membrane containing the hybridized radiolabelled probe can be measured by radiocounting. As an alternative to radiolabelling, probes can be labelled with non-radioactive materials. They can be sulphonated or labelled with digoxygenin or biotin. Hybridization is identified, in the case of sulphonated or digoxygenin-labelled probes, with enzyme-linked (e.g. peroxidase) antibodies and biotinylated probes are detected with enzyme-linked avidin. Some caution must be exercised regarding the accuracy and precision of these methods since it is not easy to ensure the uniform application or hybridization of individual samples.

As with protein analyses, it is useful to include control experiments with appropriate inhibitors. Inhibitors of DNA transcription (actinomycin, α-amanitin, novabiocin) should abolish mRNA production whereas inhibitors of translation (puromycin, anisomycin, cycloheximide) should have no effect. Cellular material is sometimes at a premium, or the numbers of mRNA transcripts are low. The RNA preparation transcripts can be increased by the polymerase chain reaction [11], but if specific

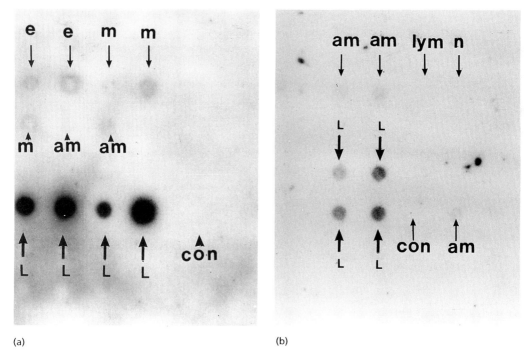

Fig. 2.6 Dot-blot hybridization for mRNA of α_1-antichymotrypsin. (a) Positive dot-blots with RNA preparations from human liver (L), alveolar macrophages (am) and bronchial epithelium (e). Liver RNA treated with RNAase was negative (con). Equivalent amounts of RNA were applied from each tissue and the strong signal obtained with liver demonstrates therefore that this tissue contains relatively more mRNA for α_1-antichymotrypsin than do alveolar macrophages or bronchial epithelium. (b) Dot-blots showing α_1-antichymotrypsin mRNA in liver (L) and alveolar macrophages (am) but not in lymphocytes (lym), neutrophils (n) or RNAase-treated liver (con).

cells are under investigation, purity of the cells is essential since low transcript numbers in contaminating cells will also be amplified.

Another method that is more sensitive than Northern blotting for detecting mRNA is an RNAase protection assay. A radiolabelled cRNA or cDNA probe is allowed to hybridize with the cell lysate and non-hybridized mRNA is digested with added ribonucleases. Non-hybridized (single-stranded) RNA is degraded by the ribonucleases, but hybridized (double-stranded) mRNA is protected from digestion and detected by autoradiography after electrophoresis in polyacrylamide gels. The transcript size can be estimated if a full-length cDNA or cRNA probe is used but non-full-length probes will leave the remaining mRNA in a single-stranded form which will be degraded subsequently (see also Chapter 1).

Just as a protein can be present within a cell in the absence of mRNA, the opposite is also true; it is possible for mRNA to be detected in cells without detectable protein product. In studies of blood monocytes from subjects with the α_1-antitrypsin genotype Null Mattawa a full-length mRNA was detected but not intracellular or excreted α_1-antitrypsin protein. This was attributed to a single nucleotide insertion causing a 3′ frameshift resulting in a premature signal for termination of translation. The translated foreshortened, or truncated, protein is unstable and degraded rapidly [12]. Alternatively, the presence of mRNA but no protein might reflect the rapid secretion of a successfully translated protein from the cell; as already described above, the prevention of intracellular translocation and secretion from the cell, with monensin or brefeldin A, would lead to the accumulation of the protein and permit detection. It is also possible that the mRNA, although transcribed efficiently, does not survive long enough for sufficient detectable protein to be translated.

Other factors causing reduced expression of a protein include those which reduce transcription of the gene or lead to a rapid turnover of mRNA. The transcriptional rate of DNA to produce mRNA can be studied by nuclear run-off [13]. Cell nuclei are isolated and labelled with radiolabelled (^{32}P) nucleoside triphosphates, which will be incorporated into newly transcribed RNA and can be detected by dot-blotting followed by measurement of incorporated radiolabel. Since the cytoplasm is absent, reduced mRNA would suggest reduced transcription, but if the mRNA run-off is constant, the results would suggest that reduced protein expression is occurring at a post-transcriptional stage. This could result from increased mRNA catabolism, reduced translation or altered post-translational processing of the protein.

Another way to study RNA stability is to treat whole cells with a transcription inhibitor (Table 2.1; Fig. 2.1) and measure the decrease of specific mRNA with time, thus obtaining the mRNA half-life.

Post-translational protein modification

More than 100 post-translational modifications of proteins have been identified although the effects of most of these are unknown. They may alter the functions of a protein and its ultimate fate within or outside the cell.

Many proteins are glycosylated. The effects of glycosylation in the Golgi and endoplasmic reticulum on protein traffic, function or catabolism can be studied in several ways. Co-culture of cells with the antibiotic tunicamycin inhibits all N-glycosylation. Alternatively, the purified proteins can be incubated with enzymes that remove selected oligosaccharides or all linked sugar residues (N-glycanase).

The most common modification of proteins is the phosphorylation, by protein kinases, of hydroxyl groups on serine, threonine or tyrosine residues. These phosphorylation events are reversible *in vivo*, due to the action of phosphatases. Phosphorylation events can be studied by

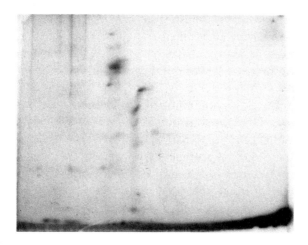

Fig. 2.7 Autoradiograph of two-dimensional electrophoresis, in polyacrylamide gel, of whole neutrophil cellular proteins following incubation of the cells with [^{32}P]-orthophosphate. The proteins were subjected to isoelectric focusing in the first dimension (left to right at top) in which proteins were separated according to the isoelectric point (charge). For the second dimension (top to bottom) the proteins were treated with the detergent SDS and separation was according to protein size. The autoradiograph reveals proteins that have been phosphorylated by the cells, thus incorporating added [^{32}P]-orthophosphate. (Photograph by courtesy of Dr Janet Lord, Department of Immunology, University of Birmingham, UK.)

incubating cell lysates with ^{32}P and newly phosphorylated proteins are identified by autoradiography of two-dimensional electrophoresis gels (Fig. 2.7) in which proteins are separated by isoelectric focusing followed by SDS-PAGE [14].

Protein sorting and secretion

Once synthesized, proteins are distributed to sites within the cell or secreted [15]. Some protein transport occurs by translocation across membranes, mediated by receptors that recognize specific sorting signals on the protein. One form of signal is a signal peptide of up to 60 amino acids on the amino terminus that is usually cleaved from the protein after recognition and receptor binding. Another form of signal is a 'signal patch' formed only after the protein has folded into its tertiary conformation. Amino acid sequences that are not adjacent to each other in the unfolded protein can become closely associated in the mature protein. A resulting three-dimensional feature on the protein may therefore be recognized as a receptor site. Different signal peptides determine different destinations in the cell. Protein transport can also be mediated by membrane vesicles, where portions of membrane from one compartment bud off, becoming transport vesicles. These contain proteins captured from the original compartment and fuse with the membrane of the target compartment, thus transferring the protein cargo. This process may also be selectively determined by sorting signals on the proteins. The significance of these processes is illustrated by the ZZ phenotype of α_1-antitrypsin, which differs from the MM phenotype in a single amino acid substitution (glutamic acid (342) lysine). Although the ZZ protein is transcribed [16] and translated [17] the protein accumulates in the cell. This suggests that the glutamic acid (342) lysine substitution results in impairment of the secretory pathway of the protein from the endoplasmic reticulum [18], presumably through the loss of the appropriate transport signal. Recent evidence, however, suggests that this accumulation is dependent upon protein polymerization [19].

Protein traffic within a cell can be studied by its identification in isolated subcellular structures following pulse—chase experiments, or by immunoelectron microscopy. In addition, recombinant DNA coding for natural mutations (as with the Z variant of α_1-antitrypsin) or produced by site-directed mutagenesis (see Chapter 6) can be expressed in a cellular expression vector system and the effects of mutagenic substitutions on protein sorting and other functional properties can be studied.

Protein catabolism

The ability of a cell to degrade proteins rapidly in response to regulatory signals is becoming recognized as an important way in which protein expression is altered. In some cases this may be of equal importance to the ability to alter expression at the transcriptional or translational stages. In addition to pathological consequences, such as those arising from the Null Mattawa α_1-antitrypsin protein, rapid degradation following translation may be important in regulating the functions of enzymes catalysing rate-limiting steps in metabolic pathways and proteins such as oncogenes that have a role in cell growth and development. Furthermore, the recognition and degradation of proteins that are misfolded, denatured or otherwise 'abnormal' are likely to be important mechanisms for the removal of useless or potentially dangerous proteins. In eukaryotic cells, degradation is dependent on the ubiquitin pathway. Ubiquitin is a polypeptide member of the heat-shock protein family that binds covalently to lysine residues of abnormal proteins and proteins with destabilizing N-terminal amino acids [20]. Once conjugated, the protein—ubiquitin complex becomes a substrate for a large adenosine triphosphate-dependent multi-enzyme complex that has a broad proteolytic specificity towards the complexes [21]. The rate of degradation of a protein can be determined by measuring its half-life after blocking translation with one of the appropriate inhibitors (Fig. 2.1; Table 2.1).

Conclusions

The identification of the cellular sources of specific proteins is merely the first step in studying the factors that determine the intracellular and extracellular expression of proteins. The cellular mechanisms controlling protein expression are complex, occurring at many levels from the signals initiating DNA transcription to the final processing, sorting, transport and degradation or secretion of the protein products. Experimental methods appear to come into and go out of fashion but it is important to utilize a variety of techniques to probe the synthetic pathways at different stages if these processes are to be understood and interpreted correctly.

References

1 Stockley RA. Measurement of soluble proteins in lung secretions. *Thorax* 1984; 39: 241–7.
2 Taylor CR. *Immunomicroscopy: A Diagnostic Tool for the Surgical Pathologist*. Philadelphia: WB Saunders, 1986.
3 Crocker J, Jenkins R, Burnett D. Immunohistochemical demonstration of leucocyte elastase in human tissues. *J Clin Pathol* 1984; 37: 1114–18.
4 Crocker J, Jenkins R, Burnett D. Immunohistochemical localization of cathepsin G in human tissues. *Am J Surg Pathol* 1985; 9: 338–43.
5 Bainton DF, Ullyot JF, Farquhar MG. The development of neutrophilic polymorphonuclear leukocytes in human bone marrow: origin and content of azurophil and specific granules. *J Exp Med* 1971; 134: 907–34.
6 Fouret P, Du Bois RM, Bernaudin J-F, Takahashi H, Ferrans VJ, Crystal RG. Expression of the neutrophil elastase gene during human bone marrow cell differentiation. *J Exp Med* 1989; 169: 833–46.
7 Hembry RM, Murphy G, Reynolds JJ. Immunolocalization of tissue inhibitor of metalloproteinases (TIMP) in human cells. Characterization and use of a specific antiserum. *J Cell Sci* 1985; 73: 105–9.
8 Towbin H, Staehelin T, Gordon J. Electrophoretic transfer of proteins from polyacrylamide gels to nitrocellulose sheets: procedures and some applications. *Proc Natl Acad Sci USA* 1979; 76: 4350–4.
9 Salvesen GS, Enghild JJ. An unusual specificity in the activation of neutrophil serine proteinase zymogens. *Biochemistry* 1990; 29: 5304–8.
10 Sambrook J, Fritsch EF, Maniatis T. *Molecular Cloning: A Laboratory Manual*, 2nd edn (three volumes). New York: Cold Spring Harbor Laboratory Press, 1989.
11 Erlich HA. *PCR Technology: Principles and Applications for DNA Amplification*. New York: Stockton Press, 1989.
12 Curiel D, Brantly M, Curiel E, Stier L, Crystal RG. α_1-Antitrypsin deficiency caused by the α_1-antitrypsin NULLmattawa gene. An insertion mutation rendering the α_1-antitrypsin gene incapable of producing α_1-antitrypsin. *J Clin Invest* 1989; 83: 1144–52.
13 Hanson RD, Connolly NL, Burnett D, Campbell EJ, Senior RM, Ley TJ. Developmental regulation of the human cathepsin G gene in myelomonocytic cells. *J Biol Chem* 1990; 265: 1524–30.
14 O'Farrell PH. High resolution two-dimensional electrophoresis of proteins. *J Biol Chem* 1975; 250: 4007–21.
15 Pugsley AP. *Protein Targetting*. San Diego: Academic Press, 1989.

16 Bathurst IC, Errington DM, Foreman RC, Judah JD, Carrell RW. Human Z alpha1-antitrypsin accumulates intracellularly and stimulates lysosomal activity when synthesized in the *Xenopus* oocyte. *FEBS Lett* 1985; 183: 304−8.

17 Foreman RC. Alpha$_1$-antitrypsin deficiency — a defect in secretion. *Biosci Rep* 1987; 7: 307−11.

18 Verbanac KM, Heath EC. Biosynthesis, processing and secretion of M and Z variant α_1 antitrypsin. *J Biol Chem* 1986; 261: 9979−89.

19 Lomas D, Evans D, Ll., Finch JT, Carrell RW. The mechanism of Z α_1-antitrypsin accumulation in the liver. *Nature* 1992; 357: 605−7.

20 Finley D, Bartel B, Varshavsky A. The tails of ubiquitin precursors are ribosomal proteins whose fusion to ubiquitin facilitates ribosome biogenesis. *Nature* 1989; 338: 394−401.

21 Mayer RJ, Doherty F. Intracellular protein catabolism: state of the art. *FEBS Lett* 1986; 198: 181−93.

3 Methods for *in situ* hybridization

GIORGIO TERENGHI AND JULIA M. POLAK

Introduction

The technique of *in situ* hybridization was first applied by Gall and Pardue [1], but it is only in recent years that it has been used with increasing frequency. The technique is based on the formation of hybrids by complementary base pairing of two single-stranded nucleic acids. By using a labelled known sequence, or probe, it is possible to recognize morphologically the target messenger RNA (mRNA) or DNA within a cell. With the identification of nucleic acid sequences, *in situ* hybridization offers the possibility to confirm many of the results obtained by immuno-histochemistry, and also it can give an indication of the cellular syn-thetic activity in physiological and pathological situations.

Recent improvements of the methodology of *in situ* hybridization have increased the reliability and the sensitivity of the technique. The current literature presents a wide range of protocols [2, 3], and this is possibly due to specific applications required in different studies. However, there are general principles and guidelines which are valid for all different types of investigations. In this chapter we give an updated overview of these principles by examining different aspects of the methodology. We also look at the application of *in situ* hybridization in the study of lung research and pathology.

Generation of probes

There are three different types of probes: DNA, RNA and oligonucleotide probes. Their use is dictated by different factors, including availability and type of application. Complementary DNA (cDNA) probes have been commonly used for molecular biology studies; consequently they were also applied for *in situ* hybridization [4–6]. A cDNA probe sequence is generally cloned into a bacterial plasmid vector, which can multiply easily producing a large supply of probes [7]. The cloned probe can be labelled using a variety of protocols [8], and kits are commercially available. DNA probes present the advantage of being stable and resistant to degradation, as specific DNA nucleases, or DNases, are easy to eliminate from the preparations. However, DNA probes are double stranded and

48

they need to be denatured before use to allow hybridization of the complementary single strand with the target sequence. Inevitably the re-annealing process of the probe competes with the hybridization reaction; hence there is an effective decrease of the amount of probe available for hybridization, which ultimately impairs the efficiency of hybrid formation [9]. Furthermore, cDNA probes are constituted generally by long sequences, which can adversely affect the penetration of the probe into the tissue.

Single-stranded complementary RNA (cRNA) probes are becoming more popular for *in situ* hybridization, as they are more sensitive compared with DNA probes [9]. To prepare RNA probes, a chosen cDNA is inserted in a plasmid vector downstream from a promoter (or RNA polymerase) sequence; RNA probes are then transcribed from the template sequence using an appropriate RNA polymerase enzyme in the presence of ribonucleotides [10, 11]. One or more of the ribonucleotides can be tagged to a reporter molecule, either isotopic or non-radioactive, ensuring an even labelling of the transcribed probe. The size of the insert can be optimized, so that the synthesized probe is within the optimal size range of 100−400 bases, which gives generally the best signal/noise ratio. Certain precautions have to be taken while working with RNA probes, as they are easily degraded by ribonuclease (RNase), which is a ubiquitous and heat-resistant enzyme. A recent development in the preparation of RNA probes has been the use of the polymerase chain reaction (PCR) in conjunction with primer containing an RNA polymerase promoter sequence. This allows the preparation of template for RNA probe transcription avoiding the subcloning of cDNA in a vector [12].

Oligonucleotide probes are in essence single-stranded DNA probes, which are prepared by solid phase synthesis according to any given sequence [13, 14]. Some care has to be taken when choosing the sequence of the oligonucleotide probe, in order to avoid cross-hybridization due to sequence homology, which can easily occur in such short probes. The small size of these probes (generally 20−50 bases) is favourable for tissue penetration during the hybridization procedure, although the conditions have to be carefully controlled to obtain sequence-specific hybrids [15]. The labelling method available allows the incorporation of only a single end label or short labelled 'tail' of reporter molecules, and this results in a limited sensitivity particularly when working with targets which are present in low copy number. It is possible to overcome the problem by synthesizing oligonucleotides which include a promoter sequence for RNA polymerase. These can be used as template for the transcription of RNA-labelled probes [16].

Isotope labelling and autoradiography

The commonly used isotopes are ^{32}P, ^{35}S and ^{3}H, and their choice is based on a balance between resolution, sensitivity and speed. Radioactive labels are considered to be the most sensitive, although resolution and rapidity do not always coincide when using different isotopes [17]. The characteristics of the three radioisotopes are summarized in Table 3.1.

For rapid results ^{32}P is the isotope of choice, as it possesses a very high specific activity and autoradiography exposure time can be as short as 24 h. However, the range of emission of its β-particle is high, which results in a wide scatter of silver grain in the autoradiographic emulsion and generally poor resolution, particularly when using tissues with high cell density. In contrast, ^{3}H has low specific activity and a short range of β-particle emission. Resolution is very good, mostly confined to the target cell, but autoradiography requires long exposure times (3−4 weeks). ^{35}S represents a suitable balance between the other two isotopes, as it gives good resolution within a relatively short time of autoradiographic exposure (5−10 days; Fig. 3.1). A problem commonly found when using ^{35}S-labelled probes is high background, mainly due to non-specific binding of the sulphur to the tissue. To overcome this problem it is important to include dithiothreitol (DTT, 100 mmol l^{-1}) in both hybridization buffer and stringency washes [18].

Autoradiography is the recording of radioactive emission within a photographic film by the formation of silver grains, and it is the method of choice to identify the hybridization site of the radiolabelled probes. Film or emulsion autoradiography can be chosen according to the need. Film autoradiography (or macro-autoradiography) can supply results rapidly when using ^{32}P- and ^{35}S-labelled probes. However, it is not possible to obtain single cell resolution, and the method gives best results when applied for the identification of cell subpopulations within a tissue.

Micro-autoradiography is the application of a thin layer of liquid photographic emulsion, which is quickly gelled on to the tissue preparation. The interaction between the emitted β-particles and the silver bromide crystals in the emulsion produces the formation of silver grains,

Table 3.1 Characteristics of the radioisotopes most commonly used for *in situ* hybridization. Note that the β-particles show a reduced range of emission in the autoradiographic emulsion, which is the result of the increased density of the dried emulsion due to the high loading of silver bromide

Isotope	Half-life	Emission type/ max energy (MeV)	β-Emission range (μm) tissue/emulsion
^{32}P	14 days	β/1.71	8000/2000
^{35}S	87 days	β/0.167	300/80
^{3}H	12 years	β/0.018	5/1

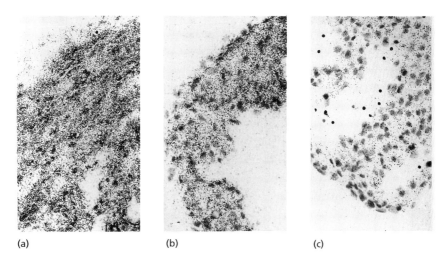

(a)   (b)   (c)

Fig. 3.1 Sections of human right atrium hybridized with atrial natriuretic peptide (ANP) cRNA probes which were labelled with (a) ^{32}P- (3 days' exposure), (b) ^{35}S- (5 days' exposure) and (c) ^{3}H-CTP cytidine triphosphate (28 days' exposure). Note the different intensity of signal and resolution with the various isotopic labels. Emulsion autoradiography and haematoxylin counterstaining ($\times$ 206.5).

which can be easily visualized under the microscope in relation to single cells. Different types of liquid emulsion are available, offering a variety of grain size, but the most commonly used are Ilford K5 or Kodak NTB2. Particular attention has to be paid during the autoradiographic procedure, as variation of emulsion thickness, of drying and exposure conditions, and of temperature can result in formation of high levels of background silver grains [19].

The use of radiolabelled probes presents some advantages such as the possibility to combine *in situ* hybridization and immunocytochemistry on the same section [20–22]. Furthermore, quantification of the hybridization reaction can be carried out using either grain counting techniques [23] or densitometric analysis of autoradiography film [22, 24, 25].

Non-radioactive labels and chromogenic detection systems

Different types of non-radioactive labelling methods have been used for *in situ* hybridization [26–30], but until now their application has been limited. The more widely used labels are biotin and digoxigenin. In the past the use of non-radioactive labels has been curbed by a lack of detection sensitivity, but recent publications have shown that the sensitivity of non-isotopic and radiolabelled probes is comparable [31–35]. Because non-radioactive probes show prolonged stability, increased resolution and rapidity of detection, they are ideally suited for clinical and diagnostic use.

Biotin-labelled probes were first introduced by Langer *et al.* [36], and the method was later modified and improved [37, 38]. Most of the published studies use biotin as marker for cDNA, although it has been used successfully for labelling cRNA and oligonucleotide probes [39−42]. The detection of biotinylated probes is based on immunocyto-chemical methods, which play an important role in determining the resolution and sensitivity of the hybridization [42]. A major problem of biotinylated probes is the high background staining, due to high levels of endogenous biotin. Blocking procedures for endogenous biotin have been described for immunocytochemistry, but they are not equally efficient for *in situ* hybridization, possibly because of the high tempera-tures and presence of formamide and other chemical reagents during the hybridization procedure.

Digoxigenin-labelled probes [43] have recently gained widespread favour, as they are not associated with background problems and show an increased sensitivity compared with biotinylated probes [33, 44]. Like biotin, the detection of digoxigenin is based on immunocytochemical techniques, with either fluorescent or enzymatic reporter labels [43]. Because of the versatility of the immunocytochemical detection methods, it is also possible to use biotinylated and digoxigenin-labelled probes for the simultaneous identification of different target sequences within the same tissue [45, 46]. Alternatively, double *in situ* hybridization can also be carried out using a combination of immunocytochemical detection and directly labelled probes [47].

Tissue preparation

To obtain good hybridization results, it is necessary that the tissue is processed correctly in order to obtain maximum retention of nucleic acid target and optimal morphological preservation. These can be achieved with fixation, which will also stop the degradation processes. Degradation of nucleic acids depends on many different factors, but it is acknowledged that endogenous nucleases play a major role [48]. In particular, when the target is mRNA or the probes are RNA sequences, the presence of ubiquitous RNase is a major concern and any contamination should be carefully avoided. Protocols are available for the preparation of RNase-free equipment and solutions [7]. It has also been observed that dehy-dration, manipulation and dissection of unfixed samples accelerate the nucleic acid degradation process, most probably because of the release of endonucleases and lysosomal products [49]. Similar problems might also be found in tissue with necrotic areas, such as tumours.

Delay between tissue collection and fixation should be kept at a minimum, as target degradation can be extremely fast [50, 51]. However, it is interesting to note that with post-mortem material successful *in situ* hybridization has been carried out on tissue collected up to 10 h after death [52, 53]. This is consistent with the finding of prolonged mRNA stability in post-mortem tissue [49, 54], reinforcing the point that untouched cooled tissue shows a slower degradation time curve than surgical or experimental tissue, which has undergone a certain amount of ischaemia and manipulation.

Different types of fixative have been tested for *in situ* hybridization [8, 18, 40, 50, 52, 55−57]. The final choice is dependent on the system under investigation and the type of probe, but for peptide mRNA hybridization paraformaldehyde appears to be the most suitable fixative. It has to be remembered that prolonged fixation might affect adversely the hybridization results [58, 59], and permeabilization treatment with protease might be necessary to increase probe penetration [18, 41, 58].

Tissue processing does not appear to be as critical as fixation, if this has been carried out in an appropriate way. Although cryostat sections seem to be favoured by many authors, good hybridization results have been obtained on paraffin-embedded tissue as this processing does not alter significantly the hybridization sensitivity [35, 41, 60, 61]. Also *in situ* hybridization can be easily carried out on cultured cells, either grown directly on to glass slides or, in the case of cells grown in suspension, cytospun on to coated slides.

Conditions for hybridization

The prerequisite for a successful hybridization result is penetration of the probe within the tissue, in order to hybridize with the target molecule. As already discussed, probe size is important, and several studies have tried to define an optimal probe size [4−6, 57, 62]. There seems to be an agreement that with cRNA probes best results are obtained with a size range of 200−500 bases. There is experimental evidence that using cDNA probes longer than 1000 bases might be advantageous, as they might form networks which result in signal amplification [6]. The intrinsic small size of oligonucleotide probes makes them ideally suited for an easy tissue penetration, although this advantage might be offset by the more limited sensitivity of these probes.

Permeabilization treatment is generally useful to improve probe penetration, although excessive permeabilization might cause loss of morphology and leakage of target nucleic acid [6, 18, 63]. Lipolytic detergents such as Triton X-100, and protease digestion with proteinase K or pronase, are the most commonly used treatments, and offer the advantage of variable dosage according to the tissue under investigation. Further treatment can be carried out to decrease non-specific binding of the probe to the tissue. This can be caused by electrostatic interaction between the probe and the positively charged moieties within the tissue, and acetylation of tissue proteins has been shown to reduce this interaction [64].

The formation and the stability of hybrids are influenced by different factors. The stability of the hybrid is enhanced by their length, by the number of G-C pairs and by high salt concentrations. Conversely, the hybrids are destabilized by formamide, base mismatching and high temperatures. These factors are often combined in an equation that predicts the melting temperature, defined as the temperature at which half the hybrids dissociate (or melt). Generally, the temperature chosen for hybridization is 25−30°C below melting temperature [65]. In order to preserve tissue morphology and minimize section loss from the slide, the hybridization temperature can be lowered by addition of formamide to the hybridization buffer [66]. Each percentage of formamide included decreases the hybridization temperature by 0.35°C for RNA/RNA hybrids [9] and by 0.65°C for DNA/DNA duplexes [67].

Following hybridization, non-specifically bound probes can be removed by serial washes with stringencies higher than those used during hybridization, thus dissociating probes which are weakly bound to non-specific sequences. When using cRNA probes, a further wash containing RNase helps in removing single-stranded RNA, while leaving the double-stranded hybrid molecule intact [9].

Lung studies

The presence of regulatory peptides can be detected by immunocyto-chemical techniques. However, the identification of cellular antigens is not confirmatory of peptide synthesis within that cell, or cannot give any information on the dynamic changes of the cellular metabolic processes. This information can be gained by using *in situ* hybridization.

Atrial natriuretic peptide (ANP) has been identified by immunocyto-chemistry in both atria and ventricles of the heart. Further studies also confirmed the presence of mRNA for this peptide in atrial and ventricular cells, both in tissue section and cultured myocytes [68]. Other tissues, such as brain, eye, salivary glands, adrenal glands, kidney and pituitary, have been shown to contain ANP. Similarly, ANP was detected in lung using the radioimmunoassay technique, although it was not possible to determine whether the presence of the peptide was due to uptake from the circulation or to local synthesis. With a combined approach of *in situ* hybridization and immunocytochemistry, it was possible to demonstrate that in lung the site of synthesis and storage of ANP was the smooth muscle cells of both extra- and intrapulmonary veins [69]. The role of ANP in the lung is still a matter of speculation, but its localization suggests a possible release caused by vein stretching, with a possible local paracrine effect, as well as a contribution to the levels of circulating peptide.

In the pathology of endocrine tumours, *in situ* hybridization has been particularly useful in the characterization of tumour types, as often peptide hypersecretion and limited peptide storage prevent the successful use of immunocytochemistry [70]. Gastrin-releasing peptide (GRP), a peptide with trophic effect on tumour cells, can be found in high levels in patients with small cell carcinoma of the lung. However, because of its quick secretion turnover, it proved very difficult to identify peptide immunoreactivity in the tumour cells. By using *in situ* hybridization it was possible to demonstrate that GRP synthesis occurs in a large number of tumour cells (Fig. 3.2), confirming the origin of the circulating peptide [71].

Endothelin-1 (ET-1) is a peptide isolated from endothelial cells [72], and subsequently localized by immunocytochemistry to endocrine cells of the lung and in bronchial epithelium [73]. Because of the distribution and a possible trophic role of this peptide, the presence of ET-1 was investigated in different types of pulmonary tumours. The results of the study showed that ET-1 is synthesized and stored in tumour cells of squamous cell carcinomas and adenocarcinomas, but not in small cell carcinomas [74]. The differential distribution of GRP and ET-1 would suggest that each peptide has a specific growth promoting effect for different cell types. It is interesting to note that preliminary results of *in vitro* binding experiments have shown ^{125}I-ET-1 binding on newly formed blood vessels within lung tumour, but not on tumour cells.

Chromogranin A (CgA) is a neuroendocrine marker identified by immunocytochemistry in normal and tumour cells. Circulating CgA can be detected in patients with neuroendocrine tumours, including small cell carcinoma of the lung. Similar to GRP, CgA immunoreactivity cannot be detected in the cell of this tumour, although CgA mRNA can be easily demonstrated by *in situ* hybridization, reaffirming the validity of CgA as a marker for neuroendocrine tumours [75].

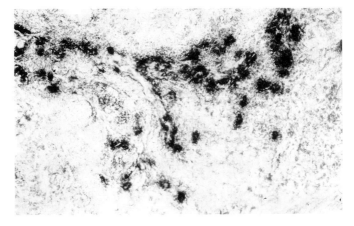

Fig. 3.2 Section of human small cell carcinoma of the lung hybridized with ^{32}P-GRP cRNA probes shown as black silver grain deposits over the tumour cells. Emulsion autoradiography, 3 days' exposure, haematoxylin counterstaining ($\times$ 187.6).

These examples confirm that *in situ* hybridization is a suitable technique for morphological investigations, which can complement, and sometimes enhance, the information gained by other morphological techniques. Because of the improved and user-friendly methodology which is now available, *in situ* hybridization represents an ideal tool in both research and pathological studies.

References

1 Gall G, Pardue HL. Formation and detection of RNA—DNA hybrid molecules in cytological preparations. *Proc Natl Acad Sci USA* 1969; 63: 378—81.

2 Valentino K, Erberwine JH, Barchas JD, eds. *In Situ Hybridization Applications to Neurobiology.* Oxford: Oxford University Press, 1987.

3 Polak JM, McGee JOD, eds. *In Situ Hybridization — Principles and Practice.* Oxford: Oxford University Press, 1990.

4 Brahic M, Haase AT. Detection of viral sequences of low reiteration frequency by *in situ* hybridization. *Proc Natl Acad Sci USA* 1978; 75: 6125—9.

5 Angerer LM, Angerer RC. Detection of poly A+ RNA in sea urchin eggs and embryos by quantitative *in situ* hybridization. *Nucleic Acids Res* 1981; 9: 2819—40.

6 Lawrence JB, Singer RH. Quantitative analysis of *in situ* hybridization methods for the detection of actin gene expression. *Nucleic Acids Res* 1985; 13: 1777—99.

7 Maniatis T, Fritsch EF, Sambrook J. *Molecular Cloning — A Laboratory Manual.* New York: Cold Spring Harbor Laboratory Press, 1989.

8 Terenghi G, Fallon RA. Techniques and applications of *in situ* hybridization. In: Underwood JCE, ed. *Current Topics in Pathology — Pathology of the Nucleus.* Berlin: Springer-Verlag, 1990: 290—337.

9 Cox KH, De Leon DV, Angerer LM, Angerer RC. Detection of mRNAs in sea urchin embryos by *in situ* hybridization using asymmetric RNA probes. *Dev Biol* 1984; 101: 485—502.

10 Melton D, Kneg P, Rabagliati M, Maniatis T, Zinn K, Green MR. Efficient *in vitro* synthesis of biologically active RNA and RNA hybridization probes from plasmids containing a bacteriophage SP6 promoter. *Nucleic Acids Res* 1984; 12: 7035—56.

11 Angerer RC, Cox KH, Angerer LM. *In situ* hybridization to cellular RNAs. *Genet Eng* 1985; 7: 43—65.

12 Young ID, Ailles L, Deugau K, Kisilevsky R. Transcription of cRNA for *in situ* hybridization from polymerase chain reaction-amplified DNA. *Lab Invest* 1991; 64: 709—12.

13 Caruthers MH, Beaucage SL, Efcavitch JW *et al.* Chemical synthesis and biological studies on mutated gene control regions. *Cold Spring Harbor Symp Quant Biol* 1982; 47: 411—18.

14 Lewis ME, Sherman TG, Watson SJ. *In situ* hybridization histochemistry with synthetic oligonucleotides; strategies and methods. *Peptides* 1985; 6 (Suppl. 2): 75—87.

15 Kajimura Y, Krull J, Miyakoshi S, Itakura K, Toyoda H. Application of long synthetic oligonucleotides for gene analysis: effect of probe length and stringency conditions on hybridization specificity. *Genet Anal Tech Appl* 1990; 7: 71—9.

16 Brysch W, Hagendorff G, Schlingensiepen K-H. RNA probes transcribed from synthetic DNA for *in situ* hybridization. *Nucleic Acids Res* 1988; 16: 2333.

17 Brady MAW, Finlan FM. Radioactive labels: autoradiography and choice of emulsion for *in situ* hybridization. In: Polak JM, McGee JOD, eds. *In Situ Hybridization — Principles and Practice.* Oxford: Oxford University Press, 1990: 31—58.

18 Singer RH, Lawrence JB, Villnave C. Optimization of *in situ* hybridization using isotopic and non-isotopic detection methods. *Biotechniques* 1986; 4: 230−50.

19 Rogers AW. *Technique of Autoradiography*. Amsterdam: Elsevier, 1979.

20 Höfler H, Putz B, Rurhi C, Wirnsberger M, Smolle J. Simultaneous localization of calcitonin mRNA and peptide in a medullary thyroid carcinoma. *Virchows Arch B* 1987; 54: 144−51.

21 Giaid A, Gibson SJ, Ibrahim NBN *et al*. Endothelin-1, an endothelium-derived peptide, is expressed in neurons of the human spinal cord and dorsal root ganglia. *Proc Natl Acad Sci USA* 1989; 86: 7634−8.

22 Steel JH, O'Halloran DJ, Jones PM, Chin WW, Bloom SR, Polak JM. Simultaneous immunocytochemistry and *in situ* hybridization of β thyroid stimulating hormone and its messenger ribonucleic acid in euthyroid and hypothyroid rat pituitary. *Mol Cell Probes* 1990; 4: 385−96.

23 Davenport AP, Nunez DJ. Quantification in *in situ* hybridization. In: Polak JM, McGee JOD, eds. *In Situ Hybridization — Principles and Practice*. Oxford: Oxford University Press, 1990: 95−112.

24 McCafferty J, Cresswell L, Alldus C, Terenghi G, Fallon R. A shortened protocol for *in situ* hybridization to mRNA using radiolabelled RNA probes. *Techniques* 1989; 1: 171−82.

25 Nunez DJ, Davenport AP, Emson PC, Brown MJ. A quantitative *in situ* hybridization method using computer assisted image analysis. *Biochem J* 1989; 263: 121−7.

26 Jablonsky E, Moomaw EW, Tullis RH, Ruth J. Preparation of oligodeoxynucleotide alkaline phosphatase conjugates and their use as hybridization probe. *Nucleic Acids Res* 1986; 14: 6115−28.

27 Hopman AHN, Wiengant J, Tesser GI, Van Duijn P. A non-radioactive *in situ* hybridization method based on mercurated nucleic acid probes and sulphydryl-hapten ligands. *Nucleic Acids Res* 1986; 14: 6471−88.

28 van der Ploeg, Landegent JE, Hopman HHN, Raap AK. Non-autoradiographic hybridocytochemistry. *J Histochem Cytochem* 1986; 34: 126−33.

29 Niedobitek G, Finn HH, Bornhoft G, Gerdes J, Stein H. Detection of viral DNA by *in situ* hybridization using bromodeoxyuridine labelled DNA probes. *Am J Pathol* 1988; 1313: 1−4.

30 Kiyama H, Emson PC, Tohyama M. Recent progress in the use of the technique of non-radioactive *in situ* hybridization histochemistry: new tools for molecular neurobiology. *Neurosci Res* 1990; 9: 1−21.

31 Bhatt B, Burns J, Flamery D, McGee JOD. Direct visualization of single copy genes on banded metaphase chromosome by non-isotopic *in situ* hybridization. *Nucleic Acids Res* 1988; 16: 3951−61.

32 Lawrence JB, Villnave CA, Singer RH. Sensitive, high-resolution chromatin and chromosome mapping *in situ*: presence and orientation of two closely integrated copies of EBV in a lymphoma line. *Cell* 1988; 52: 51−61.

33 Furuta Y, Shinohara T, Sano K, Meguro M, Nagashima K. *In situ* hybridization with digoxigenin-labelled DNA probes for detection of viral genomes. *J Clin Pathol* 1990; 43: 806−9.

34 Podell S, Maske W, Ibanez E, Jablonski E. Comparison of solution hybridization efficiencies using alkaline phosphatase-labelled and ^{32}P-labelled oligodeoxynucleotide probes. *Mol Cell Probes* 1991; 5: 117−24.

35 Unger ER, Hammer MI, Chenggis ML. Comparison of ^{25}S and biotin as labels for *in situ* hybridization: use of an HPV model system. *J Histochem Cytochem* 1991; 39: 145−50.

36 Langer PR, Waldrop A, Ward D. Enzymatic synthesis of biotin labelled polynucleotides: novel nucleic acid affinity probes. *Proc Natl Acad Sci USA* 1981; 78: 6633−7.

37 Hutchison NJ, Langer-Safer PR, Ward DC, Manikalo BA. *In situ* hybridization at the electron microscopical level: hybrid detection by autoradiography and colloidal gold. *J Cell Biol* 1982; 95: 609–18.

38 Leary JJ, Brigati DJ, Ward DC. Rapid and sensitive colorimetric method for visualizing biotin labelled DNA probes hybridized to DNA or RNA immobilized on nitrocellulose. *Proc Natl Acad Sci USA* 1983; 80: 4045–9.

39 Zabel M, Schafer H. Localization of calcitonin and calcitonin gene-related peptide mRNA in rat parafollicular cells by hybridocytochemistry. *J Histochem Cytochem* 1988; 36: 543–6.

40 Guitteny AF, Fouque B, Mongin C, Teoule R, Boch B. Histological detection of mRNA with biotinylated synthetic oligonucleotide probes. *J Histochem Cytochem* 1988; 36: 563–71.

41 Larsson L-I, Christensen T, Dalboge H. Detection of POMC mRNA by *in situ* hybridization using biotinylated oligodeoxynucleotide probes and avidin-alkaline phosphatase histochemistry. *Histochemistry* 1988; 89: 109–16.

42 Giaid A, Hamid Q, Adams C, Springall DR, Terenghi G, Polak JM. Non-isotopic RNA probes. Comparison between different labels and detection systems. *Histochemistry* 1989; 93: 191–6.

43 Kessler C. The digoxigenin anti-digoxigenin (DIG) technology — a survey on the concept and realization of a novel bioanalytical indicator system. *Mol Cell Probes* 1991; 5: 161–205.

44 Morris RG, Arends MJ, Bishop PE, Sizer K, Duvall E, Bird CC. Sensitivity of digoxigenin and biotin labelled probes for detection of human papillomavirus by *in situ* hybridization. *J Clin Pathol* 1990; 43: 800–805.

45 Herrington CS, Burns J, Graham AK, Bhatt B, McGee JOD. Interphase cytogenetics using biotin and digoxigenin labelled probes. II: simultaneous detection of two nucleic acid species in individual nuclei. *J Clin Pathol* 1989; 42: 601–606.

46 Trask BJ, Massa H, Kenwrick S, Gitschier J. Mapping of human chromosome Xq28 by two colour fluorescence *in situ* hybridization of DNA sequences to interphase cell nuclei. *Am J Hum Genet* 1991; 48: 1–15.

47 Dirks RW, van Gijlswijk RPM, Tullis RH *et al.* Simultaneous detection of different mRNA sequences coding for neuropeptide hormones by double *in situ* hybridization using FITC- and biotin-labelled oligonucleotides. *J Histochem Cytochem* 1990; 38: 467–73.

48 Nielsen DA, Shapiro DJ. Insight into hormonal control of messenger RNA stability. *Mol Endocrinol* 1990; 4: 953–7.

49 Johnson SA, Morgan DG, Finch CE. Extensive post-mortem stability of RNA from rat and human brain. *J Neurosci Res* 1986; 16: 267–80.

50 Höfler H, Childers H, Montminy MR, Lechan RM, Goodman RH, Wolfe HJ. *In situ* hybridization methods for the detection of somatostatin mRNA in tissue sections using antisense RNA probes. *Histochem J* 1986; 18: 597–604.

51 Asanuma M, Ogawa N, Mizukawa K, Haba K, Mori A. Comparison of formaldehyde-preperfused frozen and freshly frozen tissue preparation for the *in situ* hybridization for α-tubulin mRNA in the rat brain. *Res Commun Chem Pathol Pharmacol* 1990; 70: 183–92.

52 Terenghi G, Polak JM, Hamid Q *et al.* Localization of neuropeptide Y mRNA in neurons of human cerebral cortex by means of *in situ* hybridization with complementary RNA probes. *Proc Natl Acad Sci USA* 1987; 84: 7315–18.

53 Gibson SJ, Polak JM, Giaid A *et al.* Calcitonin gene-related peptide mRNA is expressed in sensory neurons of the dorsal root ganglia and also in spinal moto-neurons in man and rat. *Neurosci Lett* 1988; 91: 283–8.

54 Taylor GR, Carter GI, Crow TJ *et al.* Recovery and measurement of specific RNA species from postmortem brain tissue: a general reduction in Alzheimer's disease

detected by molecular hybridization. *Exp Mol Pathol* 1986; 44: 111–16.

55 Haase AT, Brahic M, Stowring L. Detection of viral nucleic acids by *in situ* hybridization. In: Maramorosch K, Koprowski H, eds. *Methods in Virology, VII.* New York: Academic Press, 1984: 189–226.

56 McAllister HA, Rock DL. Comparative usefulness of tissue fixatives for *in situ* viral nucleic acid hybridization. *J Histochem Cytochem* 1985; 33: 1026–32.

57 Moench TR, Gendelman HE, Clements JE, Narayan O, Griffin DE. Efficiency of *in situ* hybridization as a function of probe size and fixation technique. *J Virol Methods* 1985; 11: 119–30.

58 Brigati DJ, Myerson D, Leary JJ *et al.* Detection of viral genomes in cultured cells and paraffin-embedded tissue sections using biotin labelled hybridization probes. *Virology* 1983; 126: 32–50.

59 Wilcox JN, Gee CE, Roberts JL. *In situ* cDNA–mRNA hybridization: development of a technique to measure mRNA levels in individual cells. *Methods Enzymol* 1986; 124: 510–33.

60 Tournier I, Bernau D, Poliard A, Schoevaret D, Fedman G. Detection of albumin mRNAs in rat liver by *in situ* hybridization: usefulness of paraffin embedding and comparison of various fixation procedures. *J Histochem Cytochem* 1987; 35: 453–9.

61 Farquharson M, Harvie R, McNicol AM. Detection of mRNA using a digoxigenin end labelled oligodeoxynucleotide probe. *J Clin Pathol* 1990; 43: 424–8.

62 Gee CE, Roberts JL. A technique for the study of gene expression in single cells. *DNA* 1983; 2: 157–63.

63 Shivers BD, Schachter BS, Pfaff DW. *In situ* hybridization for the study of gene expression in the brain. *Methods Enzymol* 1986; 124: 497–510.

64 Hayashi S, Gillam IC, Delaney AB, Tener GM. Acetylation of chromosome squashes of *Drosophila melanogaster* decreases the background in autoradiographs from hybridization with ^{125}I-labelled RNA. *J Histochem Cytochem* 1978; 26: 677–9.

65 Britten RJ, Graham DE, Neufeld BR. Analysis of repeating DNA sequences by reassociation. *Methods Enzymol* 1974; 29: 363–418.

66 Kourilsky P, Leidner J, Tremblay GY. DNA:DNA hybridization on filter at low temperature in the presence of formamide or urea. *Biochimie* 1971; 53: 1111–14.

67 McConaughy BL, Laird CD, McCarthy BJ. Nucleic acid reassociation in formamide. *Biochemistry* 1969; 8: 3289–95.

68 Hamid Q, Wharton J, Terenghi G *et al.* Localization of atrial natriuretic peptide mRNA and immunoreactivity in the rat heart and human atrial appendage. *Proc Natl Acad Sci USA* 1987; 84: 6760–4.

69 Springall DR, Bhatnagar M, Wharton J *et al.* Expression of the atrial natriuretic peptide gene in the cardiac muscle of the rat extrapulmonary and intrapulmonary veins. *Thorax* 1988; 43: 44–52.

70 Bishop AE, Hamid Q, Adams C *et al.* Expression of tachykinins by ileal and lung carcinoid tumours assessed by combined *in situ* hybridization, immunocyto-chemistry and radioimmunoassay. *Cancer* 1989; 63: 1129–37.

71 Hamid Q, Bishop AE, Springall DR *et al.* Detection of human probombesin mRNA in neuroendocrine (small cell) carcinoma of the lung. *Cancer* 1989; 63: 266–71.

72 Yanagisawa M, Kurihara H, Kimura S *et al.* A novel potent vasoconstrictor peptide produced by vascular endothelial cells. *Nature* 1988; 332: 411–15.

73 Springall DR, Howarth P, Counihan H, Djukovic R, Holgate S, Polak JM. Endothelin immunoreactivity of airway epithelium in asthmatic patients. *Lancet* 1991; 337: 697–701.

74 Giaid A, Hamid Q, Springall DR *et al.* Detection of endothelin immunoreactivity and mRNA in pulmonary tumours. *J Pathol* 1990; 162: 15–22.

75 Hamid Q, Corrin B, Sheppard MN, Huttner WB, Polak JM. Expression of chromo-granin A mRNA in small cell carcinoma of the lung. *J Pathol* 1991; 163: 8293–7.

4 Finding disease genes

MICHAEL C. IANNUZZI

Introduction

Knowing the biochemical or structural abnormality responsible for an inherited disorder usually facilitates cloning the disease gene. The defective protein is isolated and purified, its amino acid sequence determined, and the gene cloned by screening genomic or complementary DNA (cDNA) libraries. When the pathogenesis of a disease is not well understood, and when standard biochemical methods fail to identify relevant proteins, positional cloning may be used. Positional cloning offers the means for not only identifying inherited disease genes in single gene disorders, but also for identifying hereditary susceptibility genes in multifactorial disorders. Positional cloning has been used to yield the genes for several single gene disorders including chronic granulomatous disease, Duchenne muscular dystrophy, retinoblastoma and neurofibromatosis, and is being used for several other Mendelian disorders [1−4]. Hereditary susceptibility genes in multifactorial disorders have also been targeted for the positional cloning strategy and include diseases such as asthma, diabetes, rheumatoid arthritis, multiple sclerosis and breast cancer [5−9].

Once a disease gene is cloned, the pathogenesis can be elucidated at an astonishing pace. The gene sequence indicates the nature of the defective protein, gives its amino acid composition and may suggest relationships to previously sequenced polypeptides. Peptides can be synthesized, antibodies raised, and the protein's location and intracellular trafficking demonstrated. The specific cells expressing the gene and the timing of expression during development may also be determined. Expressing the gene in model systems, such as cell culture and transgenic mice, greatly aids functional studies; and in many instances once the gene is cloned and expressed in model systems, treatment by gene therapy becomes a possibility. This chapter describes the main features and discusses the techniques involved in positional cloning. Figure 4.1 presents the overall positional cloning strategy.

Positional cloning

The best known example of using positional cloning to advance the understanding and treatment of disease is cystic fibrosis (CF) [10−12].

60

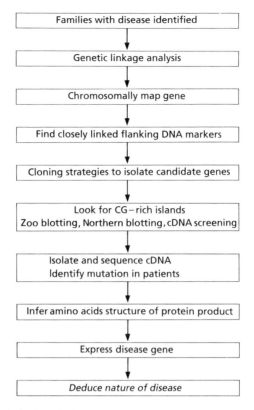

Fig. 4.1 Positional cloning strategy.

Investigators, relying on standard biochemical strategies, were unable to identify the responsible defective protein. These strategies were hindered for many reasons, including lack of information about the structure and regulation of ion channels, and the lack of functional assays. Once the CF gene, the cystic fibrosis transmembrane regulator (CFTR), was identified, several advancements promptly followed. Tests to detect carriers and for accurate DNA-based diagnosis became available [13–15]; the basic cellular defect could be probed in ways not previously possible, and an animal model created which is likely to accelerate further the understanding and treatment of the disease [16, 17]. New treatment strategies, including using recombinant CFTR protein replacement and gene therapy, are now being developed and offer the possibility of cure [18].

Positional cloning begins with establishing the chromosomal map position of the disease gene or in the case of multifactorial disorders, such as breast cancer, establishing the map position of a disease susceptibility gene. The first and simplest example of assigning a gene to a specific chromosome is the colour blindness gene. Because of its distinctive pedigree pattern and gender difference it clearly maps to the X chromosome. When a disorder is associated with a cytogenetic abnormality, such as a chromosomal deletion or rearrangement, the visualized chromosomal abnormality points to the disease locus. For example, a deletion within the long arm of chromosome 13 associated with retinoblastoma pointed to the location of the responsible gene [19]. For most inherited diseases, no observable cytogenetic abnormalities exist, so the disease locus must be established by another means, namely, genetic linkage analysis.

Genetic linkage analysis

To understand genetic linkage analysis, it is helpful to review a few terms. The human genome, which contains the instructions or genes for making tens of thousands of different proteins, consists of two sets of 23 chromosomes including the autosome chromosomes number 1 through 22 and the sex chromosomes X and Y. During the formation of gametes in the process of meiosis, the members of each pair of homologous chromosomes separate into daughter cells. The display of the human genome at meiosis, when each chromosome has its own unique pattern of bands, is the karyotype. While homologous chromosomes have the same band pattern and are the same shape and size, their DNA sequences are different. Any difference in the DNA sequence (polymorphism) that allows maternal and paternal chromosomes in a homologous chromosome pair to be distinguished is a DNA or genetic marker. The gene locus is the chromosomal address at which the gene for a particular trait resides, and is reported as the chromosome number, whether it is on the long arm (q) or short arm (p), and the chromosomal band(s) to which it has been located. For example, the human angiotensin gene has been located to 1q42−q43 [20]. An allele is one of several alternative forms of a gene occupying a given locus on a chromosome.

A gene locus, as defined by genetic linkage analysis, is generally from one million to several million base pairs (bp); and genes may range in size from a few hundred bp to as many as several hundred thousand. The length of the human genome is 3 billion bp. Applying genetic linkage analysis to finding a disease gene on a chromosome in the human genome is the same as locating a specific person in a house on Earth while standing on the moon. A task of this magnitude can be achieved because of two factors: first, the availability of cloned 'marker' DNA with assigned chromosomal locations, and second, the biological phenomenon of recombination of genetic material during meiosis.

DNA markers

Thousands of DNA segments spanning the human genome have been cloned and mapped [21]. Assignment of DNA segments to specific chromosomes is based on a variety of methods. Somatic cell hybrids, containing a single or few human chromosomes, have been used extensively to assign genes to particular chromosomes. Initially these assignments were made by demonstrating that the human chromosome present in the hybrid was concordant with a specific human gene product. This is now usually done by demonstrating concordance of the human chromosome with hybridization of cloned genomic or cDNA to DNA prepared from the hybrid.

DNA segments may also be mapped by hybridization to DNA prepared from single chromosomes obtained by fluorescence-activated cell sorting or by *in situ* hybridization to metaphase chromosome spreads. More recently, fluorescent affinity reagents have been used to label probes directed at interphase chromosomes. Interphase chromosomes, which are not as compact as metaphase chromosomes, allow for ordering DNA markers across a chromosome region separated by as little as 50−100 kilobases (kb) [22, 23].

A cloned DNA segment with assigned chromosomal position is useful as a marker for linkage analysis when it detects sequence variation (polymorphism) in the population. When the difference in sequence, which may be as small as a single base change, creates or eliminates a recognition site detected by a specific restriction endonuclease, restriction fragment length polymorphisms (RFLPs) occur (see Chapter 1). RFLPs are detected by comparing DNA from several individuals using the method of Southern blotting to reveal the pattern of specific DNA fragments (Fig. 4.2). A change in DNA sequence that affects the restriction site for a specific enzyme alters the length of the DNA fragments produced by enzymatic cleavage. Thus the cloned and mapped DNA

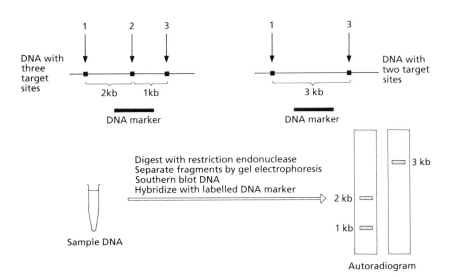

Fig. 4.2 Restriction fragment length polymorphism. The DNA sequence change affects the restriction site detected on Southern blot.

segment defines the locus, and the restriction endonuclease that recognizes and cleaves a specific sequence of bases detects the polymorphism.

Linkage analysis in the 1980s relied on RFLP detection, but improved methods for polymorphic detection have been developed. Before turning to these newer methods, we review the biological phenomenon of recombination and how measurement of recombination rates allows for gene mapping and detecting linkage.

Genes, as well as polymorphic non-coding fragments of DNA, tend to be inherited together — that is 'linked' when they are close together on the chromosome, and inherited independently when they are far apart. During meiosis, when homologous chromosomes are paired, bridges form between corresponding regions of the chromosome pair (Fig. 4.3). These chiasmas are regions in which the two chromosomes break at identical points along their length and subsequently rejoin, the segments having been switched from one homologous chromosome to the other. Chiasma formation and crossing over in humans occurs with great frequency in every meiosis. These crossing-over events can be detected by noting that polymorphic DNA segments which appear to be together in the same chromosomal region in the parents are not in the same chromosomal region in their children. The frequency of recombination between two DNA segments can be used to derive their distance apart (Fig. 4.3).

Segments far apart on the chromosome or on separate chromosomes

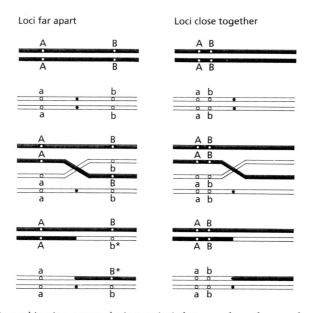

Fig. 4.3 Recombination occurs during meiosis between homologous chromosomes. Left: example showing loci far apart so that recombination in the interval A−B or a−b is likely to occur. Right: example showing loci close together so that recombination in the interval A−B or a−b is a rarer event.

have a recombination frequency of 50%: that is, the segments are inherited together 50% of the time and are unlinked (independent segregation). Linkage is detected when recombination occurs significantly less often than the 50% predicted for independent segregation. The LOD score method of statistical analysis is used to detect linkage. A LOD score (log of the odds in base 10) indicates how likely the segments are to be linked and how far apart on the chromosome they are likely to be [24]. A LOD score of greater than 3 means that there is a greater than 1000 to 1 chance that the two loci are on the same chromosome and are linked. A LOD score below -2 indicates that the loci are unlinked and well apart on a chromosome or are on different chromosomes.

The recombination frequency between a DNA marker and a disease locus in families not only provides for linkage analysis, but also gives an approximate distance between the DNA marker and the disease.

$$\text{map distance} = \frac{\text{number of recombinants}}{\text{total number of progeny}}$$

1% recombination = 1 map unit = 1 cM

Linkage studies have indicated that the length of the entire human genome in recombination or genetic distance is 3300 centimorgans (cM). By definition, the distance between two segments that cross-over in 1% of the progeny is 1 cM. Loci with a 1% recombination frequency or a genetic distance of 1 cM therefore lie 1/3300 of the human genome apart. Since the physical length of the genome is about 3 billion bp, 1 cM is about 1 million bp (1/3300 × 3 billion). The physical distance determined from genetic distance is only an estimate since recombination is not evenly spaced over the genome; there are hot spots for recombination and regions where recombination is suppressed.

Improved polymorphic detection

A recombination event can be detected by a DNA marker only when the marker detects allelic heterozygosity in the parents. If the parents are homozygous for a marker, that locus cannot reveal recombination. To illustrate this, take the example of a mother who has the homozygous haplotype for three markers ABC, ABC, and the father who has the heterozygous haplotype ABC, AXY. A crossing-over event occurring in the mother would be undetected in the children since if recombination between the two chromosomes occurred anywhere in the A−B interval or B−C interval the inherited chromosome would still demonstrate the haplotype ABC. If an ABY chromosome was found in any offspring, it could only arise from a recombination event in the father.

The maximum heterozygosity for restriction endonucleases, which detect polymorphic difference only at their DNA recognition sites, is

50% — there are only two possible alleles. To increase the heterozygosity for a locus, several enzymes can be used, but even then additional RFLPs will not always increase heterozygosity at the locus. A new class of markers, called variable number of tandem repeats (VNTR) of an oligonucleotide sequence, defines highly polymorphic loci [25]. Polymorphisms of this class are detected by polymerase chain reaction amplification using primers homologous to unique sequences flanking the repeats. Simple gel electrophoresis can be used to distinguish between alleles according to size. Examples of tandemly repeated DNA are the very short simple sequence repeats $(dC-dA)_n$ and $(CA)_n$ [26]. There are $50\,000-100\,000$ interspersed $(CA)_n$ blocks through the human genome. The precise role of CA repeats is not known, but alleles always differ in size by multiples of two bases with most blocks of repeats less than 30 bp.

Table 4.1 summarizes methods of mapping. To illustrate linkage analysis we review how the CF gene was mapped. Linkage to CF was first reported with the polymorphic serum enzyme paroxonase (PON); unfortunately, the PON gene had not been cloned and its chromosomal location was not known [27]. Shortly after that, linkage was reported to the DNA marker DOCRI-917 [28]. This was localized to the long arm of chromosome 7 (7q) using somatic cell hybrids. Subsequent studies showed that two other previously cloned DNA markers from 7q21-31, the *met* gene and J3.11 (D7S8), were closer [29, 30]. DOCRI-917, the most distant to CF, was at a recombination distance of 15 cM. A large collaborative study involving seven research groups, that had collected and typed over 200 families with CF, provided the linkage map for CF indicating that the disease gene was somewhere between *met* and D7S8 and the distance between these two markers was 1−2 cM [31].

Genetic linkage maps, such as that derived for CF, give some estimate of the physical distance between markers on the chromosome and the size of the region that must be scrutinized to find the disease gene. The resolution between DNA markers flanking a disease locus provided by the genetic linkage map is generally not better than 1−2 cM, or to about 1 or 2 million bp, because the number of affected families is not infinite

Table 4.1 Methods of mapping

Chromosomal aberrations
Somatic cell hybridization
Hybridization to flow-sorted chromosomes
In situ hybridization to metaphase chromosome spreads
In situ hybridization to interphase chromosomes
Pulsed field gel electrophoresis
Genetic linkage analysis
Hybridization to yeast artificial chromosomes

and recombination is unlikely to occur within the small chromosomal interval between a linked marker and the disease gene. For example, despite a 4-year search by several groups around the world, only one certain recombinant between D7S8 and CF was found [30]. Although the 1−2 cM distance between the flanking markers *met* and J3.11 is large in physical terms, linkage analysis did serve to provide flanking DNA segments as starting points for using various gene cloning strategies to home in on the CF gene, including chromosome walking, saturation cloning, cloning from subchromosomal sized fragments and chromosome jumping.

Cloning strategies

Chromosome walking makes use of phage and cosmid libraries that are screened with probes derived from linked markers. Overlapping clones are repeatedly isolated and the process proceeds along a stretch on the chromosome (Fig. 4.4). Cosmids, the cloning vectors with the largest capacity, carry 40−45 kb of insert DNA, and yield about 20 kb of additional DNA with each new clone. Chromosome walking with cosmid or phage is tedious, and because of repetitive or unclonable DNA present throughout the genome, seldom continues in a stretch of more than 200 000−300 000 bases in a given direction.

A tactic to help shorten the target region is saturation cloning. Saturation cloning, performed by isolating and mapping hundreds of random clones from a chromosome-specific library, aims to find a clone from within the target region. Saturation cloning is further aided by screening phage and cosmid libraries constructed from subchromosomal pieces of DNA containing the target region. There are several methods used to generate subchromosomal sized pieces of DNA. One method is to isolate subchromosomal pieces of DNA by preparative pulsed field gel electrophoresis (PFGE). Essential to this method was the discovery of 'rare cutter' restriction enzymes that cleave DNA into fragments with an average size ranging from 100 000 to 1 million nucleotides. The recognition sequences for rare cutter restriction enzymes contain the dinucleotide CpG (cytosine−guanine). This dinucleotide is under-represented in the mammalian genome and frequently methylated making it more resistant to endonuclease digestion. For example, *Not*I (which contains two CpG dinucleotides in its recognition sequence GCGGCCGC) cuts human DNA into fragments averaging about 500 000 bp. PFGE separates these large DNA fragments, generated by the rare cutter restriction enzymes, by subjecting the cleaved DNA to pulses of non-uniform opposing fields [32, 33]. This is in contrast to conventional gel electrophoresis, which uses a constant unidirectional electric field. Separation of longer DNA fragments with PFGE probably results from conformational changes, uncoiling and recoiling of DNA, that occur

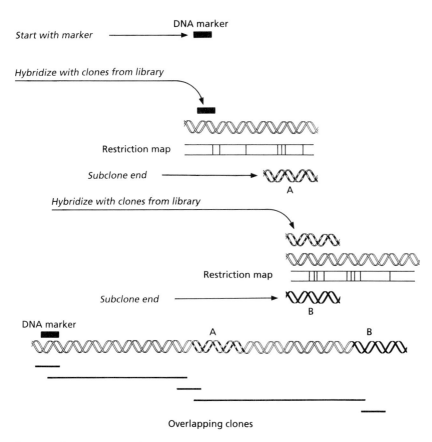

Fig. 4.4 Chromosome walking is accomplished by repeatedly isolating overlapping clones along a stretch on the chromosome. The initial DNA marker is used to identify a DNA clone from the relevant library and a restriction map is established. The distal end is then subcloned (A) and used to identify the next stretch of DNA, which has a different restriction map. Again the 3′ end is subcloned (B) and the process repeated.

by switching field directions. The shorter DNA fragments move down the gel more quickly than the larger DNA because they take less time to orient to the changing electric fields. A variety of instruments for PFGE are available and differ primarily in the geometry of the electric fields used to separate the DNA, but all separate DNA from 50 kb to more than 9 megabase pairs (1 megabase = 1 million bp = 1 Mb). The critical parameters affecting size separation are agarose concentration, voltage, buffer, temperature and pulse time.

The technology that has emerged as the method of choice for obtaining subchromosomal sized DNA is cloning in yeast artificial chromosomes (YACs) [34]. Plasmid vectors containing known yeast centromere and telomere sequences along with selectable markers are used to maintain artificial chromosomes in yeast hosts (Fig. 4.5) [35]. YAC libraries made with these vectors yield clones with inserts that are hundreds of kilobases in size that can then be subcloned into phage or cosmid libraries. PFGE

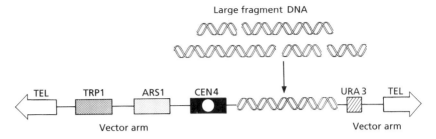

Fig. 4.5 Large inserts of DNA are ligated into plasmid vector arms to form a YAC. The vector arms contain telomere sequences at each end (TEL) and centromeres (CEN), replication origins (ARS) and selectable markers (TRP and URA3).

and cloning in YACs serve to bridge the size gap between chromosomal DNA and segments of DNA isolated by phage and cosmid cloning and not only help saturation cloning but also greatly aid mapping.

Another gene cloning strategy that addresses the general problem of cloning over large distances is chromosome jumping [36, 37]. Chromosome jumping allows the isolation of DNA segments separated in the genome by distances up to several hundred thousand base pairs without isolating all the intervening DNA as required in chromosome walking (Fig. 4.6) [38]. Chromosome jumping depends on circularizing very large DNA fragments, followed by cloning the junction fragments of these circles which bring together DNA sequences that were originally located a considerable distance apart. An additional advantage of chromosome jumping is that it avoids the problem of the presence of repetitive or unclonable DNA which prevents sequential walks.

The search for a disease gene often requires the combination of several of these molecular techniques. For CF, saturation cloning provided two markers, D7S122 and D7340, mapped to within the *met* and D7S8 interval [39]. These markers helped to narrow the search, and chromosome jumping accelerated cloning of DNA from the target region. Each jump clone traversed about 75−100 kb of DNA, and at the end of each jump, bi-directional walks were initiated to obtain DNA between the jumps. Recombination analyses with RFLPs detected by the jump and walk clones excluded more than 300 kb of DNA in the interval between D7S8 and the CF gene [40]. Because individuals recombinant in the interval between D7S122 and the CF gene were not available, it was necessary to search through more than 280 kb of continuous DNA to find the CF gene [10].

An interesting point to consider when sifting through the DNA from a chromosomal region is how to decide when an isolated clone is part of a gene? There are several signposts which help (Table 4.2). Since many genes show evolutionary conservation, one sign that suggests that an isolated clone may be part of a gene is that of detecting cross-hybridizing DNA sequences between species. If the sequence in the cloned DNA

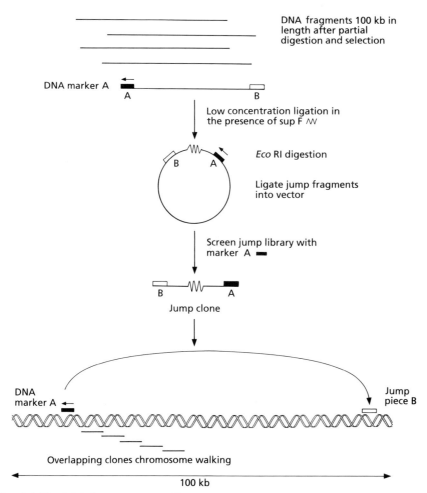

Fig. 4.6 The DNA fragment (≈100 kb) containing marker A is isolated, circularized and ligated with supF. The circle is then digested and ligated into an appropriate vector. The new jump clone is identified by marker A but now contains marker B within 200 bp and can be used to identify marker B on the original chromosome.

Table 4.2 Signposts for gene detection

Evolutionary conservation (zoo blot)
CG islands
Northern analysis of affected tissues
Screening cDNA libraries
Define mutations
Correct the defect in cell culture

segment is conserved across species, it is likely to be important and likely to be a gene. Cross-hybridizing sequences can be detected by labelling phage or cosmid clones and hybridizing to Southern blots containing DNA from a variety of species such as bovine, chicken and mouse ('zoo blot'). A second sign is the presence of CG (C = cytosine; G = guanine) islands [41]. These islands are stretches of DNA 500−2000 bp in length, which are rich in the non-methylated dinucleotide CG and often mark the 5′ end of vertebrate genes. Additional tests that aid the search include using the isolated clones to detect mRNA in Northern blot analysis and to screen cDNA libraries for evidence of transcription in affected tissues. The best evidence that the gene of interest has been found rests on finding mutations present in patients with disease that are not present in healthy individuals and in correcting the defect in affected cells.

Linkage analysis of complex disorders

How can relevant genes in complex disorders, such as breast cancer and asthma, be approached using positional cloning? Positional cloning applied to multifactorial diseases still depends on linkage analysis, but while the LOD score method is used for diseases with a clear Mendelian inheritance pattern, the search for a susceptibility gene in a multifactorial disease is based on the observation of non-random segregation at a marker locus in affected sibs. In this method, called the affected sib pair method of linkage analysis (ASP) [42, 43], a disease susceptibility locus is linked to the marker when there is genotypic concordance among affected sibs in excess of that expected. To determine genotypic concordance requires the use of highly polymorphic markers, such as dinucleotide CA repeats, or highly polymorphic genes such as the human leucocyte antigen (HLA) genes. In fact, the ASP method was initially developed to test for linkage of disease to HLA. The HLA region is so polymorphic that it is almost always possible to determine if a sib pair share none, one or two haplotypes.

The affected sib pair method has often been more powerful in detecting the presence of disease-predisposing genes than standard HLA association studies, and has been used to detect susceptibility genes for a number of diseases, including insulin-dependent diabetes mellitus, multiple sclerosis and rheumatoid arthritis [9, 44, 45]. Association studies require the existence of linkage disequilibrium between the alleles of the marker and disease-predisposing loci. Significant linkage disequilibrium values are not usually expected for loci with recombination distances greater than 1−2%, while deviations from random segregation of haplotype sharing values in affected sibs can be detected over much larger recombination distances between the marker loci and the disease-predisposing loci [46].

Weeks and Lange [47] have extended the affected sib pair method to sets of affected pedigree members, affected relative pairs (ARP). Linkage of disease to susceptibility locus then depends on the contribution of the increase in risk to relatives with a particular haplotype compared with the population prevalence of that haplotype. Linkage analyses by ASP and ARP, which only examine affected family members, are not only useful for those diseases without a clear Mendelian pattern of inheritance, but also for those diseases in which it may be difficult to exclude disease in asymptomatic family members.

The study of cloned genes

Once the disease gene is cloned, investigations from nearly all perspectives can begin. Mutational analysis provides for new diagnostic tests, carrier detection, prognostication and analysis of protein function. Direct detection of mutations is straightforward using polymerase chain reaction (PCR) amplification. DNA primers flanking the relevant DNA segments are synthesized and PCR is used to obtain an exponential increase in the target sequence copy number [48, 49]. Several methods can then be used to determine if the amplified sequence is normal or contains a mutation. These methods include allele-specific oligonucleotide screening; direct sequencing of the PCR product; denaturing gradient gel electrophoresis to compare the electrophoretic mobility of wild-type and mutant DNA strands; and cleavage mismatch methods to detect sequence differences between wild-type and mutant single-stranded molecules [50−53].

Another perspective is to examine the physiological effect of the gene by expressing it in model systems. The cDNA may be subcloned into bacterial or mammalian cell expression vectors and introduced into host cells. Which vectors and which hosts depend on the particular structure−function relationships the investigator wishes to examine. Studies in which the normal version of the gene is expressed in the cells affected by the disease could be influenced by the presence of the abnormal gene product, but a great deal of information may still be obtained. In particular, the question of potential for gene therapy may be addressed. Another approach is to use cells which do not normally express the gene. For example, expression of CFTR in *Xenopus* oocytes and in non-epithelial invertebrate cells allowed for a more rigorous testing of the hypothesis that CFTR is a regulated low conductance chloride channel [54, 55]. The effects of mutations on function, whether designed or found in nature, can also be evaluated. Functional domains may be deleted or expressed in excess and the effect on protein and cellular function determined.

The introduction of genes into the germ lines of animals particularly mice (transgenic mice) offers another strategy of analysis of gene structure and function. In only 3 years from the time the CF gene was cloned, the first animal model for CF has been reported. A gene equivalent to the human CFTR had been identified in mice [56], and the CFTR gene in mouse embryonic stem cells was disrupted. The targeted cell lines were then injected in the blastocoele cavity of embryos and the offspring mated until mice homozygous for the disrupted gene were found [16]. Another example, that has allowed detailed studies of the role of copper—zinc superoxide dismutase in preventing pulmonary oxygen toxicity, is the creation of transgenic mice made to express elevated levels of this enzyme [57].

Possibly the most important perspective is that of therapeutics. The cloned gene can be used to make recombinant protein for replacement therapy and can be directly transferred to affected cells for correcting the defect. The use of a cloned gene for gene therapy is discussed in Chapter 18.

The Human Genome Project

The Human Genome Project promises to map and sequence the entire human genome within the next 10—15 years. This map and sequence will greatly aid the process of positional cloning and will have an enormous influence on understanding and treating human disease. From a complete map, sets of markers spaced at equal intervals along the chromosomes may be used to search for genes. After discovering linkage, the location of the disease gene may be pinpointed further by selecting additional markers from the defined region. A computer search of the DNA sequence of this interval may then reveal the gene of interest. If not, all cloned DNA from the smaller target region would be immediately available for transcript searching. Assuming one character per nucleotide, the result of the Human Genome Project will fill 13 sets of the *Encyclopaedia Britannica* [58]. However, this encyclopaedia will never be out of date and will serve many future generations.

Summary

The genetic defects in several inherited diseases have been identified using the package of molecular genetic techniques called positional cloning, and several more will be found in the near future. The only limiting factor is the availability of families in which to apply genetic linkage analysis. The positional cloning approach has wide applicability because it relies on the chromosomal map position to direct the search for the disease gene, and does not require knowledge of how the gene's protein product functions. The completion of the human genome map promises to greatly accelerate the positional cloning strategy by supplying the location of all our genes. Once an inherited disease gene is cloned, the gene's sequence can be used to help define the physiological defect, to design accurate diagnostic tests and to develop new treatment strategies such as gene therapy which may offer the ultimate solution to a number of inherited diseases.

References

1 Monaco AP, Neve RL, Colletti-Feener C *et al.* Isolation of candidate cDNAs for portions of the Duchenne muscular dystrophy gene. *Nature* 1986; 323: 646–50.

2 Orkin S. Molecular genetics of chronic granulomatous disease. *Annu Rev Immunol* 1989; 7: 277–307.

3 Wallace MR, Collins FS. Molecular genetics of von Recklinghausen neurofibromatosis. *Adv Hum Genet* 1991; 20: 267–307.

4 Cawthon RM, O'Connell P, Buchberg P *et al.* Identification and characterization of transcripts from the neurofibromatosis 1 region: the sequence and genomic structure of EV12 and mapping of other transcripts. *Genomics* 1990; 7: 555–65.

5 Sibbald B. Genetic basis of asthma. *Semin Respir Med* 1986; 7: 307–15.

6 Newman B, Austin MA, Lee M, King MC. Inheritance of human breast cancer: evidence for autosomal dominant transmission in high risk families. *Proc Natl Acad Sci USA* 1988; 85: 3044.

7 Hall JM, Lee M, Newman B, Marrow JE *et al.* Linkage of early-onset familial breast cancer to chromosome 17q21. *Science* 1990; 250: 1684.

8 Olerup O, Hiller J. HLA class II-associated genetic susceptibility in multiple sclerosis: a critical evaluation. *Tissue Antigens* 1991; 38: 1–15.

9 Wordsworth P, Bell J. Polygenic susceptibility in rheumatoid arthritis. *Ann Rheum Dis* 1991; 50: 343–6.

10 Rommens JM, Iannuzzi MC, Kerem B *et al.* Identification of the cystic fibrosis gene: chromosome walking and jumping. *Science* 1989; 245: 1059–65.

11 Collins FS, Riordan JR, Tsui LC. The cystic fibrosis gene: isolation and significance. *Hosp Pract* 1990; 25: 47–57.

12 Iannuzzi MC, Collins FS. Reverse genetics and cystic fibrosis. *Am J Respir Cell Mol Biol* 1990; 2: 309–16.

13 Beaudet AL. Carrier screening for cystic fibrosis (editorial). *Am J Hum Genet* 1990; 47: 603–5.

14 Ballabio A, Gibbs RA, Caskey CT. PCR test for cystic fibrosis deletion. *Nature* 1990; 354: 220.

15 Rommens J, Kerem BS, Greer W *et al.* Rapid nonradioactive detection of the major cystic fibrosis mutation (letter). *Am J Hum Genet* 1990; 46: 395–6.

16 Snouwaert J, Brigman KK, Latour AM *et al.* An animal model for cystic fibrosis made by gene targeting. *Science* 1992; 257: 1083–8.

17 Clarke L, Grubb BR, Gabriel SE, Smithies O, Koller BH, Boucher RC. Defective epithelial chloride transport in a gene targeted mouse model of cystic fibrosis. *Science* 1992; 257: 1125–8.

18 Collins F. Cystic fibrosis: molecular biology and therapeutic implications. *Science* 1992; 256: 774–80.

19 Friend SH, Bernards R, Rogelj S *et al.* A human DNA segment with properties of the gene that predisposes to retinoblastoma and osteosarcoma. *Nature* 1986; 323: 643–6.

20 Isa M, Boyd E, Morrison N, Harrap S, Clauser E, Connor JM. Assignment of the human angiotensin gene to chromosome 1q42-43 by nonisotopic *in situ* hybridization. *Genomics* 1990; 8: 598–600.

21 McAlpine P, Shows TB, Boucheix C, Huebner M, Anderson WA. The 1991 catalog of mapped genes and report of the nomenclature committee. *Cytogenet Cell Genet* 1991; 58: 5–102.

22 Lawrence J, Villnave CA, Singer RH. Sensitive high resolution chromatin and chromosome mapping *in situ*: presence and orientation of two closely integrated copies of EBV in a lymphoma line. *Cell* 1988; 52: 51–61.

23 Lawrence J, Singer RH, McNeil JA. Interphase and metaphase resolution of different distances within the human dystrophin gene. *Science* 1990; 249: 928−32.

24 Ott J. *Analysis of Human Genetic Linkage.* Baltimore: The Johns Hopkins University Press, 1985.

25 Nakamura Y, Leppert M, O'Connell P *et al.* Variable number of tandem repeat (VNTR) markers for human gene mapping. *Science* 1987; 235: 1616−22.

26 Weber J, May PE. Abundant class of human DNA polymorphisms which can be typed using the polymerase chain reaction. *Am J Hum Genet* 1989; 44: 388−96.

27 Eiberg H, Mohr K, Schmeigelow K, Nielson LS, Williamson R. Linkage relationships of paraoxonase (PON) with other markers; indication of PON-cystic fibrosis synteny. *Clin Genet* 1985; 28: 840−5.

28 Tsui L, Buchwald M, Barker D *et al.* Cystic fibrosis locus defined by a genetically linked polymorphic DNA marker. *Science* 1985; 230: 1054−7.

29 Wainwright B, Scambler PJ, Schmidtke J *et al.* Localization of the cystic fibrosis locus to human chromosome 7cen-q22. *Nature* 1985; 318: 384−6.

30 White R, Leppert M, O'Connell P *et al.* Further linkage data on cystic fibrosis: the Utah study. *Am J Hum Genet* 1986; 39: 694−8.

31 Beaudet A, Bowcock A, Buchwald M *et al.* Linkage of cystic fibrosis to two tightly linked DNA markers: joint report from a collaborative study. *Am J Hum Genet* 1986; 39: 681−93.

32 Schwartz D, Cantor CF. Separation of yeast chromosome sized DNAs by pulsed field gradient gel electrophoresis. *Cell* 1984; 37: 67−75.

33 Barlow D, Lehrach H. Genetics by gel electrophoresis: the impact of pulsed field gel electrophoresis on mammalian genetics. *Trends Genet* 1987; 3: 167−71.

34 Burke D, Carle GF, Olson MV. Cloning of large segments of exogenous DNA into yeasts by means of artificial chromosome vectors. *Science* 1987; 236: 806−12.

35 Schlessinger D. Yeast artificial chromosomes: tools for mapping and analysis of complex genomes. *Trends Genet* 1990; 6: 251−8.

36 Poustka A, Lehrach H. Jumping libraries and linking libraries: the next generation of molecular tools in mammalian genetics. *Trends Genet* 1986; 2: 174−9.

37 Collins F, Weissman SM. Directional cloning of DNA fragments at a large distance from an initial probe: a circularization method. *Proc Natl Acad Sci USA* 1984; 81: 6812−16.

38 Collins FS, Drumm ML, Cole JL, Lockwood W, Vande WG, Iannuzzi MC. Construction of a general human chromosome jumping library, with application to cystic fibrosis. *Science* 1987; 235: 1046−9.

39 Rommens JM, Zengerling S, Burns J *et al.* Identification and regional localization of DNA markers on chromosome 7 for the cloning of the cystic fibrosis gene. *Am J Hum Genet* 1988; 43: 645−63.

40 Iannuzzi MC, Dean M, Drumm ML *et al.* Isolation of additional polymorphic clones from the cystic fibrosis region, using chromosome jumping from D7S8. [Published erratum appears in *Am J Hum Genet* 1989; 45: 342.] *Am J Hum Genet* 1989; 44: 695−703.

41 Bird A. CpG rich islands and the function of DNA methylation. *Nature* 1986; 321: 209−13.

42 Risch N. Linkage strategies for complex traits. I. Multilocus models. *Am J Hum Genet* 1990; 46: 222−8.

43 Risch N. Linkage strategies for genetically complex traits. II. The power of affected relative pairs. *Am J Hum Genet* 1990; 46: 229−41.

44 Dorman J, Trucco M, LePorte R, Kuller LH. Family studies: the key to understanding the genetic and environmental etiology of chronic disease? *Genet Epidemiol* 1988; 5: 305−10.

45 Hyer R, Julier C, Buckley JD *et al*. High resolution linkage mapping for susceptibility genes in human polygenic disease: insulin dependent diabetes mellitus and chromosome 11q. *Am J Hum Genet* 1991; 48: 243−57.

46 Payami H, Thomson G, Louis E. The affected sib method III. Selection and recombination. *Am J Hum Genet* 1984; 36: 352−62.

47 Weeks D, Lange K. The affected-pedigree-member method of linkage analysis. *Am J Hum Genet* 1988; 42: 315−26.

48 Mullis K, Faloona F, Scharf S, Saiki R, Horn G, Erlich H. Specific enzymatic amplification of DNA *in vitro*: the polymerase chain reaction. *Cold Spring Harbor Symp Quant Biol* 1986; 51: 263−73.

49 Rose E. Applications of the polymerase chain reaction to genome analysis. *FASEB J* 1991; 5: 46−54.

50 Cotton R, Rodriques NR, Campbell RD. Reactivity of cytosine and thymine in single base pair mismatches with hydroxylamine and osmium tetroxide and its application to the study of mutations. *Proc Natl Acad Sci USA* 1988; 85: 4397−401.

51 Grompe M, Muzny DM, Caskey CT. Scanning detection of mutations in human ornithine transcarbamoylase by chemical mismatch cleavage. *Proc Natl Acad Sci USA* 1989; 86: 5888−92.

52 Orita M, Suzuki Y, Sekiza T, Hayashi K. Rapid and sensitive detection of point mutations and DNA polymorphisms using the polymerase chain reaction. *Genomics* 1989; 5: 874−9.

53 Dean M, Drumm ML, Stewart C *et al*. Approaches to localizing disease genes as applied to cystic fibrosis. *Nucleic Acids Res* 1990; 18: 345−50.

54 Bear C, Duguay F, Naismith A, Karner N, Hanrahan JW, Riordan JR. Chloride channel activity in *Xenopus* oocytes expressing the cystic fibrosis gene. *J Biol Chem* 1991; 266: 19142−5.

55 Drumm ML, Wilkinson DS, Smith LS *et al*. Chloride conductance expressed by F508 and other mutant CFTRs in *Xenopus* oocytes. *Science* 1991; 254: 1979−99.

56 Tata F, Wicking C, Halford S *et al*. Cloning the mouse homolog of the human cystic fibrosis transmembrane regulator gene. *Genomics* 1991; 10: 301−18.

57 White C, Avraham KB, Shanley PF, Groner Y. Transgenic mice with expression of elevated levels of copper−zinc superoxide dismutase in the lungs are resistant to pulmonary oxygen toxicity. *J Clin Invest* 1991; 87: 2162−8.

58 McKusick V. Mapping and sequencing the human genome. *N Engl J Med* 1989; 320: 910−15.

5 Protein and gene polymorphisms

NOOR A. KALSHEKER

This chapter will focus on the nature of mutations in DNA and proteins and how DNA variations can be used as markers for disease.

Types of mutations in DNA

Mutations occur in the nucleotides of DNA. There are four types of mutations in DNA: substitution, deletion, insertion and inversion (Fig. 5.1). The commonest change is substitution where one nucleotide is replaced by another. When one nucleotide is either deleted or inserted into a coding sequence it results in a frameshift mutation as the coding sequence is altered. There are two types of substitution. A transition is a substitution of a purine (adenine or guanine) by another purine or a pyrimidine (cytosine or thymine) by another pyrimidine. If a purine replaces a pyrimidine and vice versa this is referred to as a transversion (Fig. 5.2).

Insertions and deletions occur more commonly in non-coding sequences and can vary from a few nucleotides to several thousand. Small insertions and deletions are probably caused by errors in DNA replication. Large insertions or deletions arise from unequal crossing over or via transposition when DNA sequences move from one chromosome to another (Fig. 5.3). Gene conversion is a phenomenon that is related to unequal crossing over. The total number of nucleotides is not altered but there is repair of mismatched bases in heteroduplex DNA (Fig. 5.4).

If mutations occur at random among the four nucleotides transversions would be expected to occur two times more commonly than transitions. However, in practice transitions occur more commonly than expected and the types of transitions do not occur with equal frequency. For example, the frequency of C—T change is higher than expected.

Mutations in proteins

Mutations in proteins are a direct result of mutations in DNA coding for the amino acids of proteins. Prior to the advent of DNA technology mutations were detected by examining the physicochemical properties

ACGTAT   Wild-type

ACGCAT   Substitution

ACG△AT   Deletion

ACGGTAT   Insertion

ACTGAT   Inversion

Fig. 5.1 The major types of single point mutations in DNA. The wild-type indicates the normal nucleotide sequence.

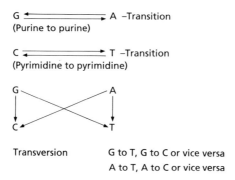

Fig. 5.2 Transitions and transversions in DNA.

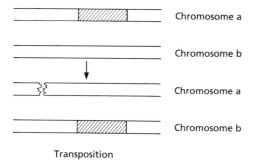

Transposition

Fig. 5.3 Transposition — transfer of DNA from one chromosome to another.

of proteins. Mutations in coding sequences of DNA do not always result in amino acid substitutions (see Chapter 1). There are 64 possible codons or triplet of bases. Some amino acids have unique codons (ATG codes for methionine) but there are three termination codons which signal the end of the protein. Of the remaining 19 amino acids there may be one to six alternative codons and this is referred to as degeneracy of the code. This simply means that there may be more than one combination of triplet bases coding for the same amino acid. Also if a mutation alters the third base in the triplet codon this is less likely to alter the amino acid than mutations occurring in either the first or second base. This

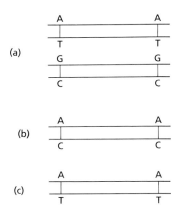

Fig. 5.4 Gene conversion. Correction of mismatched base pairs and no net change in the number of base pairs. (a) Allelic DNA sequences; (b) recombination; (c) correct base-pairing restored.

variability in the third base is referred to as 'wobble'. DNA mutations that do not alter the coding sequence of proteins are referred to as silent mutations and do not result in phenotypic changes. Missense mutations alter a codon representing one amino acid into a codon representing another amino acid, one that cannot function in the protein in place of the original residue (in practice such mutations are detected as changes in activity of the protein). The effects of the mutation can be reversed by insertion of either the original amino acid or another amino acid that is acceptable to the protein. When a point mutation creates one of three termination codons this results in premature termination of protein synthesis by the mutant codon. This usually abolishes protein function and is referred to as a nonsense mutation.

Protein differences are often studied by electrophoretic techniques that mainly rely on electrical charge differences. Under the usual conditions of electrophoresis basic amino acid residues such as lysine and arginine are positively charged whereas acidic residues such as glutamic acid and aspartic acid are negatively charged and all other amino acids are effectively neutral. It is therefore possible to compute the proportion of amino acid changes that result in a significant charge change, which has been estimated to be about 25–30% [1].

The use of isoelectric focusing (IEF) has made it possible to detect some amino acid substitutions which only cause minor charge differences. This has increased the number of protein variants that can be detected. An example of IEF in the detection of a number of α_1-antitrypsin (AAT) variants is shown in Fig. 5.5. Alternatively, mutations in protein can be detected by deficiencies in function of the protein. For example, a naturally occurring mutation of the α_1-antitrypsin gene referred to as AAT Pittsburgh results in loss of functional activity towards neutrophil elastase [2].

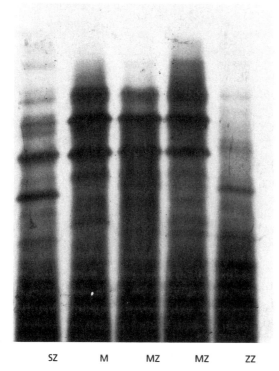

SZ   M   MZ   MZ   ZZ

Fig. 5.5 Isoelectric focusing. The detection of common deficiency variants of α_1-antitrypsin is shown. The characteristic banding patterns for the normal M and deficiency S and Z variants of α_1-antitrypsin AAT are shown.

Genes in populations and the Hardy–Weinberg equilibrium

If studies are to be made of gene and allele frequencies in patients with well-defined disease it is important to know first the frequency in a healthy population. This can be determined by direct studies of the healthy population and similar studies can be carried out in those with disease. However, it is then necessary to be able to predict whether the frequency within a disease population is at variance with the healthy group. In order to determine this an equation can be applied to deter-mine whether both populations are similar. The expected frequencies of the distribution of specific genotypes are determined by the Hardy–Weinberg equation. In a two allele locus where the alleles are A1 and A2 the possible genotypes are A1A1, A1A2 and A2A2. If the number of genotypes for A1A1 is N11, N12 for A1A2 and N22 for A2A2 the gene frequency (p) of A1 is:

$$\frac{(2N11 + N12)}{2N}$$

where $N = N11 + N12 + N22$. The frequency of A2 (q) $= 1 - p$. The expected genotype frequencies are given by:

$$(p + q)^2 = p^2 + 2pq + q^2$$

$$= \frac{N11}{N} + \frac{N12}{N} + \frac{N22}{N}$$

Observed allele frequencies should give genotype frequencies that are similar to the expected frequencies if the genotypes demonstrate Hardy−Weinberg equilibrium [3]. Several factors will influence the deviation from Hardy−Weinberg proportions. These include inbreeding and natural selection.

For codominant alleles all the genotypes are identifiable using restriction fragment length polymorphisms (RFLPs; see Chapter 1). Most protein polymorphisms are controlled by codominant alleles and since all the genotypes are usually detectable RFLPs behave as codominant alleles.

Linkage disequilibrium

Because the alleles at different loci are not always randomly combined in chromosomes the genotype frequencies in a randomly mating population are not necessarily given by the products of gene frequencies. If two loci on the same chromosome are close together, then it is likely that they will be inherited together as the likelihood of crossing over or recombination at meiosis is reduced (Fig. 5.6). The converse is also true, i.e. the further apart they are, the less likely they are to be inherited together. When two loci are inherited together they are said to be in linkage disequilibrium.

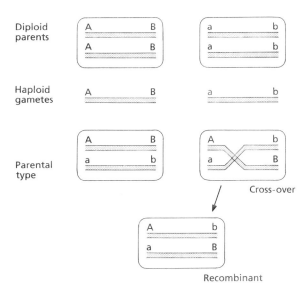

Fig. 5.6 Recombination. At meiosis homologous chromosomes may exchange genetic material. The likelihood of this taking place is related to the distance between alleles.

The principle of linkage has been used to track disease genes to particular chromosomes and subsequently to identify the gene responsible for the disease. In practice, the approach has involved tracking genetic markers in families with a particular disease and looking at the proportion of recombinants in families. If a DNA marker or RFLP segregates with a specific disease then the abnormal gene causing the disease is likely to be on the same chromosome. The search for markers segregating with disease can be a labour-intensive exercise. The probability of linkage is examined by log odds ratios or LOD scores (see Chapter 1). A LOD score of 3 or more makes it highly probable that a DNA marker is close to a disease gene. A crucial determinant of linkage analysis is recombination. The higher the proportion of recombinants the less likely is the probability that the marker segregates with the disease. Linkage was the approach used for cystic fibrosis in which the common genetic defect was eventually identified [4] and in Huntington's disease [5].

Genetic markers and disease

Linkage disequilibrium relies on using large-scale family studies. However, another approach that is commonly used is to study populations and look for disease associations. This approach is more common when investigating polygenic disorders where more than one gene and many environmental factors may be implicated in the pathological process and these groups of disorders account for considerable morbidity. The genes investigated are those that are thought to be important in the disease process and are often referred to as candidate genes. For example, in investigating the genetics of lung disease it would be reasonable to investigate the α_1-antitrypsin gene in detail. The rationale for this would be the great importance of α_1-antitrypsin as a major inhibitor of human neutrophil elastase (HNE) and its presumed function in protecting the lower respiratory tract from damage [6−8].

α_1-Antitrypsin and lung disease

The balance between proteinases such as HNE and inhibitors such as α_1-antitrypsin is thought to be critical in determining whether lung damage is likely to occur or not [6−8]. During inflammation and after cigarette smoking neutrophils accumulate in the lung and release some of their contents, including HNE, which is capable of degrading the connective tissue of the lung. This action is checked by α_1-antitrypsin. Consequently, individuals who are deficient in α_1-antitrypsin have an increased risk of developing progressive lung damage particularly if they smoke [9]. The recognition of the association between genetic deficiency of α_1-antitrypsin and predisposition to the development of lung damage has provided a major focus of interest in the pathogenesis of chronic lung damage.

α_1-Antitrypsin deficiency was recognized initially at the protein level by deficiency of the protein in the plasma [10], shown subsequently to be arising from a single point mutation in a coding sequence of the α_1-antitrypsin gene [11, 12]. In deficiency states arising from the Z allele only about 10−20% of the α_1-antitrypsin concentration is present in the serum as compared with the normal M allele. This mutation is also detected easily by IEF. A single base change in the gene alters the codon for amino acid residue 342 from an acidic residue glutamate to the basic residue lysine [11, 12]. This replacement results in the retarded migration of α_1-antitrypsin protein in an electric field (Fig. 5.5).

Since differences in protein charge will only detect about one-quarter to one-third of all possible mutations, the investigation of DNA poly-morphisms is required to look for additional variation. Given the association of α_1-antitrypsin deficiency and lung disease we initiated an extensive investigation of the α_1-antitrypsin gene to look for additional variation to see if any DNA polymorphisms may serve as markers for chronic lung disease.

Restriction fragment length polymorphisms

The simplest way to investigate DNA variation is to use a number of restriction enzymes to cut DNA into smaller fragments and analyse these fragments by Southern blotting (Fig. 5.7 and Chapter 1). Restriction enzymes recognize and cleave specific sequences in DNA which range from four to seven bases usually. The sequences that are recognized are palindromic. The loss or creation of a restriction enzyme site will generate fragments of a different size. These often arise because of alteration of a single base in the recognition sequence of the enzyme. These are referred to as RFLPs. The chances of detecting RFLPs are increased with longer probes as it has been suggested that mutations may occur on average in about 1 in 200−300 base pairs (bp) of DNA [13].

After identifying RFLPs it is possible to investigate the association, if any, of the RFLPs to disease. A number of RFLPs have been identified in the α_1-antitrypsin gene [14, 15]. The frequencies of several RFLPs were estimated in a healthy control population and in a group of patients with the disease pulmonary emphysema [15] and one was found more frequently in subjects with chronic lung disease [16]. This polymorphism arose as a consequence of the loss of a recognition site for the restriction enzyme Taq1. The mutation arose in the 3′ flanking region of the α_1-antitrypsin gene. Further studies demonstrated a strong association with both emphysema and bronchiectasis. Since α_1-antitrypsin is a major protein involved in protecting the lower respiratory tract from diseases

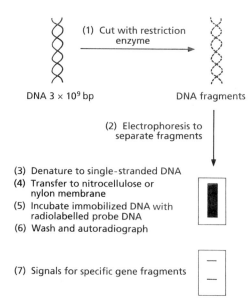

(1) Cut with restriction enzyme

DNA 3×10^9 bp

DNA fragments

(2) Electrophoresis to separate fragments

(3) Denature to single-stranded DNA
(4) Transfer to nitrocellulose or nylon membrane
(5) Incubate immobilized DNA with radiolabelled probe DNA
(6) Wash and autoradiograph

(7) Signals for specific gene fragments

Fig. 5.7 Southern blot. A common method for looking at DNA variation. This relies on digesting DNA with restriction enzymes, separating the DNA on the basis of size, transferring single-stranded DNA to a membrane and probing the DNA with a specific cloned sequence or synthetic oligonucleotide probe which is usually radiolabelled. The signals are detected by autoradiography using an X-ray film sensitive to the radiation of ^{32}P.

such as pulmonary emphysema and bronchiectasis which may share a common pathogenic mechanism [6], it was not altogether surprising to find an association with both diseases.

The Taq1 RFLP was associated with chronic lung disease in the absence of classical plasma α_1-antitrypsin deficiency. There were two possibilities for this association. The first was the inheritance of a marker in linkage disequilibrium with a mutation in a neighbouring gene or alternatively the Taq1 RFLP played a direct role in the disease process via the α_1-antitrypsin gene itself.

In order to clarify these possibilities it was thought important to characterize the mutation(s) responsible for the RFLP. The sequence of the 3' flanking region of the α_1-antitrypsin gene was not known so this was determined [17]. The mutation(s) responsible for the Taq1 RFLP was subsequently determined by generating amplification primers for the polymerase chain reaction (PCR) and sequencing the products. The polymorphism was due to a single point mutation resulting in a G to A transition. This discovery also facilitated detection of the mutation by amplification of DNA *in vitro* using the PCR and subsequent digestion by the restriction enzyme. This allows for direct visualization of the poly-morphism by staining DNA separated in an agarose gel with ethidium bromide (Fig. 5.8).

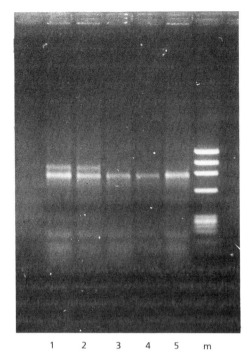

1   2   3   4   5   m

Fig. 5.8 PCR amplification of a 960 bp fragment of the α_1-antitrypsin gene. Lanes 1–5 are DNA amplification products from patient samples that have been digested with the restriction enzyme Taq1 and m corresponds to molecular weight markers (small at the bottom, large at the top). Lanes 1 and 2 show a larger band that does not digest with Taq1 whereas lanes 3–5 are all digested with Taq1. The former therefore are heterozygotes for the Taq1 polymorphism.

Of note in the DNA sequence of the normal gene was the occurrence of sequences corresponding to three potential enhancer binding elements, which regulate the expression of genes in association with promoter sequences. These may occur in any region of the gene, close to or distant to promoter regions. The sequences are orientation independent, i.e. in experimental models they will work in both orientations. At the present time the possibility that the Taq1 polymorphism influences protein expression is speculative, but we have obtained some recent evidence that seems to support this hypothesis [18]. However, this example illustrates how it is possible to use the technology to look for DNA markers in association with disease and how such studies may lead to new insights into the pathogenesis of disease.

The characterization of mutations in genes also facilitates their detection directly. The methodology primarily involves gene amplification by the PCR and detection by the use of allele-specific oligonucleotides (ASOs). By introducing a mismatch in the oligonucleotides it is possible to destabilize the hybridization of the oligonucleotide to target DNA sufficiently to distinguish between hybridization of a perfect match and one which has a single base mismatch. The combined approach of the PCR and the use of ASOs has been widely used in the detection of single point mutations. An example of this technique is demonstrated in Fig. 5.9.

Haplotypes and deficiency alleles

The presence of a combination of RFLPs or haplotypes is sometimes useful in looking at the chromosomal background from which specific mutations may have arisen. In the α_1-antitrypsin gene there is strong linkage disequilibrium between certain haplotypes and protein types. The principle of haplotype analysis is illustrated in Table 5.1. For example, if there are two variable fragments of 1 and 2 kilobases (kb) observed with a particular restriction enzyme in the same gene and another enzyme detects fragments of 3 and 4 kb there are eight possible combinations of RFLPs. Using a combination of five restriction enzymes Cox et al. [19] have demonstrated with a few exceptions that there are specific haplotypes associated with some of the α_1-antitrypsin-deficient alleles, but not the normal M alleles. Even with one of the normal alleles despite the theoretical possibility of 384 potential haplotypes only 11 were observed. There is a limitation on these studies as large numbers of samples need to be analysed to look for all possible haplotypes.

This chapter has highlighted the types of mutations that occur in DNA and proteins and how some of these are detected. It has also

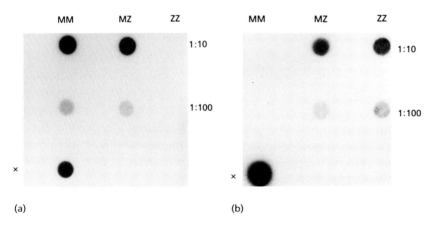

(a)   (b)

Fig. 5.9 Allele-specific oligonucleotides. Duplicate filters were spotted with DNA amplification products obtained by the PCR of a region of the α_1-antitrypsin gene containing the Z mutation. The PCR product was diluted either 1 in 10 or 1 in 100 and 5 μl was spotted on to a nylon membrane. X corresponds to an unknown sample that was being tested. (a) For the M-specific oligonucleotides only signals corresponding to the normal M allele were detected whereas (b) the Z-specific oligonucleotides only picked up signals from the Z allele. Since X was detected by both probes this sample corresponds to the MZ genotype. From Kalsheker N, Morgan K. *Thorax* 1990; 45: 759–64.

Table 5.1 Theoretical genotypes for two two-allele polymorphisms where fragments of 1 and 2 kb are obtained with one restriction enzyme and with a second enzyme fragments of 3 and 4 kb are obtained

Fragment size (kb)		
Enzyme a	Enzyme b	Haplotype
1,1	3,3	1133
1,2	3,3	1233
1,2	3,4	1234
1,2	4,4	1244
1,1	4,4	1144
2,2	3,3	2233
2,2	3,4	2234
2,2	4,4	2244

shown how DNA variation can be used in the study of disease when less specific methods fail.

References

1 Nei M, Chakraborty R. Genetic distance and electrophoretic identity of proteins between taxa. *J Mol Evol* 1973; 2: 323–8.

2 Owen MC, Brennan SO, Lewis JW, Carrell RW. Mutation of antitrypsin to antithrombin: α-1-antitrypsin Pittsburgh 358 (Met-Arg), a fatal bleeding disorder. *N Engl J Med* 1983; 309: 694–8.

3 Hardy GH. Mendelian proportions in a mixed population. *Science* 1908; 28: 49–50.

4 Kerem B-S, Rommens JM, Buchanan JA *et al*. Identification of the cystic fibrosis gene: genetic analysis. *Science* 1989; 245: 1073–80.

5 Huntington's Disease Collaborative Research Group. A novel gene containing a trinucleotide repeat that is expanded and unstable on Huntington's disease chromosomes. *Cell* 1993; 72: 971–83.

6 Janoff A. Elastase and emphysema: current assessment of the protease-antiprotease hypothesis. *Am Rev Respir Dis* 1985; 132: 417–33.

7 Stockley R. Proteolytic enzymes, their inhibitors and lung disease. *Clin Sci* 1983; 64: 119–26.

8 Crystal RG. α_1-Antitrypsin deficiency, emphysema and liver disease. *J Clin Invest* 1990; 85: 1343–52.

9 Larsson C. Natural history and life expectancy in severe alpha-1-antitrypsin deficiency Pi Z. *Acta Med Scand* 1978; 204: 345–51.

10 Laurell C-B, Eriksson S. The electrophoretic α-1-globulin pattern of serum α-1-antitrypsin deficiency. *Scand J Clin Lab Invest* 1963; 15: 132–40.

11 Yoshida A, Lieberman J, Gaidulis I, Ewing C. Molecular abnormality of human alpha-1-antitrypsin variant (Pi-ZZ) associated with plasma activity deficiency. *Proc Natl Acad Sci USA* 1976; 73: 1324–8.

12 Kidd VJ, Galbus MS, Wallace RB, Itakura K, Woo SLC. α_1-Antitrypsin deficiency detection by direct analysis of the mutation in the gene. *N Engl J Med* 1984; 310: 639–42.

13 Jeffreys AJ, Flavell RA. A physical map of the DNA regions flanking the rabbit B-globin gene. *Cell* 1977; 12: 429−39.

14 Cox DW, Woo SLC, Mansfield T. DNA restriction fragments associated with alpha$_1$-antitrypsin indicate a single origin for deficiency allele PiZ. *Nature* 1985; 316: 79−81.

15 Hodgson I, Kalsheker N. DNA polymorphisms of the human α_1-antitrypsin gene in normal subjects and in patients with pulmonary emphysema. *J Med Genet* 1987; 24: 47−51.

16 Kalsheker NA, Hodgson IJ, Watkins GL, White JP, Morrison HM, Stockley RA. Deoxyribonucleic acid polymorphism of the α_1-antitrypsin gene in chronic lung disease. *Br Med J* 1987; 294: 1151−4.

17 Morgan K, Scobie G, Kalsheker N. The characterisation of a mutation of the alpha-1-antitrypsin gene commonly associated with chronic lung disease. *Eur J Clin Invest* 1992; 22: 134−7.

18 Morgan K, Scobie G, Kalsheker NA. Point mutation in a 3′ flanking sequence of the alpha-1-antitrypsin gene associated with chronic respiratory disease occurs in a regulatory sequence. *Hum Mol Genet* 1993; 2: 253−57.

19 Cox DW, Billingsley GD, Mansfield T. DNA restriction-site polymorphisms associated with the alpha$_1$-antitrypsin gene. *Am J Hum Genet* 1987; 41: 891−906.

6   Site-directed mutagenesis

DAVID A. LOMAS AND ROBIN W. CARRELL

Introduction

The advent of site-directed mutagenesis has provided a powerful tool with which to investigate protein structure and function. This has been used to further our understanding of the role and function of proteins, including proteinase inhibitors which protect the lung from proteolytic damage. There are a variety of these inhibitors but most important are the members of a family of serine proteinase inhibitors, the 'serpins', typified by α_1-antitrypsin and α_1-antichymotrypsin [1]. Each of the family members has a unique inhibitory specificity but shares a similar overall molecular structure [2].

The pathogenesis of lung diseases such as adult respiratory distress syndrome and emphysema is thought to depend upon an imbalance between destructive leucocyte serine proteinases (such as neutrophil elastase and cathepsin G) and their serpin inhibitors, most notably α_1-antitrypsin [3–6]. Deficiency of α_1-antitrypsin is most frequently due to the Z mutation which results in the failure of protein secretion and consequently to decreased plasma proteinase inhibitory activity and progressive tissue damage [7].

The relationship of α_1-antichymotrypsin to the pathogenesis of destructive lung disease is less clear as the only abnormality so far reported is a partial, heterozygous deficiency with relatively mild and indefinite clinical consequences [8].

The aim of this chapter is to describe the technique of site-directed mutagenesis and to illustrate the way in which it has enhanced our knowledge of proteinase inhibitors and allowed the development of proteins which may have a therapeutic potential.

Site-directed mutagenesis

Mutagenesis has long been used to provide insights into biological function. Historically, mutations were performed *in vivo* and were precipitated by X-rays [9] or chemical mutagens [10]. Modern technology has led to the development of *in vitro* mutagenesis, which is much more efficient and may be targeted to the area of interest. This site-directed mutagenesis is based on the use of synthetic oligonucleotides, which are used to construct mutant alleles of isolated genes with base substitutions, insertions or deletions [11–15].

Before such techniques can be applied, the DNA coding for the protein of interest must be identified and cloned. This may be obtained from either genomic DNA selected from chromosomal gene libraries or complementary DNA (cDNA) amplified from cellular messenger RNA (mRNA). Genomic DNA has the disadvantage that the sequences which code for the protein, the exons, are interrupted by non-coding sequences, 'introns'. cDNA, however, is constructed from mRNA by reverse transcription and therefore contains only the sequence coding for the protein flanked by recognition sequences. cDNA is consequently a more common choice for site-directed mutagenesis.

Having isolated the DNA it is inserted into a single-stranded cloning vector, such as the M13 [16] or fd [17] bacteriophage.

Bacteriophages are viruses that specifically infect bacteria, a property which makes them suitable vehicles (or vectors) to transport the cloned gene into a bacterial cell. These vectors are much smaller than chromosomal DNA and are capable of extrachromosomal replication in bacterial hosts. Following the introduction of the phage vector into enteric bacteria ('transfection') the cloning phage replicates but, unlike other bacteriophages, does not lyse the host cell. Rather, transfected bacteria continue to grow at a slower rate than normal bacteria allowing them to be identified as plaques which appear as clear areas on a bacterial lawn.

The M13 phage is commonly used as a vector for mutagenesis as it has been modified to contain the lac operon marker system [16]. Following transfection into bacteria which lack the complete lac operon, the lac region of the M13 phage codes for the production of the enzyme β-galactosidase following induction with isopropylthiogalactoside (IPTG). This enzyme converts lactose to glucose and galactose and its presence may be detected by adding the lactose analogue X-gal (5-dibromo-4-chloro-3-indolylgalactoside) and IPTG to agar plates. The enzyme, if present, will cleave X-gal to produce deep blue dibromodichloroindigo which discolours the bacterial plaque. Thus bacterial plaques containing the intact vector may be selected by growing on medium containing IPTG and X-gal and choosing those plaques coloured blue.

The insertion of cloned fragments of DNA into M13 is performed using restriction sites in the lac region which will interrupt the lac DNA (Fig. 6.1). This destroys the vector's ability to code for β-galactosidase and, following growth on medium containing IPTG and X-gal, bacteria containing the vector and cDNA insert may be recognized as the plaques are colourless and no longer blue [11, 16].

Having cloned the cDNA into the vector an oligonucleotide is synthesized that is complementary to the target site apart from the designed mutation (Fig. 6.2). The oligonucleotide is allowed to anneal to a single-

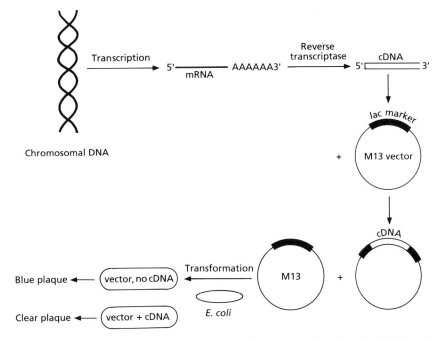

Fig. 6.1 Cloning of DNA into the M13 vector and transformation into *Escherichia coli*. The colonies containing the DNA of interest may be detected by the colour of the plaques. Those containing the M13 vector alone are blue following growth on medium containing X-gal and IPTG. Those in which the lac marker has been disrupted by the insertion of a DNA fragment fail to produce β-galactosidase and so are colourless.

	P_4	P_3	P_2	P_1	$P_{1'}$	$P_{2'}$	$P_{3'}$	$P_{4'}$
Amino acid	ala	ile	pro	Met	ser	ile	pro	pro
cDNA	GCC	ATA	CCC	ATG	TCT	ATC	CCC	CCC
Oligonucleotide	CGG	TAT	GGG	GAC	AGA	TAG	GGG	GGG
Mutated cDNA	GCC	ATA	CCC	CTG	TCT	ATC	CCC	CCC
Amino acid	ala	ile	pro	Leu	ser	ile	pro	pro

Fig. 6.2 Design of an oligonucleotide sequence to mutate the P_1 methionine of α_1-antitrypsin to leucine. The figure illustrates a portion of the active site (the P_4–P_4' residues) along with the codons which specify the amino acid sequence. The complementary oligonucleotide will anneal to the cDNA but contains a base pair mismatch. When this is subsequently used as a template for DNA replication the codon specifies leucine (CTG) and not methionine (ATG).

stranded form of the wild-type gene and acts as a primer to be further extended by DNA polymerase using the wild-type sequence as a template (Fig. 6.3). This continues around the wild-type gene until the 5′ end of the oligonucleotide is reached, at which stage the circular DNA is completed by the enzyme DNA ligase. Thus a duplex circular molecule is produced with a wild-type strand and a newly synthesized mutant strand [18–20]. If the duplex molecule is then transfected into bacteria the cell's repair mechanism will tend to correct the mutant strand and so most colonies will contain only the wild-type DNA. Several techniques have been developed to overcome this, one of which is the enzymatic degradation of the wild-type template. This is performed by specifically cleaving the circular wild-type strand with restriction endonucleases and then digesting the newly opened DNA with exonuclease III which acts to remove nucleotides one at a time from the end of non-circular DNA [21]. Following transfection into *Escherichia coli* [22] the cells containing the mutant DNA may be isolated as a pure clone.

DNA sequencing to confirm mutagenesis

Verification that the desired mutation has been introduced may be accomplished by dideoxy chain-termination sequencing of single-stranded DNA [23–25], or chemical cleavage of double-stranded DNA [26, 27]. Dideoxy chain-termination sequencing is most commonly performed

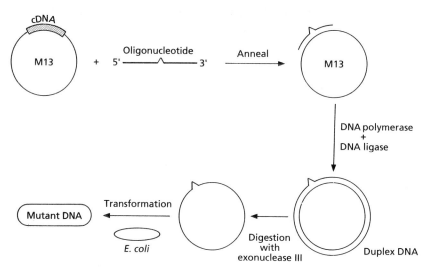

Fig. 6.3 The synthesis of mutant DNA by site-directed mutagenesis. The oligonucleotide containing the mutation is annealed to the cDNA in a cloning vector. Duplex DNA is completed by DNA polymerase and DNA ligase and the wild-type (inner) strand is then opened with a restriction endonuclease and digested with exonuclease III. Following transformation into *E. coli* the mutant DNA may be isolated as a pure clone.

and is described in more detail in Chapter 1. It is important to sequence the whole gene and not merely the newly mutated region as mutations may be inadvertently introduced into non-target sequences during the process of site-directed mutagenesis [28, 29].

Expression of mutant protein

Having confirmed that the desired mutation has occurred and that there are no new mutations in the residual cDNA sequence the mutant gene is cut out of the mutagenesis vector and inserted into the expression vector from which the protein will be produced. This vector also codes for antibiotic resistance and contains a promoter sequence upstream of the mutated gene. The vector is introduced or transformed into cells such as *E. coli* or *Saccharomyces cerevisiae*, which have been permeabilized by physical or chemical treatment [22, 30]. 'Following permeabilization', these cells are said to be competent and take up the vector. The resulting transformants containing the vector are selected by screening for antibiotic sensitivity [31]. The cells that contain the vector are then grown in large-scale culture and induced to express the mutant protein. This induction requires the use of strong promoters such as λ-phage, lac, trp or tac. These activate the transcription of the cloned gene and hence the production of the recombinant protein by adding chemicals to, or raising the temperature of, the culture medium. For example, the bacteriophage λ-promoter is usually held repressed by a heat-sensitive protein present at temperatures less than 30°C. Upon raising the temperature to 42°C the promoter is activated resulting in the production of large amounts of recombinant protein. This recombinant protein may then be isolated from the cellular proteins by standard chromatography techniques [32, 33].

Active site mutations

The inhibitory specificity of α_1-antitrypsin and other members of the serpin family is dependent upon their ability to present themselves as ideal substrates for their target proteinases. The specificity is defined by the residues at the $P_1 - P_1'$ positions of the reactive centre (Fig. 6.4 and Plate 6.1, facing p. 164) [34] as they provide the cleavage site for the target enzyme [1, 35]. In the case of α_1-antitrypsin the P_1 residue occurs at position 358 and is occupied by methionine [36]. This provides the ideal cleavage site for neutrophil elastase, which precisely fits and complexes with the active site of α_1-antitrypsin.

The importance of mutations of the P_1 residue became apparent clinically when a 14-year-old boy from Pittsburgh died of recurrent haemorrhage attributed to a phenotypically abnormal α_1-antitrypsin [37]. Further investigation [38] revealed that the methionine at the 358

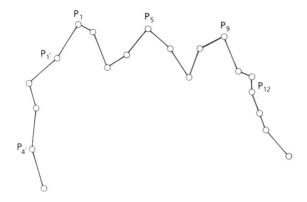

Fig. 6.4 Diagrammatic illustration of the reactive loop of α_1-antitrypsin. This has yet to be crystallized intact and so the structure shown is modelled on ovalbumin, another member of the serpin family. From Jones TA, Thirup S. *EMBO J* 1986; 5: 819–22; Unger R, Harel D, Wherland S, Sussman JL. *Proteins Struc Func Gen* 1989; 5: 355–73. The diagram shows the key P_1–P_1' residues which provide the cleavage site for the target enzyme.

position of α_1-antitrypsin had been replaced by arginine. This converted the α_1-antitrypsin from its normal function as an inhibitor of elastase [39] to an inhibitor of thrombin, thus massively enhancing the patient's natural anticoagulant activity. During intercurrent illnesses the 'acute phase' response led to an increase in the plasma concentration of this mutant α_1-antitrypsin resulting in significant haemorrhage, which was eventually fatal. Further studies on this naturally occurring mutant (α_1-antitrypsin Pittsburgh) revealed that not only was it an effective inhibitor of thrombin [40] but that it was also a potent inhibitor of other members of the clotting cascade [41].

Such an observation led to the prediction that engineered modifications of the P_1 residue of α_1-antitrypsin should result in predictable changes in inhibitory activity. The P_1 methionine of α_1-antitrypsin is susceptible to oxidation thereby inactivating the protein as an inhibitor of elastase [39, 42]. Rosenberg *et al.* [43] replaced the methionine at the 358 position with valine which was predicted to provide an elastase cleavage site and hence enzyme inhibition, but which would not be susceptible to oxidation. The resulting protein was shown to retain its activity as an inhibitor of elastase and was resistant to the oxidative inactivation characteristic of the naturally occurring α_1-antitrypsin [44]. These predictions and observations were subsequently confirmed by other workers [32, 45, 46] who also demonstrated that the elastase inhibitory activity may be attenuated by adding an alanine at the 356 position [47]. This second mutation made the protein a specific inhibitor of pancreatic elastase and illustrated that amino acid substitutions within the active centre but not necessarily of the P_1 residue also play a role in defining inhibitor specificity [48, 49].

The role of the P_1 residue in determining α_1-antitrypsin inhibitor specificity was also illustrated by Matheson *et al.* [50] who correctly predicted that substitutions of alanine and reduced cysteine at the 358 position would have no effect on the capacity of the serpin to inhibit neutrophil and pancreatic elastase. The cysteine residue was then oxidized (producing a dramatic fall in elastase inhibitory activity), carboxy-methylated (producing an acidic side chain analogous to glutamic acid) and treated with chloroethylamine (producing a basic side chain analogous to lysine). These substitutions resulted in dramatic changes in inhibitory activity as outlined in Table 6.1.

In 1990 Rubin *et al.* [33], using similar technology, produced mutations of the P_1 site of α_1-antichymotrypsin (Table 6.2). As expected the substitution of arginine for leucine at the 358 site changed the protein into an inhibitor of thrombin and trypsin but reduced the inhibition of chymotrypsin by 30-fold. Surprisingly, the substitution of methionine for leucine at the P_1 site failed to produce an inhibitor of elastase suggesting that the inhibition of this enzyme may be dependent on other aspects of protein structure.

Mutations clarifying serpin structure and function

The Z mutation of α_1-antitrypsin

α_1-Antitrypsin deficiency is an autosomal recessive disorder that occurs in 1 in 1700 Caucasians of North European descent [51, 52]. A serum level of less than 35% of normal is believed to be insufficient to inhibit all lung elastase thereby predisposing the affected individual to early-onset emphysema [3, 51, 53]. The Z mutation is of particular importance because of its allelic frequency of 2.6% in North Europeans of European descent [51, 52]. It is caused by a single base substitution (G to A) leading to an amino acid change of glutamic acid (342) to lysine in exon V of the gene [54]. This results in normal α_1-antitrypsin synthesis but an 85% reduction in protein secretion from both hepatic cells [55] and mononuclear phagocytes [56]. The residual protein accumulates in the rough endoplasmic reticulum of hepatic cells and may contribute to or be the causative factor of concomitant liver disease [57].

At the molecular level the mutation is thought to disrupt the salt bridge which exists between the positively charged lysine at position 290 and the negatively charged glutamic acid at position 342 (Plates 6.1 and 6.2, facing p. 164) [58, 59]. Interestingly, however, severance of the salt bridge by mutating lysine 290 to glutamic acid failed to inhibit protein synthesis or secretion [59−61]. Furthermore, attempts at correcting the defect by mutating the lysine 290 to glutamic acid in the hope of restoring a reversed salt bridge have met with conflicting results. Although one group have described correction of the synthetic block [62], others

Table 6.1 Manipulations of the P_1 amino acid of α_1-antitrypsin and their effect on inhibitory specificity. The modification of the residue is shown along with its new target proteinase and association rate constant

Enzyme	Wild-type k_{ass} (m^{-1}s^{-1})	Modification/substitution	k_{ass} (m^{-1}s^{-1})	Reference
Human neutrophil elastase	6.5×10^7	Oxidation P_1 methionine	3.1×10^4	[39]
Human α-chymotrypsin	5.4×10^6	Oxidation P_1 methionine	1.0×10^6	[39]
Human neutrophil elastase	6.5×10^7	P_1 methionine $\rightarrow$ valine	1.5×10^7	[32]
Human neutrophil elastase	1.1×10^7	P_1 methionine $\rightarrow$ leucine	6.7×10^6	[47]
Cathepsin G	6.5×10^4	P_1 methionine $\rightarrow$ leucine	2.7×10^4	[47]
Cathepsin G	6.5×10^4	P_1 methionine $\rightarrow$ phenylalanine	1.1×10^5	[47]
Human neutrophil elastase	1.1×10^7	P_1 methionine $\rightarrow$ alanine	2.4×10^6	[47]
Human neutrophil elastase	1.1×10^7	P_1 methionine $\rightarrow$ isoleucine	3.0×10^6	[47]
Human neutrophil elastase	6.5×10^7	P_1 methionine $\rightarrow$ cysteine	5.9×10^6	[50]
Human neutrophil elastase	6.5×10^7	P_1 methionine $\rightarrow$ oxidized cysteine	1.9×10^3	[50]
Bovine α-chymotrypsin	5.9×10^6	P_1 methionine $\rightarrow$ carboxymethylcysteine	8.5×10^5	[50]
Porcine trypsin	4.2×10^4	P_1 methionine $\rightarrow$ aminoethylcysteine	4.0×10^6	[50]
Human α-thrombin	4.8×10^1	P_1 methionine $\rightarrow$ arginine	3.1×10^5	[40]
Human α-thrombin	4.8×10^1	P_1 methionine $\rightarrow$ arginine	5.0×10^5	[47]

Table 6.2 Manipulations of the P_1 amino acid of α_1-antichymotrypsin and their effect on inhibitory specificity

Enzyme	Wild-type k_{ass} $(m^{-1}s^{-1})$	Modification/substitution	k_{ass} $(m^{-1}s^{-1})$	Reference
Cathepsin G	5.1×10^7	—	—	[39]
Bovine α-chymotrypsin	7×10^5	P_1 leucine $\rightarrow$ methionine	3×10^5	[33]
Human neutrophil elastase	$< 10^3$	P_1 leucine $\rightarrow$ methionine	$< 10^3$	[33]
Human α-thrombin	$< 3 \times 10^2$	P_1 methionine $\rightarrow$ arginine	4.3×10^3	[33]

have disputed this finding [59, 61] suggesting that a positive charge due to the amino acid change at position 342 is sufficient to block α_1-antitrypsin secretion independent of the charge at residue 290. This was confirmed by Sifers *et al.* [61] who mutated the negatively charged glutamic acid (342) to a negatively charged aspartic acid (no effect on α_1-antitrypsin secretion) and to a neutral glutamine (45% reduction in α_1-antitrypsin secretion). The lowest levels of protein secretion were apparent when a positively charged lysine was introduced at the 342 position.

More recent work has shown that the accumulation of Z antitrypsin in the liver and hence its deficiency in the plasma is the consequence of a unique polymerisation process. The mutation at position 342 is at the base of the reactive centre loop and results in a distortion that allows the insertion of the loop of one molecule into the A sheet of a second to give end-on-end polymers [63]. Additional evidence that this process of loop sheet polymerisation is the cause of the accumulation comes from the demonstration of the same process in two other antitrypsin mutants (S_{iiyama} $^{53}Ser \rightarrow Phe$ [64] and M_{malton} ^{52}Phe deleted).

The DNA-binding region of α_1-antichymotrypsin

Site-directed mutagenesis has also been used to clarify the binding region of α_1-antichymotrypsin in the cell nucleus. This protein is known to bind to DNA, an observation which has been exploited in its purification [65] and may signal a physiological role in the inhibition of DNA polymerase-α [66] and DNA primase [67]. The crystallographic deduction that the DNA-binding region centres on the three positively charged lysine residues on the s4C and s3C turn [68] was confirmed *in vitro* by Rubin, (reference 68) who substituted increasing numbers of glutamic acids for the lysine residues and demonstrated the abolition of protein binding to DNA.

'Designer' proteins for therapeutic use

It is now widely accepted that patients with α_1-antitrypsin deficiency are susceptible to the development of early-onset emphysema [3, 51] and as a consequence it is logical to redress the deficiency by parenteral replacement therapy. Gadek *et al.* [69] and Wewers *et al.* [53] demonstrated that weekly injections of α_1-antitrypsin could restore lung inhibitor concentrations to acceptable levels and at the time of writing several uncontrolled trials assessing the efficacy of α_1-antitrypsin replacement therapy in patients with congenital deficiency are under way.

Assuming that replacement therapy does slow the progression of emphysema it is possible that it may also have a role in patients with emphysema but normal α_1-antitrypsin concentrations. It has been suggested that such patients may develop progressive destructive lung disease by a smoking-induced oxidation and inactivation of α_1-antitrypsin [42, 40, 41] although this hypothesis is far from proven. However, with these thoughts in mind and in view of the observation that α_1-antitrypsin Pittsburgh may protect against septicaemic shock [72], several authors have speculated on the role of recombinant preparations for use in patients with emphysema or infection. Rosenberg *et al.* [43] suggested that valine (P_1) α_1-antitrypsin may be useful as this is resistant to oxidative inactivation and shows a greater capacity to protect against tissue damage than the native protein [7, 73]. Jallat *et al.* [47] proposed a role for leucine (P_1) α_1-antitrypsin as this acts as an inhibitor of cathepsin G as well as elastase. This combines the advantages of resistance to oxidation with a broader inhibitory activity towards other leucocyte proteinases.

The recombinant α_1-antitrypsin preparations are, however, not a therapeutic panacea for, although they are as effective as proteinase inhibitors [32, 47, 74], they are potentially more antigenic and have a shorter half-life [32, 73] than plasma α_1-antitrypsin. This probably reflects the fact that they are not glycosylated. Moreover, although oxidized plasma α_1-antitrypsin is a poor inhibitor of elastase it retains activity against other proteinases such as chymotrypsin [39], which may be lost with mutated proteins. Furthermore, while inactivation of α_1-antitrypsin by oxidation of the active site methionine may be disadvantageous in 'systemic inflammation', it may on the other hand confer physiological advantage in allowing tissue breakdown and repair at sites of local inflammation [7].

α_1-Antichymotrypsin unlike α_1-antitrypsin is not susceptible to inactivation by cigarette smoke [42] but the recombinant protein is less active as a proteinase inhibitor [33]. Moreover, no α_1-antichymotrypsin inhibitor of both neutrophil elastase and cathepsin G has been produced and its role in the pathogenesis of disease has yet to be clarified.

Summary

The role of replacement therapy is controversial and patients must be selected carefully [75] as capricious use of these agents may be unrewarding, potentially dangerous and very expensive. Despite these reservations recombinant proteins offer interesting prospects for therapy for those patients with progressive destructive lung disease.

Acknowledgements

We wish to thank Dr Craig Marshall for modelling Figs 6.4−6.6 and Paul Hopkins for his helpful comments. David Lomas is an MRC Training Fellow.

References

1 Carrell RW, Boswell DR. Serpins: the superfamily of plasma serine proteinase inhibitors. In: Barrett A, Salvesen G, eds. *Proteinase Inhibitors*. Amsterdam: Elsevier Science Publishers BV (Biomedical Division), 1986: 403—20.

2 Huber R, Carrell RW. Implications of the three-dimensional structure of α_1-antitrypsin for structure and function of serpins. *Biochemistry* 1989; 28: 8951—66.

3 Laurell CB, Eriksson S. The electrophoretic α_1-globulin pattern of serum in α_1-antitrypsin deficiency. *Scand J Clin Lab Invest* 1963; 15: 132—40.

4 Eriksson S. Proteases and protease inhibitors in chronic obstructive lung disease. *Acta Med Scand* 1978; 203: 449—55.

5 McGuire WW, Spragg RG, Cohen AB, Cochrane CG. Studies on the pathogenesis of the adult respiratory distress syndrome. *J Clin Invest* 1982; 69: 543—53.

6 Stockley RA. Proteolytic enzymes, their inhibitors and lung diseases. *Clin Sci* 1983; 64: 119—26.

7 Carrell RW, Jeppsson JO, Laurell CB, Brennan SO, Owen MC, Vaughan L, Boswell DR. Structure and variation of human α_1-antitrypsin. *Nature* 1982; 298: 329—34.

8 Lindmark BE, Arborelius M, Eriksson SG. Pulmonary function in middle-aged women with heterozygous deficiency of the serine protease inhibitor alpha$_1$-antichymotrypsin. *Am Rev Respir Dis* 1990; 141: 884—8.

9 Muller HJ. Artificial transmutation of the gene. *Science* 1927; 66: 84—7.

10 Auerbach C, Robson JM. The production of mutations by chemical substances. *Proc R Soc Edin* 1947; 62: 271—83.

11 Messing J. New M13 vectors for cloning. *Methods Enzymol* 1983; 101: 20—89.

12 Zoller MJ, Smith M. Oligonucleotide-directed mutagenesis of DNA fragments cloned into M13 vectors. *Methods Enzymol* 1983; 100: 468—500.

13 Itakura K, Rossi JJ, Wallace RB. Synthesis and use of synthetic oligonucleotides. *Annu Rev Biochem* 1984; 53: 323—56.

14 Botstein D, Shortle D. Strategies and applications of *in vitro* mutagenesis. *Science* 1985; 229: 1193—201.

15 Craik CS. Use of oligonucleotides for site-specific mutagenesis. *Biotechniques* 1985; 3: 12—19.

16 Messing J, Groneneborn B, Muller-Hill B, Hofschneider PH. Filamentous coliphage M13 as a cloning vehicle: insertion of a HindII fragment of the lac regulatory region in M13 replicative form *in vitro*. *Proc Natl Acad Sci USA* 1977; 74: 3642—6.

17 Wasylyk B, Derbyshire R, Guy A, Molko D, Roget A, Teoule R, Chambon P. Specific *in vitro* transcription of conalbumin gene is drastically decreased by single-point mutation in T-A-T-A box homology sequence. *Proc Natl Acad Sci USA* 1980; 77: 7024—8.

18 Hutchinson CA, Phillips S, Edgell MH, Gillam S, Jahnke P, Smith M. Mutagenesis at a specific position in a DNA sequence. *J Biol Chem* 1978; 253: 6551—60.

19 Razin A, Hirose T, Itakura K, Riggs AD. Efficient correction of a mutation by use of chemically synthesized DNA. *Proc Natl Acad Sci USA* 1978; 75: 4268—70.

20 Gillam S, Smith M. Site-specific mutagenesis using synthetic oligodeoxyribo-nucleotide primers: I. Optimum conditions and minimum oligodeoxyribo-nucleotidëlength. *Gene* 1979; 8: 81—97.

21 Taylor JW, Ott J, Eckstein F. The rapid generation of oligonucleotide-directed mutations at high frequency using phosphorothioate-modified DNA. *Nucleic Acids Res* 1985; 13: 8765—85.

22 Dagert M, Ehrlich SD. Prolonged incubation in calcium chloride improves the competence of *Escherichia coli* cells. *Gene* 1979; 6: 23—8.

23 Sanger F. Determination of nucleotide sequences in DNA. *Science* 1981; 214: 1205–10.

24 Sanger F, Coulson AR, Barrell BG, Smith AJH, Roe BA. Cloning in single-stranded bacteriophage as an aid to rapid DNA sequencing. *J Mol Biol* 1980; 143: 161–78.

25 Sanger F, Nicklen S, Coulson AR. DNA sequencing with chain-terminating inhibitors. *Proc Natl Acad Sci USA* 1977; 74: 5463–7.

26 Maxam AM, Gilbert W. A new method for sequencing DNA. *Proc Natl Acad Sci USA* 1977; 74: 560–4.

27 Gilbert W. DNA sequencing and gene structure. *Science* 1981; 214: 1305–12.

28 Osinga KA, Van der Bliek AM, Van der Horst G, Groot Koerkamp MJA, Tabak HF. *In vitro* site-directed mutagenesis with synthetic DNA oligonucleotides yields unexpected deletions and insertions at high frequency. *Nucleic Acids Res* 1983; 11: 8595–608.

29 Villafranca JE, Howell EE, Voet DH, Strobel MS, Ogden RC, Abelson JN, Kraut J. Directed mutagenesis of dihydrofolate reductase. *Science* 1983; 222: 782–8.

30 Beggs JD. Transformation of yeast by a replicating hybrid plasmid. *Nature* 1978; 275: 104–8.

31 Chevallier MR, Aigle M. Qualitative detection of penicillinase produced by yeast strains carrying chimeric yeast–coli plasmids. *FEBS Lett* 1979; 108: 179–80.

32 Travis J, Owen M, George P, Carrell R, Rosenberg S, Hallewell RA, Barr PJ. Isolation and properties of recombinant DNA produced variants of human α_1-proteinase inhibitor. *J Biol Chem* 1985; 260: 4384–9.

33 Rubin H, Wang Z, Nickbarg EB *et al*. Cloning, expression, purification and biological activity of recombinant native and variant human α_1-antichymotrypsins. *J Biol Chem* 1990; 265: 1199–207.

34 Schechter I, Berger A. On the size of the active site in proteases. 1. Papain. *Biochem Biophys Res Commun* 1967; 27: 157–62.

35 Carrell R, Travis J. α_1-Antitrypsin and the serpins: variation and countervariation. *Trends Biochem Sci* 1985; 10: 20–4.

36 Johnson D, Travis J. Structural evidence for methionine at the reactive site of human α-1-proteinase inhibitor. *J Biol Chem* 1978; 253: 7142–4.

37 Lewis JH, Iammarino RM, Spero JA, Hasiba U. Antithrombin Pittsburgh: an α_1-antitrypsin variant causing hemorrhagic disease. *Blood* 1978; 51: 129–37.

38 Owen MC, Brennan SO, Lewis JH, Carrell RW. Mutation of antitrypsin to antithrombin. α_1-Antitrypsin Pittsburgh (358 Met to Arg), a fatal bleeding disorder. *N Engl J Med* 1983; 309: 694–8.

39 Beatty K, Bieth J, Travis J. Kinetics of association of serine proteinases with native and oxidised α-1-proteinase inhibitor and α-1-antichymotrypsin. *J Biol Chem* 1980; 225: 3931–4.

40 Travis J, Matheson NR, George PM, Carrell RW. Kinetic studies on the interaction of α_1-proteinase inhibitor (Pittsburgh) with trypsin-like serine proteinases. *Biol Chem Hoppe-Seyler* 1986; 367: 853–9.

41 Scott CF, Carrell RW, Glaser CB, Kueppers F, Lewis JH, Colman RW. Alpha-1-antitrypsin-Pittsburgh. A potent inhibitor of human plasma factor XIa, kallikrein, and factor XIIf. *J Clin Invest* 1986; 77: 631–4.

42 Carp H, Miller F, Hoidal JR, Janoff A. Potential mechanism of emphysema: α_1-proteinase inhibitor recovered from lungs of cigarette smokers contains oxidised methionine and has decreased elastase inhibitory capacity. *Proc Natl Acad Sci USA* 1982; 79: 2041–5.

43 Rosenberg S, Barr PJ, Najarian RC, Hallewell RA. Synthesis in yeast of a functional oxidation-resistant mutant of human α_1-antitrypsin. *Nature* 1984; 312: 77–80.

44 George PM, Vissers MCM, Travis J, Winterbourne CC, Carrell RW. A genetically

engineered mutant of α_1-antitrypsin protects connective tissue from neutrophil damage and may be useful in lung disease. *Lancet* 1984; 1426−8.

45 Courtney M, Jallat S, Tessier LH, Benavente A, Crystal RG, LeCocq JP. Synthesis in *E. coli* of α_1-antitrypsin variants of therapeutic potential for emphysema and thrombosis. *Nature* 1985; 313: 149−51.

46 Janoff A, George-Nascimento C, Rosenberg S. A genetically engineered, mutant human alpha-1-proteinase inhibitor is more resistant than the normal inhibitor to oxidative inactivation by chemicals, enzymes, cells, and cigarette smoke. *Am Rev Respir Dis* 1986; 133: 353−6.

47 Jallat S, Carvallo D, Tessier LH *et al.* Altered specificities of genetically engineered α_1-antitrypsin variants. *Protein Eng* 1986; 1: 29−35.

48 Stephens AW, Siddiqui A, Hirs CHW. Site-directed mutagenesis of the reactive center (serine 394) of antithrombin III. *J Biol Chem* 1988; 263: 15 849−52.

49 Matheson N, Bathurst I, Travis J. The primary role of the P_1' residue (ser^{359}) of alpha-1-proteinase inhibitor. *Biochem Biophys Res Commun* 1989; 159: 271−7.

50 Matheson NR, Gibson HL, Hallewell RA, Barr PJ, Travis J. Recombinant DNA-derived forms of human α_1-proteinase inhibitor. Studies on the alanine 358 and cysteine 358 substituted mutants. *J Biol Chem* 1986; 261: 1040−9.

51 Eriksson S. Studies in α_1-antitrypsin deficiency. *Acta Med Scand* 1965; Suppl. 432: 1−85.

52 Sveger T. Liver disease in alpha$_1$-antitrypsin deficiency detected by screening of 200 000 infants. *N Engl J Med* 1976; 294: 1316−21.

53 Wewers MD, Casolaro MA, Sellers SE, Swayze SC, McPhaul KM, Wittes JT, Crystal RG. Replacement therapy for alpha$_1$-antitrypsin deficiency associated with emphysema. *N Engl J Med* 1987; 316: 1055−62.

54 Jeppsson JO. Amino acid substitution Glu to Lys in α_1-antitrypsin PiZ. *FEBS Lett* 1976; 65: 195−7.

55 Jeppsson JO, Larsson C, Eriksson S. Characterization of α_1-antitrypsin in the inclusion bodies from the liver in α_1-antitrypsin deficiency. *N Engl J Med* 1975; 293: 576−9.

56 Mornex JF, Chytil-Weir A, Martinet Y, Courtney M, LeCocq JP, Crystal RG. Expression of the alpha-1-antitrypsin gene in mononuclear phagocytes of normal and alpha-1-antitrypsin-deficient individuals. *J Clin Invest* 1986; 77: 1952−61.

57 Eriksson S, Carlson J, Velez R. Risk of cirrhosis and primary liver cancer in alpha$_1$-antitrypsin deficiency. *N Engl J Med* 1986; 314: 736−9.

58 Loebermann H, Tokuoka R, Deisenhofer J, Huber R. Human α_1-proteinase inhibitor. Crystal structure analysis of two crystal modifications, molecular model and preliminary analysis of the implications for function. *J. Mol. Biol.* 1984; 177: 531−56.

59 McCracken AA, Kruse KB, Brown JL. Molecular basis for defective secretion of the Z variant of human alpha-1-proteinase inhibitor: secretion of variants having altered potential for salt bridge formation between amino acids 290 and 342. *Mol Cell Biol* 1989; 9: 1406−14.

60 Foreman RC. Disruption of the Lys-290−Glu-342 salt bridge in human α_1-antitrypsin does not prevent its synthesis and secretion. *FEBS Lett* 1987; 216: 79−82.

61 Sifers RN, Hardick CP, Woo SLC. Disruption of the 290−342 salt bridge is not responsible for the secretory defect of the PiZ α_1-antitrypsin variant. *J Biol Chem* 1989; 264: 2997−3001.

62 Brantly M, Courtney M, Crystal RG. Repair of the secretion defect in the Z form of α_1-antitrypsin by addition of a second mutation. *Science* 1988; 242: 1700−2.

63 Lomas DA, Evans DL, Finch JT, Carrell RW. The mechanism of Z α_1-antitrypsin accumulation in the liver. *Nature* 1992; 357: 605−7.

64 Lomas DA, Finch JT, Seyama K, Nukiwa T, Carrell RW. α_1-antitrypsin S_{iiyama} ($Ser^{53} \rightarrow$ Phe); further evidence for intracellular loop-sheet polymerisation. *J Biol Chem* 1993; 268: 15333−35.

65 Abdullah M, Siddiqui AA, Hill JA, Davies RJH. The purification of α_1-antichymotrypsin from human serum using DNA−cellulose chromatography. *Arch Biochem Biophys* 1983; 225: 306−12.

66 Tsuda M, Umezawa Y, Masuyama M, Nozaki SF, Yamaguchi K, Katsunuma T. Inhibition of DNA synthesis by α_1-antichymotrypsin. *Tokai J Exp Clin Med* 1988; 13: 329−36.

67 Takada S, Tsuda M, Matsumoto M, Fujinami S, Yamamura M, Katsunuma T. Incorporation of alpha-1-antichymotrypsin into human stomach adenocarcinoma cell nuclei and inhibition of DNA primase activity. *Tokai J Exp Clin Med* 1988; 13: 321−7.

68 Baumann U, Huber R, Bode W, Grosse D, Lesjak M. Crystal structure of cleaved human α_1-antichymotrypsin at 2.7 Å resolution and its comparison with other serpins. *J Mol Biol* 1991; 218: 595−606.

69 Gadek JE, Klein HG, Holland PV, Crystal RG. Replacement therapy of alpha-1-antitrypsin deficiency. Reversal of protease−antiprotease imbalance within the alveolar structures of PiZ subjects. *J Clin Invest* 1981; 68: 1158−65.

70 Gadek JE, Fells GA, Crystal RG. Cigarette smoking induces functional antiprotease deficiency in the lower respiratory tract of humans. *Science* 1979; 206: 1315−16.

71 Colman RW, Flores DN, De La Cadena RA *et al*. Recombinant α_1-antitrypsin Pittsburgh attenuates experimental gram-negative septicemia. *Am J Pathol* 1988; 130: 418−26.

72 Janoff A, Carp H, Lee DK, Drew RT. Cigarette smoke inhalation decreases α_1-antitrypsin activity in rat lung. *Science* 1979; 206: 1313−14.

73 George PM, Pemberton P, Bathurst IC *et al*. Characterization of antithrombins produced by active site mutagenesis of human α_1-antitrypsin expressed in yeast. *Blood* 1989; 73: 490−6.

74 Avron A, Reeve FH, Lickorish JM, Carrell RW. Effect of alanine insertion (P'5) on the reactive centre of α_1-antitrypsin. *FEBS Lett* 1991; 280: 41−3.

75 Cohen AB. The clinical usefulness of different forms of alpha-1-protease inhibitor. *Am Rev Respir Dis* 1986; 133: 349−50.

7 Tissue specificity

KEVIN MORGAN AND NOOR A. KALSHEKER

Introduction

Eukaryotic gene expression is a highly regulated process as exemplified by the ordered and programmed development of different tissues from a single cell precursor. Clearly, the factors that determine gene regulation are important. This chapter will discuss some of the processes involved in regulating tissue-specific gene expression using the α_1-antitrypsin (AAT) gene to illustrate some of these mechanisms. Regulation of gene expression can take place at two stages:

1 Primary control occurs at the transcriptional level due to interaction of regulatory proteins with specific DNA sequences. Activation of a gene requires binding of a protein factor to its promoter together with the interaction of defined regulatory proteins (*trans*-activating factors) with specific DNA recognition sequences (*cis*-elements) adjacent to the gene.

2 Further control occurs at the post-transcriptional level due to alternative RNA splicing.

We will initially describe this latter process briefly and then discuss the first in greater detail.

Post-transcriptional regulation

The majority of mammalian genes consist of alternating exons (protein coding sequence) and introns (non-coding sequence), which must be removed before a gene can be translated. They are present in the primary transcript but removed by the process of RNA splicing to yield a mature messenger RNA (mRNA) product (see Chapter 1). Consensus base sequences are found at intron/exon boundaries and are recognized by small nuclear ribonucleoprotein particles (snRNPs), which together with other proteins constitute the spliceosome complex responsible for the removal of non-coding introns and the contiguous assembly of the exons [1]. There may be variation in the number of exons assembled giving rise to the phenomenon of alternative splicing. This permits different tissues to generate more than one mRNA from a single gene. An example of this is described for the α_1-antitrypsin gene.

104

Alternative splicing at the 5′ end of the α₁-antitrypsin gene

Full-length α_1-antitrypsin complementary DNA (cDNA), prepared from liver mRNA, contains 1434 base pairs (bp) consisting of 49 bp of 5′ untranslated sequence, 1254 bp of coding region and a further 79 bp of 3′ non-coding sequence as well as a poly(A) tail after the stop codon [2]. The gene is composed of seven exons separated by six introns [3], and there are two promoter regions, one for hepatocytes (Ph) and one for monocytes/macrophages (Pm) (Fig. 7.1). The major site of α_1-antitrypsin gene expression is the liver [4], but small amounts (about 1% of that produced by hepatocytes) are also synthesized by monocytes [5]. The two promoters are mutually exclusive: the monocyte promoter does not function in hepatocytes and vice versa [3]. This suggests the presence of *trans*-activating transcription factors that activate the process in a tissue-specific manner. The mRNA produced by monocytes differs from hepatocyte mRNA in that it contains additional exons and is present as two distinct mRNA species (Fig. 7.1).

In the hepatocyte, transcription starts in the middle of exon 1C to produce 1.4 kilobases (kb) RNA. On the other hand, monocyte transcription begins 2 kb upstream of the hepatocyte promoter and the

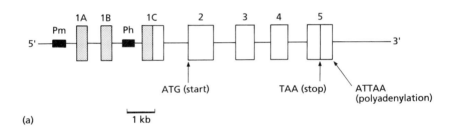

(a)

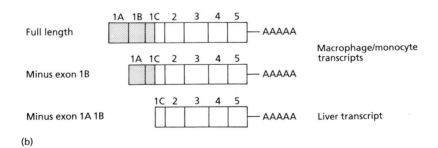

(b)

Fig. 7.1 (a) Structure of the α_1-antitrypsin gene. The coding sequences (exons) are represented by boxes and the intervening sequences (introns) by lines. Pm and Ph represent the monocyte- and hepatocyte-specific promoters. (b) The mRNA species of monocytes and hepatocytes (alternative transcripts) are shown below. Two monocyte mRNA species are shown; exon 1B may or may not be present. A,T,G — nucleotide bases adenine, thymine, guanine. The shaded areas represent the segments of exon 1 that are alternatively spliced.

transcript includes exon 1A (207 bp), exon 1B (209 bp) and all of 1C (101 bp), and alternative splicing results in the removal of exon 1B. Both monocyte transcripts are present under basal conditions but the smaller form predominates after stimulation with cytokines [6, 7]. Exons 1A and 1B contain non-coding sequences so they are transcribed but not translated; consequently, the α_1-antitrypsin protein arising from all transcripts is probably identical. The additional exons could well influence the rate of α_1-antitrypsin synthesis since the presence of 5' untranslated mRNA reduces translational efficiency. This is also observed with the mouse α-amylase gene where there are two independent promoters in the salivary gland and the liver. Expression of amylase protein varies almost 100-fold in the tissues and the only difference in the mRNA species is in the length of the 5' untranslated region suggesting that this region may have a profound effect on expression [8].

As well as the monocyte transcripts having extra exons, within these exons are additional short open reading frames; one in exon 1B and the other at the beginning of exon 1C before it joins the first liver-specific exon. These start sites are 37 bp apart [3]. Similar situations exist in other genes including the human [9] and chicken oestrogen receptors [10], the human transferrin receptor [11] and the yeast regulatory protein GCN4 [12]. In the latter case there is convincing evidence to suggest that the short upstream open reading frames are essential for translational repression [12]. It can be envisaged that if α_1-antitrypsin translation is initiated in exon 1B/C there may be competition with the recognized site in exon II which would ultimately influence the rate of synthesis of the mature protein.

Alternative splicing at the 3' end of genes

After the primary transcript has been produced it is capped at the 5' end (7-methylguanosine) and rapidly cleaved at a point downstream of the protein-coding sequence where the poly(A) tail is added. In many genes the process of cleavage and polyadenylation can occur at varying positions within the primary transcript in different tissues resulting in alternative mRNA species (and hence expressed protein), which can then be differentially spliced. Examples of alternative 3' splicing include the synthesis of membrane-bound and secretory forms of immunoglobulin M [13, 14] and calcitonin and calcitonin gene-related peptide (CGRP) [15].

The best understood example is seen in the genes that code for the immunoglobulin heavy chain of the antibody molecule which plays an important role in the regulation of the immune response. Early in the immune response binding of antigen to membrane-bound immunoglobulin receptors triggers B-cell proliferation and produces more antibody-producing cells. These cells secrete immunoglobulin which interacts with antigen and activates other cells of the immune system.

The production of membrane-bound and secreted forms of immunoglobulin is controlled by alternative splicing of different RNA molecules which differ in their 3' ends. The larger of the two messages produced contains two exons which code for the part of the molecule that anchors it in the membrane. When this molecule is spliced these two exons are included but the region coding for the last 20 amino acids of the secreted form is excluded. In the shorter message the two exons encoding the membrane anchor are absent and the region specific for the secreted form is included. This choice of splicing pattern is dependent on which polyadenylation site is used; deletion of the upstream site results in use of the downstream one and increased message for the membrane-bound form. With α_1-antitrypsin the primary regulatory event is differential promoter usage whereas with immunoglobulin it is the site of cleavage and polyadenylation.

Another type of alternative 3' splicing is seen with the gene encoding the calcium-regulating protein, calcitonin [15]. When the gene coding for calcitonin was isolated it was discovered that it also had the potential to produce message for an entirely different peptide, CGRP. Calcitonin is produced by the thyroid gland whereas CGRP is present in the hypothalamus. These two peptides are produced by alternative splicing of two distinct transcripts, which differ in their 3' ends. However, this case is different from that seen with immunoglobulin M in that deletion of the polyadenylation site used for the shorter calcitonin messages does not result in an increase of CGRP expression in these cells. Instead large unspliced transcripts utilizing the downstream (CGRP) polyadenylation site accumulate. In CGRP-producing cells such transcripts could normally be spliced to yield CGRP mRNA but this does not happen in calcitonin-producing cells and the unspliced precursors accumulate. With the calcitonin−CGRP gene the use of different polyadenylation sites is secondary to the differential RNA splicing. This suggests the existence of tissue-specific splicing factors whose presence or absence regulates the splicing pattern [16]. In the rat skeletal muscle troponin T gene alternative splicing of four combinational exons (exons 4−8) and two mutually exclusive exons (exons 16 and 17) can result in up to 64 distinct mRNAs depending on muscle cell type [17].

The amount of protein a given message produces will depend on its stability in the cytoplasm once it leaves the nucleus. If it is rapidly degraded it will only produce low levels of protein. If a regulatory signal alters the stability of mRNA then it provides an effective means of gene regulation. The mRNA for the milk protein casein has a half-life of 1 h in untreated mammary gland cells. However, when stimulated with prolactin the half-life increases to over 40 h and this results in accumulation of casein mRNA with a concomitant rise in protein levels in response to the hormone [18]. The sequences involved in the regulation of degradation of specific mRNA species have been localized to the 3' untranslated region [19, 20]. These sequences have the potential to form secondary stem—loop structures, which are more stable, and this folding may occur in response to a specific signal [19]. As with alternative RNA processing, cases where RNA stability is regulated represent adaptation to the requirements of a particular situation, i.e. the need to generate two closely related proteins from one gene or to respond rapidly to some form of stimulation.

Transcriptional regulation

The section above describes briefly how post-translational events can influence gene expression. However, regulation of gene expression occurs primarily at the level of transcription. Prior to the onset of transcription various changes must occur in the chromatin structure of genes.

In eukaryotic cells DNA is tightly complexed with proteins (histones) to form nucleosomes, which then fold on themselves to form a more compact solenoid structure (chromatin) [21, 22]. This structure must be modified in order to expose sites to which regulatory proteins can readily gain access and bind before transcription can take place [23]. Another change that occurs in DNA associated with active or potentially active genes is methylation, the most common base being 5-methylcytosine [24]. A number of genes exhibit a tissue-specific methylation pattern being unmethylated in tissues where the gene is active and methylated in other tissues [25]; there is some evidence (from the chicken globin gene) that *trans*-acting factors may not bind to the gene in tissues where it is methylated [26].

It is clear that a number of changes occur in the chromatin structure of genes during the process of activation and commitment to tissue specificity. These changes include modification of the DNA itself (under-methylation) and to the way the DNA is packaged. The way in which tissues respond differently to inducers of gene expression is probably due to the fact that in one tissue certain genes will be inaccessible within the solenoid to bind factors necessary for activation. In other genes, which are more accessible due to a relaxed structure, binding of factors to defined sequences will occur. In turn, this will allow other regulatory proteins to interact with their specific DNA recognition sequences and cause transcription to proceed.

DNA recognition sequences (*cis*-elements) and regulatory proteins (*trans*-factors)

Promoters

Eukaryotic mRNA is transcribed by RNA polymerase II which has a specific recognition DNA sequence, referred to as the promoter, located upstream from the initiation codon (see Chapter 1). Each promoter contains characteristic sets of short conserved sequences that are recognized by appropriate transcription factors and/or RNA polymerase and are modular in design [27]. These *cis*-acting sites are normally within 100 bp upstream of the start site; the sequence between them is probably not important but the distance is. Some of these modules and the factors that recognize them are common, i.e. they are found in constitutive promoters, whereas others are tissue-specific and their use is regulated. Transcription factors bind to the promoter sequence elements to form a complex in which protein−protein interactions are also important. RNA polymerase binds as part of this complex and initiation can then proceed.

Sequence components of the promoter are defined in that they are required for initiation and are located close to the start point. Another group of DNA sequences enhance transcription but these can be located a long way (up to several thousand base pairs) from the start site, either upstream or downstream of it, and in either orientation; these sequences constitute enhancer elements. Enhancers resemble promoters in that they consist of a variety of modular elements; they can be targets for tissue-specific or temporal regulation. It is becoming increasingly difficult to distinguish between promoters and enhancers on the basis of consensus sequences since some modules are common to both; the best definition remains an operational one. Table 7.1 lists some common consensus sequences and the factors which bind to them.

Most eukaryotic protein-coding genes (Fig. 7.2) contain the canonical TATA sequence in their promoters at about position -25 with the consensus being $TATA^T/_AA^T/_A$. A mutation or loss of any base in this consensus sequence effectively reduces transcription [29]. The transcription factor TFIID is a protein that binds to the TATA box and is the first stage in the assembly of the transcription complex. Two other proteins TFIIA then TFIIB become incorporated before RNA polymerase II is able to join the complex; finally, TFIIE joins to form the competent transcription unit. The sequence of the events described above is probably similar in all promoters that contain TATA sequences. These protein factors can be regarded as general transcription factors. Other common promoter DNA elements are the CAAT box and GC box. Studies in yeast promoters indicate that there are upstream activation sequences (UAS), which specifically bind protein and influence transcription. In higher eukaryotes the first recognized upstream sequence was CAAT (consensus sequence GGCCAATCT) which binds the protein nuclear factor 1 (NF1/CTF). It is often located at about -80 but can function at considerable distances from the start point and in either orientation. Mutations in the CAAT box influence transcription markedly and thus indicate that this sequence is important in determining the efficiency of the promoter [30]. Increasing numbers of eukaryotic promoters are being found that lack a TATA box but instead have multiple copies of the GC box (con-

Table 7.1 Some promoter and enhancer consensus sequences and the regulatory proteins which bind to them. For a more complete list see the article by Faisst and Mayer [28]

Module	Consensus	Factor	Promoter/ enhancer	Gene
TATA box	TATA$^T/_A$A$^T/_A$	TFIID	P	Many
CAAT box	GGCCAATCT	CTF/NFI	P	α, β-globulin, HSV, TK, c-*ras*, c-*myc*, albumin, etc.
GC box	GGGCGG	SP1	P	TK, dihydrofolate reductase, phosphoglycerate kinase, type II procollagen, etc.
AP1	TGTGTCA	AP1	E	SV40, α_1-antitrypsin, metallothionein-11A
AP2	CCCCAGGC	AP2	P/E	SV40, collagenase, human growth hormone
AP3	AGGGTG	AP3	E	SV40
AP4	GCTGTGG	AP4	E	SV40
Octamer	ATTTGCAT	OCT-1/OCT-2	P/E	Many including immunoglobulin, SV40
$_\kappa$B	GGGACTTTCC	NF$_\kappa$B/H2-TFI	P/E	Immunoglobulin
Core	TGTGG$^T/_A$$^T/_A$$^T/_A$TAG	EBP	E	Immunoglobulin, α_1-antitrypsin, antithrombin III, tyr aminotransferase
E	TTNNGCAAT	C/EBP	E	α_1-antitrypsin

sensus GGGCGG) located within 100 bp of the start site, which can also occur in either orientation. The GC box binds the transcription factor SP1 and appears to be a feature of 'housekeeping' genes, i.e. genes that are expressed in all cells.

The occurrence of a number of DNA sequence modules in the promoter region would argue for each of these modules having different roles. Indeed, the thymidine kinase (TK) promoter provides a good example (Fig. 7.3). Proceeding upstream from the initiation codon there is a TATA box, a GC box, a CAAT box and then a second GC box. The GC boxes are in opposite orientation and the CAAT box is reversed but nevertheless the promoter conveys directional information and tran-

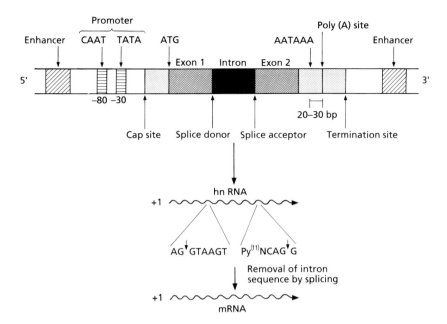

Fig. 7.2 Typical structure of a eukaryotic protein encoding gene. The promoter is located at the 5′ end while enhancers can be at the 5′ and/or 3′ end of the gene. Intronic (non-coding) sequence is removed by a splicing reaction; the splice site consensus sequences are shown together with the splice sites (↓).

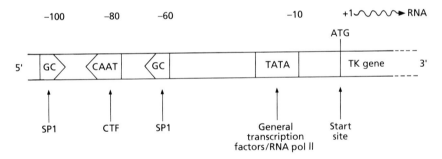

Fig. 7.3 Organization of *cis*-elements in the thymidine kinase promoter. Orientation of the conserved sequences is shown by arrows together with their corresponding transcription factors.

scription only proceeds in a downstream direction. The CAAT and GC boxes serve to bring the RNA polymerase into the general vicinity of the start site but do not actually align the enzyme; these upstream elements may make the initial contacts that start the assembly of the transcription complex at the promoter. Choice of the start point depends on the TATA box, it aligns RNA polymerase so that it starts at the right point; this explains why its location is fixed with respect to the initiation codon. None of these elements are uniquely essential for function since some promoters lack a TATA box and others have no CAAT box and/or

GC boxes. Promoters are constructed from the same sets of modules but they can differ in number, location and orientation to each other and essentially provide a specific isolated region for binding of RNA polymerase.

Enhancers

Eukaryotic promoters do not function alone; the activity of a promoter can be increased manyfold by the presence of an enhancer [31, 32]. Operationally, the promoter is best described as a sequence or sequences of DNA that must be in a relatively fixed location with regard to the start site. Thus, the TATA box, CAAT box and other upstream elements are included but the enhancer excluded, since this location is variable. Enhancers, like promoters, are modular in nature but a difference is that the modules can be contiguous rather than spaced apart. The same modules can be in promoters or enhancers (Table 7.1) and since in either case some are capable of operating in an orientation-independent manner, distinction between the two is becoming more difficult to make. Transcription factors recognize consensus sequences whether they are in promoters or enhancers.

Probably the best characterized eukaryotic transcriptional control sequence is the simian virus 40 (SV40) enhancer (Fig. 7.4). The SV40 enhancer is located at about 200 bp upstream of the start point and contains two identical 72 bp sequences repeated in tandem [33, 34]. The SV40 enhancer binds a number of proteins. AP1 binds to the right end, octamer-1 (OCT-1) binds to the octamer-like motif (ATGCAAAG) gen-

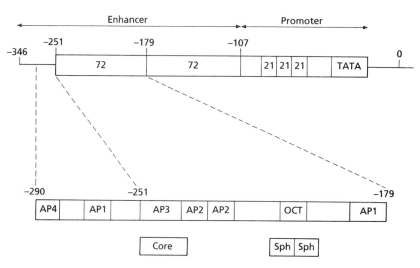

Fig. 7.4 SV40 regulatory region. The 72 bp (base pair) repeats of the enhancer and the 21 bp repeats of the promoter together with the TATA box are shown. O indicates the origin of replication. The lower portion depicts the modular organization of various motifs in the distal 72 bp enhancer repeat.

erated by the direct repeats of the Sph motif ($AAG^T/_CATGCA$), and AP2 and AP3 bind at the left end and together recognize a sequence over-lapping the core region. Another molecule of AP1 and AP4 binds to the left of the 72 bp repeat. Thus, the SV40 enhancer can be separated into two 72 bp halves; they function poorly individually but together constitute a very effective enhancer. In DNA constructs containing the β-globin gene and the 72 bp SV40 enhancer sequence the latter could activate correct initiation of transcription from heterologous promoters [35].

Tissue-specific enhancers

Many genes expressed in specific tissues also contain enhancers. These enhancers frequently exhibit tissue-specific activity; they only activate promoters in the tissue in which the gene is expressed and not in other tissues. It appears, therefore, that the situation resembles the characteristic of promoters in that some modules needed for enhancer function may be recognized by ubiquitous factors whereas others only respond to tissue-specific factors. Tissue-specific enhancers have been detected in genes expressed specifically in the liver (α-fetoprotein, albumin, $α_1$-antitrypsin), the cells of the pancreas (insulin, pancreatic elastase, pancreatic amylase), the pituitary gland (prolactin, growth hormone) and many other tissues. The tissue-specific activity of these enhancer elements plays a crucial role in the pattern of gene expression. In the case of the insulin gene, experiments linking various upstream elements of the gene to a marker gene identified a region 250 bp from the start point that was essential for high level expression in pancreatic endocrine cells [36]. This position corresponds exactly to the position of the tissue-specific enhancers [37]. Mutation of conserved sequences within the tissue-specific enhancers of the pancreatic elastase and chymotrypsin genes abolishes their tissue-specific pattern of expression [38] indicating the importance of this element in gene regulation. The binding of cell-type-specific proteins to the enhancer element has been demonstrated for many different enhancers, including those in the immunoglobulin [39] and insulin [40] genes. Promoters and enhancers can contain similar motifs and one particular motif which is present in both has been studied in detail. This is referred to as the octamer site.

Octamer site

The octamer motif is interesting in that it is an example of a consensus sequence that is found in both promoters and enhancers. It is present in the promoter for the immunoglobulin heavy and light chain [41] where it is required for lymphocyte-specific expression. As well as its presence in other promoters it is also found in the SV40 [42] and immunoglobulin heavy chain enhancers [43]. This suggests that similar protein−DNA and protein—protein interactions may be involved in both promoters and enhancers containing these elements. Once the motif has bound a protein factor it may be able to interact with other proteins of the transcriptional apparatus independent of whether its DNA-binding site lies within a promoter or enhancer, i.e. the modules function as 'scaffolding' on to which a complex of DNA-bound proteins that influence transcription can be built.

The octamer module is also recognized by more than one factor. A ubiquitous octamer-binding factor (OCT-1) has been found in all mammalian cells analysed so far [44, 45]. In lymphoid cells, a different factor, OCT-2, is present. Presumably, this latter factor can interact with the octamer motif in the heavy and light chain promoters and in the heavy chain enhancer; this would make OCT-2 a tissue-specific activator of more than one gene. A recent study has demonstrated that the octamer motif can be ubiquitous or cell-type specific depending on the binding affinity of the site and the octamer factor concentration [46]. The high affinity octamer site directs ubiquitous expression whereas those that behave in a B-cell-specific manner tend to have a weak octamer-binding site. Another example of important regulatory sequences is the response element which reacts to a specific signal, e.g. steroid response element.

Response elements

Groups of genes that are under common control share modules in their promoters and/or enhancers that are able to confer response to a specific stimulus. A number of response elements have been identified [47]. Some of these sequences are shown in Table 7.2. These modules are usually within 200 bp of the start point and act by binding specific transcription factors, which are synthesized or activated in response to the inducing signal. Steroid-inducible transcription is regulated by the hormone receptor complex, which binds to DNA via its respective response element. The responses to different hormones are mediated by distinct sequences that are related to each other (see Table 7.2). It is now believed that binding of the hormone to its receptor releases the receptor from a high molecular weight cytoplasmic protein (hsp90) allowing it to dimerize, move to the nucleus and bind to its DNA recognition sequence. As well as activating genes, steroid hormones are capable of inhibiting expression; this is achieved by binding of the receptor hormone complex, which activates steroid-inducible genes to a related but distinct negative response element. One gene can have more than one response element, thus allowing multiple patterns of regulation. Flexibility is provided by the presence of an element in one gene but not another, thus allowing one gene to respond to a particular stimulus while the other does not.

The elements shown in Table 7.2 are involved in the response of

Table 7.2 Response element sequences and their corresponding transcription factors

Module	Consensus	Factor	Stimulus
HSE	CNNGAANNTCCNNG	Heat shock transcription factor	Heat shock
CRE	$^T/_G{}^T/_A$CGTCA	CREB/ATF	Cyclic AMP
TRE	TGACTCA	AP1	Phorbol esters
GRE	TGGTACAAATGTTCT	Glucocorticoid, progesterone receptors	Glucocorticoid, progesterone
SRE	CCATATTAGG	Serum response factor	Serum growth factors
MRE	CGNCCCGGNCNC	Not known	Heavy metals
ORE	AGGTCANNNTGACCT	Oestrogen receptor	Oestrogen

genes to a particular regulatory agent. However, only a limited number of tissues will respond to a given stimulus. Some sequences present in promoters and enhancers, such as the B-cell-specific octamer motif (discussed previously) and DNA sequences which bind liver-specific transcription factors in the rat albumin and α_2-globulin genes, can also behave as response elements [48]. The behaviour of all of these sequences is determined by interaction with transcription factors.

Transcription factors

Transcription factors and other regulatory proteins must recognize specific sequences in promoters and enhancers and, once bound to DNA, either bind RNA polymerase or other factors for transcription to occur. Studies of eukaryotic transcription factors have identified several structural elements (Fig. 7.5), which either bind to DNA directly or which facilitate binding by adjacent regions of the protein molecule [49, 50].

Helix–turn–helix motif (Fig. 7.5a)

The realization that some gene products of the fruit-fly *Drosophila* were important in the regulation of development and specifically bound DNA led to studies to identify the protein structures responsible. Sequence analysis identified a 180 bp region of homology (encoding 60 amino acids), which was named the homeobox or homeodomain [51, 52], in all these genes indicating a potentially crucial role. Structural predictions of the 60 amino acid region revealed that it contained a highly conserved helix–turn–helix motif. In this structure a short region which can form an α-helix is followed by a β-turn and then another α-helix. X-Ray crystallographic studies show that one helix lies across the DNA major

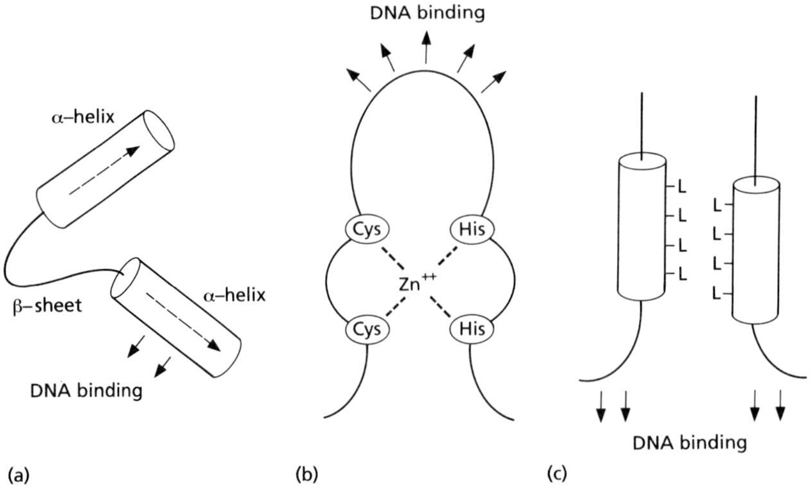

Fig. 7.5 Transcription factor motifs. (a) Helix—turn—helix; (b) zinc finger; and (c) leucine zipper.

groove while the second helix (recognition helix) lies partly within the major groove where it can make specific contact with DNA bases [49]. Subtle differences in the precise sequence of the helix—turn—helix motif in different homeoboxes can control the DNA sequence to which these proteins bind [53].

The obvious importance of the homeobox in *Drosophila* and yeast prompted a search for similar proteins in other organisms and these have been identified in *Xenopus* and mammals [54]. However, another class of regulatory proteins has been identified which contains the homeobox as part of a 160 amino acid conserved region known as the POU domain [55, 56]. These regulatory proteins were characterized as transcription factors having a particular pattern of activity. When the genes encoding mammalian OCT-1 and OCT-2 were cloned they were found to contain a stretch of 160 amino acids that was also present in Pit-1 (a transcription factor that functions on prolactin and growth hormone genes in the pituitary) and nematode UNC-86 (involved in neuroblast development). This POU (*Pit—Oct—Unc*) domain contains both a homeobox-like sequence and a second conserved POU-specific domain, which forms numerous α-helices as opposed to a typical helix—turn—helix motif.

Zinc finger motif (Fig. 7.5b)

This motif was first characterized in transcription factor TFIIIA, which binds to the promoter of the gene encoding for 5S RNA that utilizes RNA polymerase III. Pure TFIIIA has a periodic 30 amino acid repeated structure (nine repeats) and each molecule is associated with seven to

11 zinc atoms [57]. The consensus sequence of a zinc finger is $Cys-X_{2/4}-$ $Cys-X_3-Phe-X_5-Leu-X_2-His-X_3-His$ (where X represents any other amino acid). The motif takes its name from the loop of 12 amino acids that projects from the surface of the protein and is anchored at its base by the conserved Cys and His residues, which coordinate a zinc atom. Each zinc finger binds in the major groove of the DNA helix and interacts with half a helical turn (five bases) with successive fingers binding on opposite sides of the helix [58]. Three contiguous copies of the 30 amino acid zinc finger motif are found in transcription factor SP1. As well as zinc finger proteins of the Cys−His type another class has been found and designated Cys−Cys; these have the zinc-binding consensus sequence $Cys-X_2-Cys-X_{13}-Cys-X_2-Cys-X_{15/17}-Cys-X_5-$ $Cys-X_9-Cys-X_2-Cys-X_4-Cys$ [59]. Among the proteins with such structures are the steroid hormone and thyroid hormone receptors. However, unlike Cys−His fingers which are present in multiple copies, the Cys domain of steroid receptors is present only once in each receptor but is capable of making a pair of fingers.

Leucine zippers (Fig. 7.5c)

Leucine zippers consist of a stretch of amino acids with a leucine residue every seventh position. A leucine zipper in one polypeptide may interact with one in another polypeptide and dimerize. Adjacent to each zipper is a stretch of positively charged residues that are involved in DNA binding [60]. The leucine zipper has been identified in the transcription factor C/EBP where it was noted that in a stretch of 35 amino acids every seventh was a leucine [61]. Similar runs of leucine residues have been found in AP1, the yeast regulatory protein GCN4 and the proto-oncogenes Myc, Fos and Jun. The ability of the leucine zipper to dimerize allows for the possible formation of heterodimers (two different factors) as well as homodimers. Indeed, this is observed with the oncoproteins Fos and Jun. Jun binds as a homodimer to the AP1 recognition sequence to confer inducibility by phorbol esters. Fos cannot bind to DNA but forms a heterodimer with Jun, which then binds to the AP1 site with greater affinity than the Jun homodimer [62, 63]. The ability of leucine zippers to form dimeric complexes between different transcription factors introduces further versatility in the regulation of gene expression.

Regulation of α_1-antitrypsin gene expression

α_1-Antitrypsin is an acute phase protein and plasma concentrations increase three- to fourfold during inflammation or as a result of tissue injury. α_1-Antitrypsin gene expression in hepatoma cells is controlled by a combination of 5′ and 3′ regulatory sequences and *trans*-acting nuclear proteins (Fig. 7.6). Basal concentrations are probably maintained by the

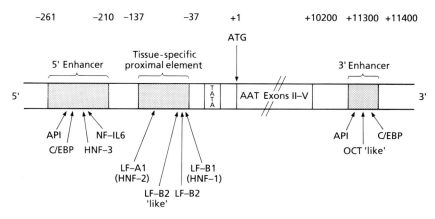

Fig. 7.6 Organization of *cis*-acting DNA elements and the *trans*-acting proteins which bind to them, responsible for regulating expression of the α_1-antitrypsin gene in the liver. A more detailed description of the interactions is provided in the text.

promoter and neighbouring sequences whereas the response during inflammation more than likely involves the use of enhancer elements. The TATA box is located at nucleotide position -25 to -20 but no homology for an upstream CAAT consensus has been found [64]. There is a GC-rich sequence at -402 to -398 [65], which could be a potential binding site for SP1. However, this region is too far removed from the start site to be considered part of a classical promoter module.

The region 300 bp upstream from the transcription start site contains two elements essential for transcription. A proximal element located at -137 to -37 appears to direct high level tissue-specific expression [66]; this region is capable of activating other promoters in hepatic cells [64, 65, 67] and mutational analysis has shown that it has two domains. Hepatocyte nuclear factor 1 (HNF-1/LF-B1), isolated from rat liver nuclei, binds across a region (-80 to -61) in one domain of the proximal element [66, 68]. This consensus site (GTTAATNATTAAC) is also found in a number of other genes expressed in the liver [69]. Part of this element also operates as a tissue-specific repressor in non-hepatic cells [70] possibly involving an LF-B2-like factor. Another protein(s) (HNF-2/LFA1) binds to a site (-125 to -100) in the second domain of the proximal element [66, 71]. These transcription factors are believed to be tissue-specific and as such are not found at comparable levels in HeLa, brain or spleen cells.

A second distal enhancer element is located between nucleotides -261 and -210 that is capable of activating transcription but not in a tissue-specific manner. This element contains sequences that are found in other plasma protein gene regulatory regions. At the centre of this region there is a sequence similar to the core enhancer (GTGGTTTC) [65] flanked on one side by an AP1 site and on the other by 11 bp identical to that flanking the haptoglobin gene [72]. Within this region there are also sites for other hepatocyte nuclear factors (HNF-3 and HNF-4) as well as another liver nuclear protein (C/EBP) [73, 74].

Another enhancer element has been found in the 3' flanking sequence located between 1.2 and 1.3 kb from the end of α_1-antitrypsin exon V ([75] and unpublished observations). Within these 100 bp there is an AP1 site, an octamer-like motif, and an overlapping region which shows remarkable similarity to the core enhancer and C/EBP binding site. Thus, there is an enhancer element at the 3' end of the gene that contains some of the modules seen in the 5' distal enhancer element.

The α_1-antitrypsin acute phase response is regulated by cytokines such as interleukin-6 (IL-6). NF-IL-6 (a nuclear factor from glioblastoma cells that activates IL-6 expression) shows sequence homology to hepatocyte C/EBP; both proteins have a leucine zipper motif and recognize similar DNA consensus sequences. Sequence comparisons show that in α_1-antitrypsin and other acute phase genes, the NF-IL-6, C/EBP and IL-6 response elements are either identical or overlapping [74, 76, 77]. A proposed model for the regulation of α_1-antitrypsin gene expression in the basal state involves competition for binding at the C/EBP enhancer elements, C/EBP is then displaced by IL-6 factors to up-regulate the gene [72].

Promoter and enhancer interactions

In order to understand regulation of gene expression we must have some understanding of: (1) the way signals are integrated between modules in promoter and enhancer elements; and (2) how signals are transmitted between promoters and enhancers when they are located apart from each other.

To carry out their functions, the proteins that bind to consensus sequences within a promoter/enhancer element must be able to interact with each other or with additional components of the transcriptional apparatus. In much the same way that cooperative interactions occur in multisubunit enzymes one can imagine that an interaction at one protein-binding site might confer to other proteins the ability to bind cooperatively at adjacent sites. This has been shown to occur for binding to modules in the SV40 enhancer [78] and the stromelysin promoter [79]. Cooperative, multiple interactions between proteins and between protein and DNA ensure that the overall specificity of the transcription complex is high even if some of the individual interactions are of low specificity. If factors were to bind too tightly they would be difficult to displace, and hence would regulate and also interfere with the use of a combination of factors. Thus, large cooperatively interacting complexes give rise to greater flexibility of control [80]. However, this type of interaction cannot explain what happens when the modules are separated by distances too large and variable to be able to accommodate direct contact between bound proteins. Transcription factors located apart within an element may be brought into direct contact by bending of the DNA. If DNA bending does occur then it must be induced by the bound proteins since the distance between adjacent modules (20−50 bp) is too small for spontaneous 'looping out' of DNA to occur. Also, the DNA must be aligned to allow the proteins to come together and not move apart. Alternatively, the proteins could interact via a separate integrator molecule [27]. This type of interaction would be favoured when multiple recognition sites in close proximity to each other allowed many protein factors to bind to adjacent sites and assembled a protein surface to which the integrator molecule could bind. It is not known whether a component such as the integrator molecule exists. However, the HSV protein VP16 provides an example of a protein that contains an activation domain but cannot bind directly to DNA. In this instance VP16 forms a complex with the octamer-binding protein, OCT-1, which provides the DNA-binding site; hence DNA-binding and activation motifs are located on separate molecules [81].

The mechanisms used to integrate signals within promoters and enhancers (over 100−200 bp) are distinct from those used to integrate signals between promoters and enhancers located some distance apart (up to several kilobases). The most attractive model for long-range signalling involves looping out of the DNA between the two regions [82, 83]. This model proposes that enhancer-driven promoter activation is a consequence of direct protein−protein interaction between the proteins bound at the end of these regions accompanied by 'looping out' of the intervening DNA sequence (Fig. 7.7). If this is the case then there

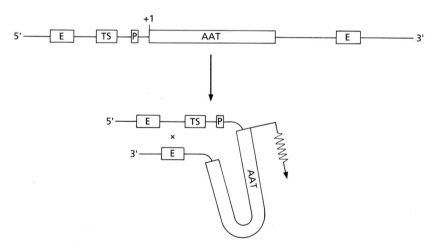

Fig. 7.7 Possible alignment of enhancer/promoter regions of the α_1-antitrypsin gene during activation according to the DNA 'looping' model. P represents the promoter, E the enhancers and TS the tissue-specific proximal element. X indicates the proposed site for protein−protein interactions, which induce 'looping out' of the gene sequence.

must be regions within the proteins which induce protein–protein contact (activator regions). Like the interactions that occur within modules this type of interaction could also be cooperative with the presence of a protein at one DNA element increasing the concentration of a second protein near its binding site [84]. A recent modification of this model [85] proposes an allosteric mechanism of enhancer action whereby different conformations of the binding proteins exist with masked and unmasked activator regions.

Collectively, all of the above interactions will give rise to a stabilized transcription complex capable of being regulated in response to diverse intracellular signals. In some instances the behaviour of the region can be predicted from the properties of its component parts but more complicated, interactive patterns of control are likely.

Experimental approaches

Identification of DNA regions that bind regulatory proteins

As discussed above, control of gene expression involves the binding of proteins to specific sites in regulatory regions (promoters and enhancers) of the gene. If a certain DNA fragment is suspected as having a regulatory role, e.g. from its location and similarity of sequence to known consensus regions, then techniques are available to investigate whether that region of DNA binds proteins (mobility shift assay) and to identify the precise sequences to which they are binding (DNase I footprinting).

A sensitive method of identifying DNA-binding proteins is provided by the DNA mobility shift or gel retardation assay [86, 87]. A radioactively labelled DNA sequence (ideally 100–200 bp), whose binding properties are under investigation, is incubated with a nuclear [88] or whole cell [89] extract under conditions which allow DNA–protein complexes to form. HeLa cell nuclear extract provides a good source of ubiquitous regulatory proteins. The DNA–protein mixtures are then electrophoresed on a non-denaturing polyacrylamide gel (4%) and the position of radioactive DNA visualized by autoradiography. The assay relies on the principle that a fragment of DNA which has bound protein will migrate more slowly than unbound DNA. Thus, the free probe (unbound DNA) will migrate further whereas a DNA–protein complex will exhibit slower mobility (Fig. 7.8). However, the mobility shift assay is capable of detecting non-specific protein–DNA binding as well as specific interactions. To help overcome this problem the nuclear proteins are pre-incubated with either heterogeneous (e.g. *Escherichia coli*) or homogeneous (poly (dI-dC)) DNA prior to addition of labelled probe, which reduces the formation of non-specific high molecular weight aggregates [90]. The precise sequence specificity of binding can be investigated by performing competition experiments. In this instance a large molar excess (100 ×) of

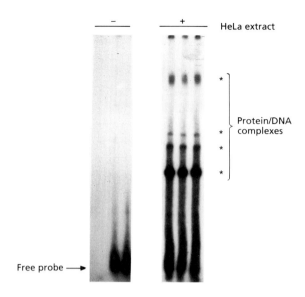

Fig. 7.8 Mobility shift assay using a 100 bp probe from the 3′ flanking sequence of the α_1-antitrypsin gene. The probe was incubated either in the presence (+) or absence (−) of HeLa nuclear protein extract. The faster moving probe is shown at the bottom of the gel (arrow) together with the protein−DNA complexes which exhibit reduced mobility (starred).

competitor DNA is included in the binding reaction. This competitor can be either unlabelled probe or, better still, synthetic oligonucleotide sequences which contain the binding sites for previously described transcription factors. If these competitor DNA sequences are capable of binding protein, since they are present in such excess, less will bind to the radiolabelled probe. Consequently, the retarded band seen on autoradiography will diminish or even disappear. By using specific oligonucleotides containing known consensus sequences it is possible to determine if the protein which binds is the same or closely related to known regulatory proteins.

While the gel retardation assay provides information about DNA−protein interaction it does not provide any detail of the region of DNA to which binding occurs; however, this can be achieved by using DNase I footprinting [91]. DNA and protein are permitted to bind as before except in this case the DNA fragment is labelled on only one strand of the double-stranded molecule. Using a radiolabelled oligonucleotide in the polymerase chain reaction provides a convenient means of generating fragments suitable for footprinting [92]. Ideally, the fragment needs to be 100−200 bp in length with the suspected site located towards the middle. After binding (similar buffer and conditions as used for the mobility shift assay can be employed) the DNA is digested with varying amounts of DNase I. The precise digestion conditions are obtained by titration so as to allow each molecule of DNA to be cut at only one site;

this is determined empirically and varies depending on the DNA fragment and the concentration of protein used in the binding reaction. Following digestion the bound protein is removed and the DNA fragments separated by electrophoresis on a 12% polyacrylamide denaturing gel, which is capable of resolving a single nucleotide. This results in a ladder of bands due to the DNase I cutting at single base pair intervals from the labelled end. Any region that has bound protein will be protected from digestion and the bands corresponding to this area will be absent and appear as a 'hole' on the gel (Fig. 7.9). The electrophoresis of a non-protein control (i.e. DNA fragment alone) with the products generated from a reaction where nuclear extract has been added, together with a DNA sequencing reaction, allows the precise sequence to which binding occurs to be identified. In some instances the bands at the boundaries of the recognition sites appear more intense; this hypersensitivity is due to changes in DNA structure, resulting from binding of protein, rendering the DNA more susceptible to cleavage. The specificity can be verified using unlabelled

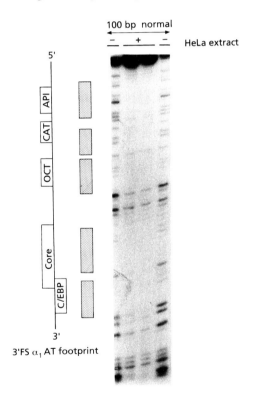

Fig. 7.9 DNase I footprinting of a 100 bp fragment from the 3′ flanking sequence of the α_1-antitrypsin gene. The 100 bp probe was generated by polymerase chain reaction, with one of the amplimers radiolabelled, and incubated either in the presence (+) or absence (−) of HeLa nuclear protein extract. DNase I digestion produces a ladder of fragments with 'holes' appearing at sites where proteins bind (shown by boxes); these match the potential regulatory sites identified by comparison with consensus sequences (shown on the left-hand side of the figure).

competitor sequences (as in the mobility shift assay) to see if it is possible to remove a particular footprint.

Isolation of the transcription factor

Once a region of DNA has been shown to bind a regulatory protein it is necessary to find out the nature of the factor. In some instances it can be identified by using competitor oligonucleotides specific for factors described previously. However, the factor may be binding to a unique sequence and if so there are a number of techniques which allow the factor to be characterized. Most binding studies are performed using crude extracts but ultimately these experiments need to be accompanied by studies with the pure protein itself.

Standard protein purification techniques, e.g. conventional chromatography and high performance liquid chromatography, do not yield transcription factors with a high degree of purity. However, the use of a DNA affinity column to which a DNA sequence containing multiple binding sites was linked to an activated Sepharose support proved to be very useful for the purification of the transcription factor SP1 [93]. Total cellular extract was applied to such a column permitting SP1 to bind specifically with its recognition site while other proteins were eluted. SP1 was harvested by increasing the buffer ionic strength to separate it from the DNA affinity column; two successive passages through this column resulted in 90% pure SP1. In this type of experiment addition of the correct amount of carrier DNA to remove non-specific binding proteins is critical. Too much will result in SP1 binding to the carrier, whereas too little will not absorb non-specific proteins which will thus bind to the column.

When purifying NF1 the majority of cellular protein and the material which bound non-specifically to *E. coli* DNA was removed before being applied to an NF1-binding column [94]. The progress of the factor through the purification protocol was monitored using the mobility shift assay. Since the abundance of transcription factors was so low these procedures only yielded small amounts of protein. However, from this approach it is possible to produce enough protein to determine molecular weight or to obtain some preliminary sequence data.

To isolate a gene coding for a particular protein factor a cDNA library is prepared from mRNA isolated from a cell type that expresses the protein [95]. The library must then be screened to identify a clone containing the gene of interest. If part of the protein sequence has been obtained, then oligonucleotide probes can be synthesized, which will code for the relevant region. However, due to the redundancy of codon usage (variable third base) a mixture of probes needs to be made. A stretch of six amino acids, i.e. 18 bp, is usually sufficient to isolate a unique sequence. The mixture of oligonucleotides is radiolabelled and used for screening; the clone containing the gene encoding the transcription factor will hybridize to the probe and can be identified by autoradiography. This approach has been used successfully to isolate the cDNA clones of purified factors such as SP1 [96], NF1 [97] and serum response factor [98].

Alternatively, if no purified protein is available, a cDNA expression library can be screened with a probe corresponding to the DNA recognition site for the protein [99]. Using this procedure the cDNAs coding for C/EBP [100] and OCT-1/OCT-2 [101, 102] have been isolated.

Functional assays

Transcriptional regulatory sequences can be detected by transfecting cells with a construct containing the fragment of DNA suspected of having a regulatory role together with a reporter gene, e.g. chloramphenicol acetyltransferase (CAT) or luciferase. Transfection systems allow exogenous DNA to be introduced into cells in culture. The recombinant plasmid can be transfected into a cell line by calcium phosphate−DNA coprecipitation or electroporation. Using this approach it is possible to assay genomic DNA fragments for enhancer or promoter activity [103]. A series of pCAT™ plasmids are commercially available (Promega Ltd, Delta House, Enterprise Road, Chilworth Research Centre, Southampton SO1 7NS, UK), which are specifically designed to test whether stretches of DNA have a regulatory role. The pCAT promoter plasmid contains the SV40 promoter and can be used when testing for putative enhancer elements, and the pCAT enhancer (SV40 enhancer) can be used for verification of promoter sequences. The putative regulatory sequences can be inserted in either orientation upstream or downstream of the reporter gene by use of multiple cloning sites. CAT activity is measured by the ability to acetylate chloramphenicol with radioactive ^{14}C. The effect of the regulatory sequence on CAT gene expression can therefore be monitored by liquid scintillation counting. Using CAT expression assays, enhancer elements have been identified in the human erythropoietin gene [104], the mouse cytokeratin Endo A gene [105] and the mouse immunoglobulin heavy chain locus [106]. The recent availability of luciferase as a reporter gene has increased the sensitivity almost 100-fold and this should prove useful when investigating the effects of weak enhancers or promoters.

Transgenic mice

Another approach which has met with some success when looking at the role of regulatory signals is the use of transgenic mice. This involves the introduction of foreign DNA sequences into the germ line cells of experimental mammals, usually mice, although sheep, rabbits and pigs have also been used. Cloned genes are injected into the pronucleus of a fertilized egg cell, which is then transplanted into a pseudopregnant foster mother [107]. The cloned segment (transgene) usually contains the gene of interest plus various promoter/enhancer elements and sequences important for tissue-specific gene expression. The transgene integrates into the recipients' genome early enough in development to transform both germ line and somatic cell lineages and is therefore transmitted on to the next generation. The copy number of the integrated sequence varies between one and several hundred in different transgenic animals and the chromosomal location is variable.

The transgenic approach has provided some useful insights into the way genes are regulated. Expression of the insulin gene is restricted to the β-cells of the pancreas and is regulated by *cis*-acting elements in the 5′ flanking region. A transgene was constructed consisting of the 5′ flanking region of the insulin gene joined to the coding region of the SV40 oncogene and introduced into mouse embryos. The oncogene product was produced exclusively in the pancreatic cells of the mice resulting in the formation of insulinomas demonstrating that the insulin gene regulatory signals dictate tissue-specific expression [108]. Other experiments have been performed in which the mouse metallothionein-1 gene promoter, which is induced by heavy metals, and other upstream elements have been fused to different coding sequences. Linkage to the SV40 thymidine kinase gene resulted in thymidine kinase activity that could be induced by heavy metals [109]. Construction of a hybrid gene with the promoter attached to rat growth hormone genomic DNA produced a transgenic mouse that demonstrated accelerated growth when placed on a zinc diet [110]. Similar experiments repeated with the human growth hormone gene showed that the synthesis of growth hormone was inducible by heavy metals [111].

The similarities between tissue distribution of these transgenes and normal expression gave rise to the hope that transgenic mice would provide a general assay for functionally dissecting DNA sequences responsible for tissue-specific/developmental regulation of genes. Transgenic mice which have incorporated the chicken transferrin gene (active in the liver) retain tissue-specific regulation. The cloned gene, together with 5′ and 3′ flanking sequences, was injected into fertilized eggs; the resulting transgenic mice expressed chicken transferrin mRNA in several tissues but it was highest in the liver [112]. However, incorporation of a cloned rabbit β-globin gene has resulted in abnormal expression [113] with no β-globin mRNA detectable in mouse erythroid cells in any of the transgenic lines examined. It has been suggested that these inappropriate patterns of expression are due to integration at abnormal chromosome positions [114]. More encouraging results have been obtained with the mouse immunoglobulin K gene. In this instance, high expression was restricted to B lymphocytes, suggesting that the microinjected gene contained gene activation target sequences specific for B lymphocytes, which were functionally independent of integration site [115]. Fusion of the milk protein gene (β-lactoglobulin) to the α_1-antitrypsin gene (including the 3' enhancer region) resulted in high level expression of biologically active human α_1-antitrypsin in the milk of transgenic mice [116]. Because of the labour intensiveness of transgene experiments, these are often restricted to highly specialized centres.

Clearly, there is an array of techniques available to the investigator wishing to characterize gene regulatory sequences. These range from the relatively simple gel mobility assay to the more complex use of transgenic animals. Over the past few years our understanding of how different factors interact with DNA has improved, but little is understood about the way in which the factors interact with each other once they are bound to the DNA. Future research should help unravel these interactions and lead to an understanding of the way in which highly complex processes such as tissue-specific expression and ultimately mammalian development are controlled.

References

1 Maniatis T, Reed R. The role of small ribonucleoprotein particles in pre-mRNA splicing. *Nature* 1987; 35: 673−8.

2 Long GL, Chandra T, Woo SLC, Davie EW, Kurachi K. Complete sequence of the cDNA for human α_1-antitrypsin and the gene for the S variant. *Biochemistry* 1984; 23: 4828−37.

3 Perlino E, Cortese R, Ciliberto G. The human α_1-antitrypsin gene is transcribed from two different promoters in macrophages and hepatocytes. *EMBO J* 1987; 6: 2767−71.

4 Carrell RW, Jeppsson JD, Laurell CB, Brennan SO, Owen MC, Vaughan L, Boswell DR. Structure and variation of human α_1-antitrypsin. *Nature* 1982; 298: 329−34.

5 Mornex JF, Chytil-Weir A, Martinet Y, Courtney M, LeCocq JP, Crystal RG. Expression of the alpha-1-antitrypsin gene in mononuclear phagocytes of normal and alpha-1-antitrypsin-deficient individuals. *J Clin Invest* 1986; 77: 1952−61.

6 Perlmutter DH, May LT, Sehgal PB. Interferon β2/interleukin 6 modulates synthesis of α_1-antitrypsin in human mononuclear phagocytes and in human hepatoma cells. *J Clin Invest* 1989; 84: 138−44.

7 Kalsheker N, Swanson T. Exclusion of an exon in monocyte alpha-1-antitrypsin mRNA after stimulation of U937 cells by interleukin-6. *Biochem Biophys Res Comm* 1990; 172: 1116−21.

8 Shaw P, Sordat B, Schibler U. The two promoters of the mouse alpha-amylase gene Amy-1a are differentially activated during parotid gland differentiation. *Cell* 1985; 40: 907−12.

9 Green S, Walker P, Kumar V, Krust A, Bornet JM, Argos P, Chambon P. Human oestrogen receptor cDNA: sequence, expression and homology to V-erb-A. *Nature* 1986; 320: 134−9.

10 Krust A, Green S, Argos P, Vijay K, Walter P, Bornet JM, Chambon P. The chicken oestrogen receptor sequence: homology with V-erb-A and the human oestrogen and glucocorticoid receptors. *EMBO J* 1986; 5: 891−7.

11 Schneider C, Williams JG. Molecular dissection of the human transferrin receptor. *J Cell Sci* 1985; 96 (Suppl 3): 139–49.

12 Mueller PP, Hinnebush AG. Multiple upstream AUG codons mediate translational control of GCN4. *Cell* 1986; 45: 201–7.

13 Sitia R, Neuberger MS, Milstein C. Regulation of membrane IgM expression in secretory B cells: translational and post-translational events. *EMBO J* 1989; 6: 3969–77.

14 Danner D, Leder P. Role of an RNA cleavage/poly (A) addition site in the production of membrane bound and secreted IgM mRNA. *Proc Natl Acad Sci USA* 1985; 82: 8658–62.

15 Rosenfeld MG, Amara SG, Evans PM. Alternative RNA processing: determining neuronal phenotype. *Science* 1984; 225: 1315–20.

16 Emerson RB, Hedjran F, Yeakley JM, Guise JW, Rosenfeld MG. Alternative production of calcitonin and CGRP mRNA is regulated at the calcitonin-specific splice acceptor. *Nature* 1989; 341: 76–80.

17 Breitbart RE, Andreadis A, Nadal-Ginard B. Alternative splicing: a ubiquitous mechanism for the generation of multiple protein isoforms from different genes. *Annu Rev Biochem* 1987; 56: 467–95.

18 Guyette WA, Matusick RA, Rosen JM. Prolactin-mediated transcriptional and post-transcriptional control of casein gene expression. *Cell* 1979; 17: 1013–23.

19 Mullner EW, Kuhn LC. A stem-loop in the 3' untranslated region mediates iron-dependent regulation of transferrin receptor mRNA stability in the cytoplasm. *Cell* 1988; 53: 815–25.

20 Shaw G, Kamen R. A conserved AU sequence from the 3' untranslated region of GM-CSF mRNA mediates selective mRNA degradation. *Cell* 1986; 46: 659–67.

21 Kornberg RD, Klug A. The nucleosome. *Sci Am* 1981; 244: 48–64.

22 Morse RH, Simpson RT. DNA in the nucleosome. *Cell* 1988; 54: 285–7.

23 McKnight SL, Bustin M, Miller OL. Electron microscope analysis of chromosome metabolism in the *Drosophila melanogaster* embryo. *Cold Spring Harbor Symp Quant Biol* 1978; 42: 741–54.

24 Razin A, Riggs AD. DNA methylation and gene function. *Science* 1980; 210: 604–10.

25 Ceder H. DNA methylation and gene activity. *Cell* 1988; 53: 3–4.

26 Becker PB, Ruppert S, Schutz G. Genomic fingerprinting reveals cell type-specific binding of ubiquitous factors. *Cell* 1987; 51: 435–43.

27 Dynan WS. Modularity in promoters and enhancers. *Cell* 1988; 58: 1–4.

28 Faisst S, Mayer S. Compilation of vertebrate-encoded transcription factors. *Nucleic Acids Research* 1992; 20: 3–26.

29 Breathnach R, Chambon P. Organisation and expression of eukaryotic split genes coding for proteins. *Annu Rev Biochem* 1981; 52: 441–66.

30 McKnight S, Tjian R. Transcriptional selectivity of viral genes in mammalian cells. *Cell* 1986; 46: 795–805.

31 Serfling E, Jasin M, Schaffner W. Enhancers and eukaryotic gene transcription. *Trends Genet* 1985; 1: 224–30.

32 Hatzopoulos AK, Schlokat U, Gruss P. Enhancers and other *cis*-acting sequences. In: Hanes BD, Glover DM, eds. *Transcription and Splicing*. Oxford: IRL Press, 1988: 43–96.

33 Zenke M, Grundstrom T, Matthes H *et al.* Multiple sequence motifs are involved in SV40 enhancer function. *EMBO J* 1986; 5: 387–97.

34 Herr W, Clarke J. The SV40 enhancer is composed of multiple functional elements that can compensate for one another. *Cell* 1986; 45: 461–71.

35 Banerji J, Rusconi S, Schaffner W. Expression of a β-globin gene is enhanced by remote SV40 DNA sequences. *Cell* 1981; 27: 299–306.

36 Walker MD, Edlund T, Boulet AM, Rutter WJ. Cell specific expression controlled by the 5' flanking region of the insulin and chymotrypsin genes. *Nature* 1983; 306: 557−61.

37 Edlund T, Walker MD, Barr J, Rutter WJ. Cell-specific expression of the rat insulin gene: evidence for role of two distinct 5' flanking elements. *Science* 1985; 230: 912−16.

38 Boulet AM, Erwin CR, Rutter WJ. Cell-specific enhancers in the rat endocrine pancreas. *Proc Natl Acad Sci USA* 1986; 83: 3599−603.

39 Sen R, Baltimore D. Multiple nuclear factors interact with the immunoglobulin enhancer sequences. *Cell* 1986; 46: 224−30.

40 Ohlsson H, Edlund T. Sequence specific interactions of nuclear factors with the insulin gene enhancer. *Cell* 1986; 45: 35−44.

41 Wirth TL, Staudt L, Baltimore D. An octamer oligonucleotide upstream of a TATA motif is sufficient for lymphoid specific promoter activity. *Nature* 1987; 329: 174−8.

42 Nomiyama H, Fromental C, Xiao JH, Chambon P. Cell-specific activity of the constituent elements of the simian virus 40 enhancer. *Proc Natl Acad Sci USA* 1987; 84: 7881.

43 Gerster TP, Matthias M, Thali J, Jiricny J, Schaffner W. Cell type-specific elements of the immunoglobulin heavy chain gene enhancer. *EMBO J* 1987; 6: 1323−30.

44 Singh H, Sen R, Baltimore D, Sharp PA. A nuclear factor that binds to a conserved sequence motif in transcriptional control elements of immunoglobulin genes. *Nature* 1986; 319: 154−8.

45 Sturm R, Baumruker T, Franza BR, Herr W. A 100-kD HeLa cell octamer binding protein (OBP100) interacts differently with two separate octamer-related sequences within the SV40 enhancer. *Genes Dev* 1987; 1: 1147−60.

46 Kemler I, Bucher E, Seipel K, Muller-Immergluck MM, Schaffner W. Promoters with the octamer DNA motif (ATGCAAAT) can be ubiquitous or cell type-specific depending on binding affinity of the octamer site and Oct-factor concentration. *Nucleic Acids Research* 1991; 19: 237−42.

47 Davidson EH, Jacobs HT, Britten RJ. Very short repeats and coordinate induction of genes. *Nature* 1983; 301: 468−70.

48 Lichtsteiner S, Wuarin J, Schibler U. The interplay of DNA binding proteins on the promoter of the mouse albumin gene. *Cell* 1987; 51: 9963−73.

49 Schleif R. DNA binding by proteins. *Science* 1988; 241: 1182−7.

50 Struhl K. Helix−turn−helix, zinc finger, and leucine zipper motifs for eukaryotic transcriptional regulatory proteins. *Trends Biochem Sci* 1989; 14: 137−40.

51 Gehring WJ. Homeoboxes in the study of development. *Science* 1987; 236: 1245−52.

52 Scott MP, Tamkun JW, Hartzell GW. Structure and function of the homeodomain. *Biochim Biophys Acta* 1989; 989: 25−48.

53 Hanes SD, Brett R. DNA specificity of the bicoid activator protein is determined by homeodomain recognition helix 9. *Cell* 1989; 57: 1275−83.

54 Akam M. Hox and HOM: homologous gene clusters in insects and vertebrates. *Cell* 1989; 57: 347−9.

55 Herr W, Sturm RA, Clerc RG *et al*. The POU domain: a large conserved region in the mammalian pit-1, oct−1, oct-2 and *Caenorhabditis elagans* unc-86 gene products. *Genes Dev* 1988; 2: 1513−16.

56 Levine M, Hoey T. Homeobox proteins as sequence-specific transcription factors. *Cell* 1988; 55: 537−40.

57 Miller J, McLachlan AD, Klug A. Repetitive zinc-binding domains in the protein transcription factor IIIA from *Xenopus* oocytes. *EMBO J* 1985; 4: 1609−14.

58 Klug A, Rhodes D. Zinc-fingers: a novel protein motif for nucleic acid recognition.

Trends Biochem Sci 1987; 12: 464−9.

59 Freedman LP, Luisi BF, Korszin ZR, Basavappa R, Gigler PB, Yamamoto KR. The function and structure of the metal coordination sites within the glucocorticoid receptor binding domain. *Nature* 1988; 334: 543−6.

60 Abel T, Maniatis T. Action of leucine zippers. *Nature* 1989; 341: 24−5.

61 Landschultz WH, Johnson PF, McKnight SL. The DNA binding domain of the rat liver nuclear protein C/EBP is bipartate. *Science* 1989; 243: 1681−8.

62 Kouzarides T, Ziff E. The role of the leucine-zipper in the *fos−jun* interaction. *Nature* 1988; 336: 646−51.

63 Turner R, Tjian R. Leucine repeats and an adjacent DNA binding domain mediate the formation of functional cfos−cjun heterodimers. *Science* 1989; 243: 1689−94.

64 Ciliberto G, Dente L, Cortese R. Cell-specific expression of a transfected human α_1-antitrypsin gene. *Cell* 1985; 41: 531−40.

65 Shen RF, Li Y, Sifers RN *et al.* Tissue-specific expression of the human α_1-antitrypsin gene is controlled by multiple *cis*-regulating elements. *Nucleic Acids Research* 1987; 15: 8399−415.

66 Hardon EM, Frain M, Paonessa G, Cortese R. Two distinct factors interact with the promoter regions of several liver-specific genes. *EMBO J* 1988; 7: 1711−19.

67 DeSimone V, Ciliberto G, Hardon E. *et al.* Cis and *trans*-acting elements responsible for the cell-specific expression of the human α_1-antitrypsin gene. *EMBO J* 1987; 6: 2759−66.

68 Courtois G, Morgan JG, Campbell LA, Fourel G, Crabtree, GR. Interaction of a liver-specific nuclear factor with the fibrogen and α_1-antitrypsin promoters. *Science* 1987; 238: 688−92.

69 Courtois G, Baumhutter S, Crabtree GR. Purified hepatocyte nuclear factor 1 interacts with a family of hepatocyte-specific promoters. *Proc Natl Acad Sci USA* 1988; 85: 7937−41.

70 DeSimone V, Cortese R. A negative regulatory element in the promoter of the human α_1-antitrypsin gene. *Nucleic Acids Research* 1989; 17: 9407−15.

71 Li Y, Shen RF, Tsai SY, Woo SLC. Multiple hepatic *trans*-acting factors are required for *in-vitro* transcription of the human alpha-1-antitrypsin gene. *Mol Cell Biol* 1988; 8: 4362−9.

72 Wu Y, Foreman RC. The molecular genetics of α_1-antitrypsin deficiency. *BioEssays* 1991; 13: 163−9.

73 Costa RH, Grayson DR, Darnell JE. Multiple hepatocyte-enriched nuclear factors function in the regulation of transthyretin and α_1-antitrypsin gene. *Mol Cell Biol* 1989; 9: 1415−25.

74 Akira S, Isshiki H, Sugita T *et al.* A nuclear factor for IL-6 expression (NF-IL6) is a member of a C/EBP family. *EMBO J* 1990; 9: 1897−906.

75 Morgan K, Scobie G, Kalsheker N. The characterization of a mutation of the 3' flanking sequence of the α_1-antitrypsin gene commonly associated with chronic obstructive airways disease. *Eur J Clin Invest* 1992; 22: 134−7.

76 Costa RH, Grayson DR, Xanthopoulos KG, Darnell JE. A liver-specific DNA binding protein recognises multiple nucleotide sites in the regulatory regions of transthyretin, α_1-antitrypsin, albumin and simian virus 40 genes. *Proc Natl Acad Sci USA* 1988; 85: 3840−44.

77 Won KA, Baumann H. The cytokine response element of the rat α_1-acid glycoprotein gene is a complex of several interacting regulatory sequences. *Mol Cell Biol* 1990; 10: 3965−78.

78 Davidson I, Xiao JH, Rosales R, Staub A, Chambon P. The HeLa cell protein TEF-1 binds specifically and cooperatively to two SV40 enhancer motifs of unrelated sequence. *Cell* 1988; 54: 931−42.

79 Sirum-Connolly K, Brinckerhoff CE. Interleukin-1 or phorbol induction of the stromolysin promoter requires an element that cooperates with AP-1. *Nucleic Acids Research* 1991; 19: 335−41.

80 Frankel AD, Kim PS. Modular structure of transcription factors: implications for gene regulation. *Cell* 1991; 65: 717−19.

81 Sadowski I, Ma J, Treizenberg S, Ptashne M. GAL4-VP16 is an unusually potent transcriptional activator. *Nature* 1988; 335: 563−4.

82 Ptashne M. Gene regulation by proteins acting nearby and at a distance. *Nature* 1986; 322: 697−701.

83 Ptashne M. How eukaryotic transcriptional activators work. *Nature* 1988; 335: 683−9.

84 Schleif R. Why should DNA loop? *Nature* 1987; 327: 369−70.

85 Staditsky VM. Allosteric mechanism of enhancer action? *FEBS Lett* 1991; 280: 5−7.

86 Fried M, Crothers DM. Equilibria and kinetics of lac repressor−operator interactions by polyacrylamide gel electrophoresis. *Nucleic Acids Research* 1981; 9: 6505−25.

87 Garner MM, Revzin A. A gel electrophoresis method for quantifying the binding of proteins to specific DNA regions: applications to components of the *Escherichia coli* lactose operon regulatory system. *Nucleic Acids Research* 1981; 9: 3047−60.

88 Dignam JD, Lebovitz RM, Roeder RG. Accurate transcription initiation by RNA polymerase II in a soluble extract from isolated mammalian nuclei. *Nucleic Acids Research* 1983; 11: 1575−89.

89 Manley JL, Fire A, Cano A, Sharp PA, Gefter ML. DNA-dependent transcription of adenovirus genes in a soluble whole-cell extract. *Proc Natl Acad Sci USA* 1980; 77: 3855−9.

90 Hennighausen L, Lubon H. Interaction of protein with DNA *in vitro*. *Methods Enzymol* 1987; 152: 721−35.

91 Galas D, Schmitz A. DNase footprinting: a simple method for the detection of protein−DNA binding specificity. *Nucleic Acids Research* 1978; 5: 3157−70.

92 Krummel B. DNaseI footprinting. In: Innis MA, Gelfand DH, Sninsky JJ, White TJ, eds. *PCR Protocols*. Academic Press San Diego, California, 1990: 184−8.

93 Kadonga JT, Tjian R. Affinity purification of sequence-specific DNA binding proteins. *Proc Natl Acad Sci USA* 1986; 83: 5889−93.

94 Rosenfeld PJ, Kelly TJ. Purification of nuclear factor I by DNA recognition site affinity chromatography. *J Biological Chemistry* 1986; 261: 1398−408.

95 Maniatis T, Fritsch EF, Sambrook J. *Molecular Cloning: A Laboratory Manual*. New York: Cold Spring Harbor Laboratory Press, 1982: 211−46.

96 Kadonga JT, Carner KR, Masiarz FR, Tjian R. Isolation of cDNA encoding the transcription factor Sp1 and functional analysis of the DNA binding domain. *Cell* 1987; 51: 1079−90.

97 Santoro C, Mermod N, Andrews PC, Tjian R. A family of human CCAAT box binding proteins active in transcription and replication: cloning and expression of multiple cDNAs. *Nature* 1988; 334: 218−24.

98 Norman C, Runswick M, Pollock R, Treisman R. Isolation and properties of cDNA clones encoding SRF, a transcription factor that binds to the c-*fos* serum response element. *Cell* 1988; 55: 989−1003.

99 Singh H, Le Bowitz JH, Baldwin AS, Sharp PA. Molecular cloning of an enhancer binding protein: isolation by screening an expression library with a recognition site DNA. *Cell* 1988; 52: 415−29.

100 Vinson CR, La Marco KL, Johnson PF, Landschulz WH, McKnight SZ. *In situ* detection of sequence-specific DNA binding activity specified by a recombinant bacteriophage. *Genes Dev* 1988; 2: 801−6.

101 Sturm RA, Das G, Herr W. The ubiquitous octamer-binding protein OCT-1 contains a POU domain with a homeobox subdomain. *Genes Dev* 1988; 2: 1582—99.

102 Staudt LM, Clerc RG, Singh H, Le Bowitz JH, Sharp PA, Baltimore D. Cloning of a lymphoid-specific cDNA encoding a protein binding the regulatory octamer DNA motif. *Science* 1988; 241: 577—80.

103 Rosenthal N. Identification of regulatory elements of cloned genes with functional assays. *Methods Enzymol* 1987; 152: 704—20.

104 Semenza GL, Nejfelt MK, Chi SM, Antonarakis SE. Hypoxia-inducible nuclear factors bind to an enhancer element located 3' to the human erythropoietin gene. *Proc Natl Acad Sci USA* 1991; 88: 5680—4.

105 Takemoto Y, Fujimura Y, Matsumoto M *et al*. The promoter of the *endoA* cytokeratin gene is activated by a 3' downstream enhancer. *Nucleic Acids Research* 1991; 19: 2761—5.

106 Lieberson R, Giannini SL, Birshtein BK, Eckhardt LA. An enhancer at the 3' end of the mouse immunoglobulin heavy chain locus. *Nucleic Acids Research* 1991; 19: 933—7.

107 Gordon JW, Ruddle FH. Integration and stable germ line transmission of genes injected into mouse pronuclei. *Science* 1981; 214: 1244—6.

108 Hanahan D. Heritable formation of pancreatic beta-cell tumours in transgenic mice expressing recombinant insulin/simian virus 40 oncogenes. *Nature* 1985; 315: 115—23.

109 Brinster RL, Chen HY, Trumbauer M, Senaer AW, Warren R, Palmiter RD. Somatic expression of herpes thymidine kinase in mice following injection of a fusion gene into eggs. *Cell* 1981; 27: 223—31.

110 Palmiter RD, Brinster RL, Hammer RE *et al*. Dramatic growth of mice that develop from eggs microinjected with metallothionein—growth hormone fusion genes. *Nature* 1982; 300: 611—15.

111 Palmiter RD, Brinster RL. Germ-line transformation of mice. *Annu Rev Genet* 1986; 20: 465—99.

112 McKnight GS, Hammer RE, Kuenzel EA, Brinster RL. Expression of the chicken transferrin gene in transgenic mice. *Cell* 1983; 34: 335—41.

113 Wagner TE, Hoppe PC, Jollick JD, Scholl DR, Hodinka RL, Gault JB. Microinjection of a rabbit β-globin gene into zygotes and its subsequent expression in adult mice and their offspring. *Proc Natl Acad Sci USA* 1981; 78: 6376—80.

114 Lacy E, Roberts S, Evans EP, Burtenshaw MD, Constantini FD. A foreign β-globin gene in transgenic mice: integration at abnormal chromosomal positions and expression in inappropriate tissues. *Cell* 1983; 34: 343—58.

115 Storb U, O'Brien RL, McMullen MD, Gollahon KA, Brinster RL. High expression of cloned immunoglobulin kappa gene in transgenic mice is restricted to B lymphocytes. *Nature* 1984; 310: 238—41.

116 Archibald AL, McClenaghan M, Hornsey V, Simons JP, Clark AJ. High-level expression of biologically active human α_1-antitrypsin in the milk of transgenic mice. *Proc Natl Acad Sci USA* 1990; 87: 5178—82.

8 Applications of molecular biology to lung disease: bacterial infection

RORY J. SHAW

Introduction

When faced with a pyrexial patient, most clinicians have at some time wished they could perform a simple blood test, send the sample to the laboratory and a few hours later be told the nature of the causative organism, whether or not the organism was resistant to any antibiotics, and where or who the organism was caught from. The techniques of molecular biology, at least theoretically, are capable of offering this service. To the practising clinician, it is in the area of infection that molecular biology may have the first major impact on day-to-day clinical practice. In addition, the epidemiologist and those trying to decide new approaches to prevention and treatment of infection are also increasingly using molecular biology tools.

In the majority of applications discussed the major question is whether a sample of DNA contains a sequence or gene of interest.

Identification of a specific DNA sequence or gene in a sample of DNA

Bacteria include specific DNA and RNA sequences that can be identified using conventional hybridization technology with relevant probes (see Chapter 1). Thus, providing the sequence sought is unique to the bacterium, the technology offers a rapid and specific method for characterizing the organism.

Simple methodology such as Southern or Northern blotting requires relatively large amounts of bacterial extract as starting material. Thus these techniques (though useful) may be less useful when numbers of organisms being studied are few (see Chapter 1).

However, in this instance, the polymerase chain reaction (PCR) amplifies the amount of specific DNA or RNA within the starting material (see Chapter 1). Two complementary sequences (primers) bind to opposite strands of native DNA straddling the sequence of interest. The enzyme, Taq polymerase, then rebuilds the DNA adjacent to these primers such that two copies of the DNA sequence of interest are made. This process is repeated until there is enough of the amplified fragment to be seen by

133

direct visualization following ethidium bromide staining. Alternatively, the amplified DNA can be immobilized on a membrane, and a third radiolabelled sequence of DNA can act as a probe to identify the amplified DNA.

Pathogenesis of infection

Molecular biology has allowed us to ask how genes in bacteria cause them to be pathogenic and how genes in the host may confer resistance to infection.

Bacterial virulence

Many bacteria are commensals, while others, even within the same species, cause disease. In most cases the pathogenicity is related to the acquisition of one or more special features such as toxin production or invasive ability. In many cases the genes encoding these properties have been identified, and it is thus possible by demonstrating that a particular bacterium contains one of these genes to determine its disease-causing potential. For example, enterotoxic *Escherichia coli* producing heat-labile toxin [1] can be identified specifically on the basis of the presence of this gene, as determined by PCR amplification. Furthermore, the presence of *E. coli* or *Shigella* species with enteroinvasive potential in food can be confirmed by PCR amplification of a plasmid which confers invasive ability [2]. Similarly, cytotoxic *Clostridium difficile* can be identified by the presence of the toxin A gene [3].

Host resistance

The ability of molecular biology to alter our thinking about host resistance to infection is illustrated by the discovery of the Bcg gene in mice [4]. Certain strains of mice have long been known to be more susceptible than others to mycobacterial infection. It is now recognized that there are two allelic forms. There is the dominant resistance (Bcg^r) allele and the recessive susceptibility (Bcg^s) allele. The gene encoding these alleles is located on chromosome 1 in the mouse and is near to genes conferring resistance or susceptibility to other organisms, namely, *Leishmania donovani* and *Salmonella typhimurium*. It is believed that at an early stage after infection, macrophages express the Bcg gene. The gene product is thought to influence macrophage function, especially the interaction of macrophages with lymphocytes. Thus, following bacterial challenge, macrophages from mice with the Bcg^r allele exhibit greater respiratory burst and hexose monophosphate shunt activity. In addition, the Bcg^r macrophages have greater Ia antigen expression and show a greater increase in Ia antigen expression and expression of the surface marker

AcM.1 after exposure to Bcg. Furthermore, Bcg^r spleen macrophages demonstrate improved antigen-presenting ability, and Bcg^r mice develop more antigen-specific T-cell proliferation and interleukin-2 (IL-2) production during Bcg infection compared with Bcg^s mice. These major differences in host defences explain the relative susceptibility of Bcg^s mice to mycobacterial disease.

In human studies, in addition to the HLA haplotype which is implicated in the clinical manifestations of tuberculosis (Tb) and leprosy, there may be other genetic factors. There is close homology between the 35 centimorgan (cM) fragment of the murine chromosome 1 and human chromosome 2q. According to the rules of comparative gene mapping a human homologue for the Bcg resistance/susceptibility locus should be located on human chromosome 2, region q32−37. If this is the case, the identification of such a locus, as well as the characterization of the gene sequence and the functional abilities of its protein product, are likely to improve greatly our understanding of how host immunity prevents infection by mycobacteria from developing into disease which is clinically overt.

Mechanism of disease

The combination of techniques to identify both proteins and DNA sequences confers a new level of sophistication to the tools used to investigate the pathogenesis of disease. An example is the study of the rheumatological disease of Yersinia reactive arthritis, in which immunofluorescence identified bacterial proteins in synovial fluid cells whereas PCR amplification failed to identify any Yersinia DNA [5]. These studies suggest that only parts of the causative agent, and not the whole microbe, are present in the joint and may play a role in the inflammation that results in reactive arthritis.

Epidemiology

Monitoring the environment

The enormous sensitivity of the PCR allows the presence of single copies of specific DNA and hence even a single organism to be detected. It is thus possible to identify organisms in the environment, which are present at such low numbers that they are unlikely to be identified by conventional culture techniques. Thus, *E. coli* and enteric pathogens (*Salmonella* and *Shigella* species) can be identified at a level of one to five organisms per 100 ml in the water supply on the basis of PCR amplification of the *lacZ* and *lamB* genes, respectively [6]. This method has been extended to identify *Legionella pneumophilia* [7, 8] in water seeded with as few as 35 colony-forming units. Application of this technique to environmental water samples may thus help in identifying the natural reservoirs of *Legionella pneumophilia* infection (see below).

Conversely, valuable information may be obtained from failing to identify the DNA of a particular pathogen in an environmental situation. Thus, PCR for HIV has been used on samples from endoscopes to confirm the efficiency of cleaning and sterilization techniques [9].

Identifying the source of the infection

Molecular biology is likely to prove a useful tool to the epidemiologist studying the spread of infection. The specific DNA sequence of a particular bacterial gene can be compared with a DNA sequence of the same gene from a similar bacterium isolated from a different patient. If the sequences are identical, it is likely that the isolates had a recent common ancestor, thus both infections may be part of the same outbreak. Conversely, if there are subtle differences in the sequence, then the common ancestor must have existed some time previously indicating that the organism and the illnesses are not related to the same epidemic. This analysis can be relatively simple to perform using restriction fragment analysis (Fig. 8.1). If the DNA of an organism is digested by restriction enzymes, the subsequent sizes of the DNA fragments relate to the distances along the DNA between each of these restriction enzyme digestion sites. If a mutation occurs at a particular enzyme digestion site such that the DNA is not cut or a new restriction site is introduced, there will be a change in the sizes of the DNA fragments (see Chapter 1). If two

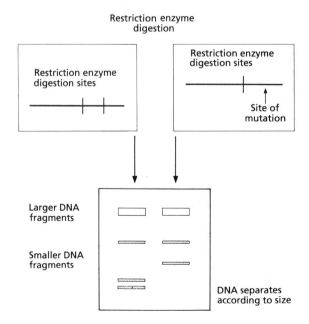

Fig. 8.1 Restriction enzyme analysis.

organisms are compared and their DNA is digested by a range of these enzymes, it is possible to compare the sizes of the DNA fragments after each digestion. An alteration in the pattern of bands formed when the DNA is separated on a gel on the basis of size indicates that there are differences in the enzyme digestion sites between the two organisms, and hence that the organisms are not identical genetically. This technique has been used by Shoemaker *et al.* [10], who have compared 15 strains of *Mycobacterium tuberculosis* by restriction fragment analysis and phage typing. There was close agreement between both techniques. There were only two examples where restriction fragment analysis did not separate strains with different phage types, and two examples where phage typing did not separate strains with different DNA restriction patterns.

Restriction enzyme analysis of other respiratory pathogens has shown that mycoplasma pneumonia can exhibit strain-specific spread in closed populations [11], whereas there are between-strain and within-serogroup differences in *Legionella pneumophilia* [12]. This latter observation has been used in an epidemiological study. Restriction endonuclease analysis of *Legionella pneumophilia* from six patients, three air conditioning- and cooling tower-derived strains and three hot water supply-derived strains demonstrated that the patient isolates were indistinguishable from the air conditioning- and cooling tower-derived strains but differed markedly from the hot water supply-derived isolates [13]. These studies were thus able to identify the environmental source of this cluster of cases of legionnaire's disease.

Antibiotic resistance

Antibiotic resistance is a growing clinical problem. Bacterial resistance to an antibiotic occurs as a result of acquiring a gene, which encodes a protein, that breaks down the antibiotic, or which allows the organism's metabolism to bypass the block conferred by the antibiotic. These genes can be identified by purification of the DNA, restriction enzyme digestion and subsequent Southern blotting, or more rapidly by PCR.

Erythromycin resistance is uncommon but may occur in a range of organisms where it is associated with the presence of erythromycin methylases, encoded by erythromycin resistance genes. Identification of these genes provides evidence of potential resistance to erythromycin, which can develop if the genes are expressed. These genes have substantial nucleotide sequence diversity, but using oligonucleotides to conserved areas within these genes in combination with PCR amplification, erythromycin resistance can be identified [14]. Similarly, the genes for the aminoglycoside-modifying enzymes AAC(3)-I, AAC(3)-II, AAC(3)-IV can be identified by PCR [15].

Antibiotic resistance plasmids have yet to be identified in mycobacteria, although antibiotic resistance is well recognized. In 1990, Martin *et al.* [16] were the first to identify, clone and sequence a genetic region in the DNA of *Mycobacterium fortuitum* which is responsible for resistance to sulphonamides. This region shared homology with a sequence termed Tn 1696 which is associated with gentamicin resistance [17]. It is thus likely that it will soon be possible to identify antibiotic resistance patterns on the basis of gene identification, as opposed to culture characteristics.

An appreciation of the mechanism of action of some antibiotics also requires an understanding of molecular biology concepts. For example, one of the major actions of the quinolone family of antibiotics is to inhibit the enzyme DNA gyrase [18]. This enzyme cleaves and rejoins bacterial double-stranded DNA so as to introduce negative supercoils into the DNA and allow the accommodation of the long circular chromosome within the limited space provided by the cell envelope. The complete process is necessary for bacterial replication and hence specific inhibition of this single metabolic step provides a successful therapeutic approach. Other treatments based upon similar concepts are likely to be developed in the future.

Taxonomy

Every organism within a species shares a large number of genes which are essentially homologous. Minor variations in base pair sequence in regions not encoding critical amino acids may develop over many generations allowing the epidemiological studies described above. However, the genetic differences between species are considerably greater. Advantage can be taken of this when trying to classify organisms. *Pneumocystis carinii* was originally suspected of being a unicellular organism with trophozoite and cystic forms. Sequencing of the DNA encoding the ribosomal RNA showed this to be homologous with some genes in fungi. This has allowed *P. carinii* to be recognized now as a fungus and not a unicellular parasite [19].

Diagnosis

Tuberculosis

Tb is one of the diseases where the diagnostic possibilities of PCR have great potential. Conventional techniques to diagnose Tb are based on visualization of the organism by staining, which requires a large number of organisms to be present and does not differentiate between subtypes of mycobacteria. Alternatively, the organism can be grown in culture and the species identified on the basis of cultural requirements and antibiotic sensitivities. This has the disadvantage that culture may take many months before a definite answer is obtained. The process may be accelerated by Bactec, which utilizes sensitive detection of ^{14}C released in the form of CO_2 from metabolized sugars in the medium. Although more rapid, Bactec also requires at least $1-2$ weeks. The clinician faced with a patient with suspected pulmonary or meningeal Tb may thus be forced to start empirical therapy while waiting for bacteriological confirmation. The problem of identifying the particular species of mycobacterium and hence likely antibiotic resistance pattern is of particular importance in samples from HIV-infected patients where both *Mycobacterium tuberculosis* and *M. avium complex* are common pathogens.

The application of molecular biology techniques to the diagnosis of Tb has taken three approaches. In the first approach, the bacterium was cultured in the usual manner taking a number of weeks. The DNA was then extracted, digested by appropriate restriction enzymes and the fragments separated on a Southern gel. The DNA was then blotted on to a nylon membrane and hybridized with a mycobacterial-specific probe. The probe was usually labelled with ^{32}P, although recently non-radioactive labelling systems have been used (see Chapter 1). Binding of the probe indicated the presence of the relevant mycobacterial gene and hence the organism [20−24].

The second approach has been to perform the more rapid Bactec culture and then extract DNA from those yielding positive growth. This DNA was then examined as above to determine the exact identity of the organism [25, 26].

The third approach took advantage of the PCR. Primers specific to the mycobacterial gene of interest were used to amplify minute quantities of DNA obtained from samples prior to culture. The presence of an amplified segment of DNA, as detected by Southern blotting, indicated the presence of mycobacterial DNA in the original sample. This technique had the advantage of speed and the requirement of only a few organisms to be present initially. For certain genes with very unique DNA sequences, the binding of the primers was sufficiently specific that amplification, followed by separation on a Southern gel and visualization by ethidium bromide staining, provided a positive result alone. In the case of genes which share homology with many other bacterial genes, further specificity could be obtained by probing the blots of the DNA with shorter oligonucleotides specific to sequences of genes unique to a particular subspecies. If required, a combination of restriction fragment digestion and probing conferred further specificity (Fig. 8.2).

Mycobacteria have a number of genes which when amplified by PCR serve as candidates for a diagnostic test as outlined earlier (see Chapter 1). The mycobacterial gene encoding the 65 kD heat shock protein (65 kDa antigen), which is expressed as a surface antigen on mycobacteria, was sequenced in 1987 [27]. The 65 kDa antigen gene has two relative disadvantages as a target for PCR. First, it is present as a single copy in mycobacteria. Thus, for every mycobacterium present

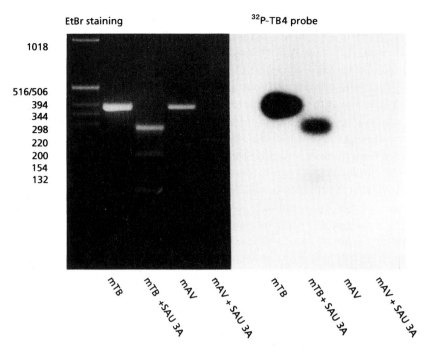

EtBr staining   **^{32}P-TB4 probe**

1018

516/506
394
344
298
220
200
154
132

mTB   mTB +SAU 3A   mAV   mAV +SAU 3A   mTB   mTB +SAU 3A   mAV   mAV +SAU 3A

Fig. 8.2 Digestion of *Mycobacterium tuberculosis* and *M. avium intracellulare* DNA by the enzyme SAU 3A. PCR-amplified 65 kD antigen DNA from *M. tuberculosis* and *M. avium intracellulare* was digested by SAU 3A. The products were separated on a gel and stained with ethidium bromide (left). The DNA was transferred to a nylon membrane by Southern blotting and probed (right). The results show that *M. tuberculosis* and *M. avium intracellulare* 65 kD antigen DNA were different on the basis of restriction enzyme analysis and ability to bind to a radiolabelled probe.

there is only one sequence of target DNA. Second, the 65 kDa antigen gene shows significant homology with a 65 kDa heat shock protein of other organisms including *Mycobacterium leprae* [27], the Gro EL protein gene of *E. coli* [28] and even mammalian heat shock proteins. Furthermore, the 65 kDa gene sequence is identical in *Mycobacterium tuberculosis*, *M. africanum* and *M. bovis* [29]. Despite these disadvantages, combined amplification by PCR and probing has been used directly on sputum and respiratory samples [30, 31] as well as cerebrospinal fluid [32] to confirm the diagnosis of Tb.

A second mycobacterial DNA sequence IS6110 has two advantages over the 65 kDa antigen gene as a target for PCR. First, it is present in multiple copies in the mycobacterium, thus providing multiple targets for PCR amplification [33−37]. This improves the sensitivity, such that in theory it is possible to detect even fragments of one organism in the sample. Second, the IS6110 sequence is very specific for a small group of *Mycobacterium tuberculosis* like organisms. IS6110 DNA has been found in *M. tuberculosis*, *M. bovis* and *M. simiae*, but not in *M. kanansasii*, *M. avium* complex, *M. scrofulaceum*, *M. fortuitum*, *M. cheloni* or *M. gordonae* [34].

We have compared PCR amplification of these two mycobacterial genes (65 kD and IS6110 sequence) as a diagnostic test for Tb [38]. Sputum, bronchoscopy washings and bronchoalveolar lavage samples from 90 patients were examined. Both tests confirmed the diagnosis of Tb in all patients with active pulmonary Tb. In cases with no evidence of disease related to Tb, IS6110 DNA was detected by amplification in 9% and the 65 kDa antigen DNA in 33%. Of greater interest, IS6110 DNA and 65 kDa antigen DNA were found in samples of 83% and 100% of cases of past Tb and 56% and 100% of contacts of Tb. This study raises concerns about the ability of this sensitive test to discriminate active from non-active disease. Furthermore, it raises questions about host immunity which appears to control the organism in one patient while leaving it to cause disease in another.

The diagnostic ability of this approach clearly needs further refinement before it can be used in routine clinical practice. However, PCR may have different diagnostic potential according to the biological fluid examined. Thus, examination of cerebrospinal fluid for 65 kDa antigen DNA was not associated with an appreciable false-positive rate [32]. Alternatively, we need to quantify the amount of *Mycobacterium tuberculosis* DNA in a biological fluid more accurately by refining the methodology in order to discriminate between a few isolated organisms rendered non-pathogenic by host immunity and those present in sufficient number to cause disease.

IS6110 DNA is an example of a gene with multiple copies in mycobacterial DNA. As indicated, this offers multiple targets for PCR amplification. An alternative approach to providing multiple targets for PCR is to use ribosomal RNA as there are multiple ribosomes in each organism. This approach may have the additional theoretical advantage that the presence of intact ribosomes may correlate more closely with organism viability. Such an approach has technical difficulties as RNA is more liable to degradation than DNA during isolation, thus requiring more complex extraction procedures. In addition, RNA has to be converted to complementary DNA (cDNA) by reverse transcriptase prior to PCR amplification, which adds further steps and expense to the assay system.

Pneumocystis carinii pneumonia

Pneumocystis carinii pneumonia is a common complication of HIV infection. At present, diagnosis relies on microscopic identification of the pathogen in induced sputum or lung secretion samples obtained at bronchoscopy. Using a specific sequence of *P. carinii* ribosomal RNA as a template, three oligonucleotides have been synthesized and two used as primers for PCR, while the third is used as an internal probe to label the amplified products [39]. In ref. 39, the ribosomal RNA itself was not used as a target but rather the DNA in the chromosome which encodes the ribosomal RNA. In an initial study of bronchoalveolar lavage samples from 47 bronchoscopies, no *P. carinii* DNA was found in 10 immunocompetent patients, and only low levels in three of 13 samples from immunosuppressed individuals without clinical evidence of *P. carinii* pneumonia. On the other hand, high levels were detectable, even by ethidium bromide staining of amplified products without the need for additional probing, in all 16 samples from patients with a clinical diagnosis of *P. carinii* pneumonia. This study suggested that when the amount of amplified *P. carinii* DNA was taken into account, clinically useful information could be obtained. More experience with this technique applied to induced sputum is required, but potentially PCR offers a rapid sensitive test for *P. carinii* pneumonia. The absence of detectable quantities of *P. carinii* DNA in non-immunocompromised patients and in HIV-seropositive patients without previous *P. carinii* pneumonia suggests that *P. carinii* pneumonia is not the result of activation of latent *P. carinii* in the lungs, but rather that it is the result of new infection. The use of PCR may now allow the epidemiology and natural reservoir of this organism to be identified.

Bordetella pertussis

Bordetella pertussis is an example of a fastidious organism which may take several days to grow in culture. The possibility of diagnosis by PCR was aided by the discovery of reiterated chromosomal sequences which are present in about 50–100 copies per cell [40–46]. The repeated sequence is 1046 base pairs long and PCR using oligonucleotides to a 153 base pair segment of the repeated element provided a 5-hour method for detection of *B. pertussis* in nasopharyngeal secretions [46]. Using this assay in samples from 332 children, PCR yielded a positive result in 98 samples compared with 66 for culture and 33 for direct immunofluorescence. Two hundred and thirty-one samples were negative for all tests. Of concern were the 33 culture and immunofluorescence negative specimens which proved to be positive using the PCR assay. However, these were thought to be biologically relevant positives, as opposed to false-positives, since the samples were collected from subjects liable to have a subclinical pertussis infection. These subjects included close contacts of culture proven pertussis patients, follow-up samples from the patients, or were from patients with serological evidence of pertussis infection [46].

Mycoplasma pneumonia

A commercially available cDNA probe homologous to ribosomal RNA of *Mycoplasma pneumonia* has been used in two studies employing samples obtained from throat swabs. To date these studies have been performed without amplification of DNA by PCR. Hata *et al.* [47] studying 163 children were able to identify *Mycoplasma pneumonia* DNA with a sensitivity of 76% and specificity of 95% when compared with a subsequent rise in specific antibodies (taken as positive evidence of infection). In a similar study of 160 army recruits in Finland, there was a sensitivity of 95% and a specificity of 85%, when comparing the probe test on sputum and throat swabs with positive serology and/or sputum culture [48].

Other

Preliminary studies have also used PCR amplification of specific bacterial genes or DNA sequences successfully to identify a wide range of organisms including *Leptospira* [49], *Listeria monocytogenes* [50], *Rickettsia Rickettsii* [51] and *Chlamydia trachomatis* [52−54]. An alternative approach is to identify the presence of the organism by DNA *in situ* hybridization on tissue samples (see Chapter 1). In this technique, the probe is applied directly to histological sections to identify the presence of specific DNA sequences. An example of this technique comes from studies on the upper gastrointestinal tract, when endoscopic biopsies have been shown to contain *Campylobacter pylori* sequences following *in situ* hybridization [55].

Limitations of technique

Contamination of reagents by target DNA derived from amplified products of a previous PCR amplification is a common problem with PCR [56, 57]. Various techniques have been employed to ensure that products of one reaction do not come into contact with the reagents of the next. For example, the laboratory equipment and surfaces need to be checked for contamination by the 'wipe test' [58]. In the 'wipe test' surfaces are swabbed and the material on the swab is examined by PCR to determine if target DNA is present as a contaminant on laboratory equipment. A recent modification is to include uridine instead of thymidine in the PCR reaction mixture. This ensures that all amplified DNA contains uridine in place of thymidine. It is then possible at the start of any PCR amplification to incubate reagents with an enzyme which digests any molecules containing uridine. This should in theory eliminate any products from previous PCR amplifications, and prevent them from being reamplified in subsequent assays. This additional step, however, adds considerable expense to an already expensive technique.

A second major limitation of the technique is that identification of DNA by whatever means does not necessarily imply organism viability or pathogenicity. This was suggested by our own study in which Tb DNA was identified in many patients with treated Tb or in contacts of cases of

Tb [38] as well as the study by Glare *et al.* [46] in which *Bordetella pertussis* DNA was identified in treated patients or contacts of patients.

Treatment of infection

Active immunization

The principle in active immunization is to vaccinate the patient with a peptide or peptides from a pathogen, such that the patient develops antibodies which will subsequently bind to and thus initiate killing of the organism if it is contracted. Using molecular biology techniques this process can be significantly refined. The strategy involves a number of stages. First, antigens which elicit a large antibody response are determined by examining various membrane antigens with human sera from patients who have recovered from an infection. Second, an attempt is made to characterize a particular outer membrane peptide molecule which is conserved antigenically, such that one antiserum will recognize all serotypes and strains. Third, the gene encoding this molecule is identified, sequenced and cloned into an expression vector such as a plasmid containing a promoter, which is constitutively activated (Fig. 8.3). When the new gene is introduced downstream from this promoter, and the plasmid reinserted into a bacterium such as *E. coli*, the organism will make large amounts of the peptide. The peptide in its pure form can then be used to develop antisera and the cytotoxic ability of this antisera against the organism can be confirmed. Subsequently, the new peptide can serve as a vaccine for immunization.

An example of this strategy comes from efforts to develop a vaccine to *Haemophilus influenzae* [59]. Two similar membrane molecules termed PAL and PCP are antigenically conserved and elicit antibody responses. The gene encoding PCP has been cloned and biosynthetic PCP used to obtain a polyclonal antiserum. This in turn has been shown to kill nine of 11 clinical strains of *H. influenzae* in a complement-mediated bactericidal assay. It is thus possible that one or both of these proteins may prove useful components in a subunit vaccine against *H. influenzae* although clinical trials have yet to be performed.

Passive immunization

Passive immunization is hampered by lack of a ready supply of safe specific antibody. To date antibody derived from humans has carried the risk of introducing infectious agents. Monoclonal antibodies are in limited supply and antibodies derived from animals may be associated with the development of host immunity and subsequent anaphylaxis. New ways of making antibodies have recently been demonstrated using gene technology. Immunoglobulin variable (V) genes have been amplified from

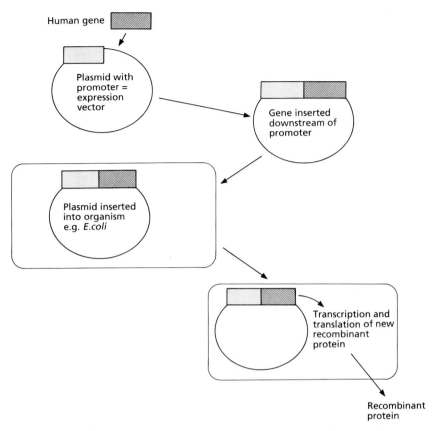

Fig. 8.3 Insertion of a human gene into an expression vector allows synthesis of recombinant proteins.

hybridomas using PCR and then cloned into expression vectors [60, 61]. These vectors are then inserted into yeast or bacteria and the DNA is transcribed and translated such that the organism produces large volumes of the appropriate variable region of the immunoglobulin. This technique should in future provide a ready source of cheap antibodies which will be suitable for passive immunization and will not stimulate a host immune response.

Modulating the host response to infection

There has been a great increase in our understanding of the role of cytokines in inflammation and the response to infection. Certain cytokines such as interferon-γ may promote the ability of macrophages to kill microorganisms, e.g. *Toxoplasma gondii* [62] or *P. carinii* [63], thereby enhancing host defences. As a result of molecular biology technology, recombinant human interferon-γ has now been produced. Jaffe *et al.* [64] have now administered recombinant human interferon-γ directly to the lungs of normal human subjects by nebulization. This route of administration did not cause side effects and yet caused appropriate biological responses in the lung, in that they documented an increase in messenger RNA of interferon-inducible genes in alveolar macrophages. This study opens the new therapeutic area of targeted cytokine therapy to augment respiratory tract defences.

Conclusions

Molecular biology includes a large number of techniques used to study DNA and RNA. In this review, applications of only a few of these have been discussed as they are the closest to having an impact on day-to-day clinical practice. At the simplest, the techniques demonstrate whether a particular gene is present. In the case of the host this may indicate resistance to disease, whereas in the case of the organism this DNA fingerprint may allow the organism to be identified and toxin or antibiotic resistance gene expression to be identified. The other major technique reviewed is the synthesis of recombinant proteins by placing a gene into an expression vector, which can be used to transfect another organism. This organism will then make large quantities of the gene product which may serve as a vaccine or drug. There are many other molecular biology techniques such as those which investigate how a particular gene is regulated and those which introduce changes into the DNA sequence of genes to alter function (site-directed mutagenesis). These have yet to have immediate clinical application to bacterial infection but in future may improve the management of patients with infection.

References

1 Olive DM. Detection of enterotoxigenic *Escherichia coli* after polymerase chain reaction amplification with a thermostable DNA polymerase. *J Clin Microbiol* 1989; 27: 261–5.

2 Lampel KA, Jagow JA, Tracksess M, Hill WE. Polymerase chain reaction for detection of invasive *Shigella flexneri* in food. *Appl Environ Microbiol* 1990; 56: 1536–40.

3 Kato N, Ou CY, Kato H *et al.* Identification of toxigenic *Clostridium difficile* by the polymerase chain reaction. *J Clin Microbiol* 1991; 29: 33–7.

4 Schurr E, Buschman E, Malo D, Gros P, Skamene E. Immunogenetics of mycobacterial infections: mouse–human homologies. *J Infect Dis* 1990; 161: 634–9.

5 Viitanen AM, Arstila TP, Lahesmaa R, Granfors K, Shurnik M, Toivanen P. Application of the polymerase chain reaction and immunofluorescence techniques to the detection of bacteria in Yersinia-triggered reactive arthritis. *Arthritis Rheum* 1991; 34: 89–96.

6 Bej AK, Steffan RJ, Di Cesare J, Atlas RM. Detection of coliform bacteria in water by polymerase chain reaction and gene probes. *Appl Environ Microbiol* 1990; 56: 307–14.

7 Starnbach MN, Falkow S, Tompkins LS. Species-specific detection of *Legionella pneumophilia* in water by DNA amplification and hybridization. *J Clin Microbiol*

1989; 27: 1257−61.

8 Bej AK, Mahbubani MH, Miller R, Di Cesare JL, Haff L, Atlas RM. Multiplex PCR amplification and immobilized capture probes for detection of bacterial pathogens and indicators in water. *Mol Cell Probes* 1990; 4: 353−65.

9 Hanson PJ, Gor D, Clarke JR *et al*. Contamination of endoscopes used in AIDS patients. *Lancet* 1989; ii: 86−8.

10 Shoemaker SA, Fisher JH, Jones WD, Jr, Scoggin CH. Restriction fragment analysis of chromosomal DNA defines different strains of *Mycobacterium tuberculosis*. *Am Rev Respir Dis* 1986; 134: 210−13.

11 Chandler DKF, Razin S, Stephens EB *et al*. Genomic and phenotypic analysis of *Mycoplasma pneumoniae* strains. *Infect Immun* 1982; 38: 604−9.

12 van Ketel RJ. Similar DNA restriction endonuclease profiles in strains of *Legionella pneumophilia* from different serogroups. *J Clin Microbiol* 1988; 26: 1838−41.

13 van Ketel RJ, de Wever B. Genetic typing in a cluster of *Legionella pneumophilia* infections. *J Clin Microbiol* 1989; 27: 1105−7.

14 Arthur M, Molinas C, Mabilat C, Courvalin P. Detection of erythromycin resistance by the polymerase chain reaction using primers in conserved regions of erm rRNA methylase genes. *Antimicrob Agents Chemother* 1990; 34: 2024−6.

15 Vliegenthart JS, Ketelaar-van-Gaalen PA, van-de-Klundert JA. Identification of three genes coding for aminoglycoside-modifying enzymes by means of the polymerase chain reaction. *J Antimicrob Chemother* 1990; 25: 759−65.

16 Martin C, Timm J, Rauzier J, Gomez-Lus R, Davies J, Gicquel B. Transposition of an antibiotic resistance element in mycobacteria. *Nature* 1990; 345: 739−43.

17 Martinez E, de la Cruz F. Transposon Tn21 encodes a RecA-independent site-specific integration system. *Mol Gen Genet* 1988; 211: 320−5.

18 Furet YX, Pechere JC. Usual and unusual antibacterial effects of quinolones. *J Antimicrob Chemother* 1990; 26 (Suppl. B): 7−15.

19 Edman JC, Kovacs JA, Masur H, Santi DV, Elwood HJ, Sogin ML. Ribosomal RNA sequence shows *Pneumocystis carinii* to be a member of the fungi. *Nature* 1988; 334: 519−22.

20 Gonzales R, Hanna BA. Evaluation of Gen-Probe DNA hybridization systems for the identification of *Mycobacterium tuberculosis* and *Mycobacterium avium-intracellulare*. *Diagn Microbiol Infect Dis* 1987; 8: 69−77.

21 Roberts MC, McMillan C, Coyle MB. Whole chromosome DNA probes for rapid identification of *Mycobacterium tuberculosis* and *Mycobacterium avium complex*. *J Clin Microbiol* 1987; 25: 1239−43.

22 Drake TA, Hindler AJA, Berlin OG, Bruckner DA. Rapid identification of *Mycobacterium avium complex* in culture using DNA probes. *J Clin Microbiol* 1987; 25: 1442−5.

23 Musial CE, Tice LS, Stockman L, Roberts GD. Identification of mycobacteria from culture by using the Gen-Probe rapid diagnostic system for *Mycobacterium avium complex* and *Mycobacterium tuberculosis complex*. *J Clin Microbiol* 1988; 26: 2120−3.

24 Sherman I, Harrington N, Rothrock A, George H. Use of a cutoff range in identifying mycobacteria by the Gen-Probe rapid diagnostic system. *J Clin Microbiol* 1989; 27: 241−4.

25 Kiehn TE, Edwards FF. Rapid identification using a specific DNA probe of *Mycobacterium avium complex* from patients with acquired immunodeficiency syndrome. *J Clin Microbiol* 1987; 25: 1551−2.

26 Ellner PD, Kiehn TE, Cammarata R, Hosmer M. Rapid detection and identification of pathogenic mycobacteria by combining radiometric and nucleic acid probe methods. *J Clin Microbiol* 1988; 26: 1349−52.

27 Shinnick TM. The 65-kilodalton of *Mycobacterium tuberculosis*. *J Bacteriol* 1987; 169: 1080−8.

28 Shinnick TM, Vodkin MH, Williams JC. The *Mycobacterium tuberculosis* 65-kilodalton antigen is a heat shock protein which corresponds to common antigen and to the *Escherichia coli* groEL protein. *Infect Immun* 1988; 56: 446–51.

29 Lu MC, Lien MH, Becker RE *et al.* Genes for immunodominant protein antigens are highly homologous in *Mycobacterium tuberculosis*, *Mycobacterium africanum*, and the vaccine strain *Mycobacterium bovis BCG. Infect Immun* 1987; 55: 2378–82.

30 Hance AJ, Grandchamp PB, Levy-Febault VJ, Lecossier D, Rauzier J, Bocart D, Gicquel B. Detection and identification of mycobacteria by amplification of mycobacterial DNA. *Mol Microbiol* 1989; 3: 843–9.

31 Brisson-Noel A, Gicquel B, Lecossier D, Levy-Febault V, Nassif X, Hance AJ. Rapid diagnosis of tuberculosis by amplification of mycobacterial DNA in clinical samples. *Lancet* 1989; ii: 1069–71.

32 Shanker P, Manjunath N, Mohan KK, Prasud K, Behari Shrinwas M, Ahuja GK. Rapid diagnosis of tuberculous meningitis by polymerase chain reaction. *Lancet* 1991; 337: 5–7.

33 Eisenach KD, Crawford JT, Bates JH. Repetitive DNA sequences as probes for *Mycobacterium tuberculosis. J Clin Microbiol* 1988; 26: 2240–5.

34 Eisenach KD, Cave MD, Bates JH, Crawford JT. Polymerase chain reaction amplification of a repetitive DNA sequence specific for *Mycobacterium tuberculosis. J Infect Dis* 1990; 161: 977–81.

35 Patel RJ, Freis WU, Piessens WF, Wirth DF. Sequence amplification by polymerase chain reaction of a cloned DNA fragment for identification of *Mycobacterium tuberculosis. J Clin Microbiol* 1990; 28: 513–18.

36 Thierry D, Brisson-Noel A, Vincent-Levy-Frebault V, Nguyen S, Guesdon JL, Gicquel B. Characterization of a *Mycobacterium tuberculosis* insertion sequence, IS 6110, and its application in diagnosis. *J Clin Microbiol* 1990; 28: 2668–73.

37 Thierry D, Cave MD, Eisenach KD *et al.* IS6110, an IS-like element of *Mycobacterium tuberculosis* complex. *Nucleic Acids Res* 1990; 18: 188–9.

38 Walker DA, Taylor I, Mitchell DM, Shaw RJ. Comparison of polymerase chain reaction (PCR) amplification of 2 mycobacterial DNA sequences, IS6110 and the 65 kD antigen gene, in the diagnosis of tuberculosis. *Thorax* 1992; 47: 690–94.

39 Wakefield AE, Pixley FJ, Banerji S *et al.* Detection of *Pneumocystis carinii* with DNA amplification. *Lancet* 1990; 336: 451–3.

40 McPheat WL, McNally T. Phase I and phase IV strains of *Bordetella pertussis* carry a repeated DNA sequence not found in other *Bordetella* species. *FEMS Microbiol Lett* 1987; 41: 357–60.

41 McPheat WL, McNally T. Isolation of a repeated DNA sequence from *Bordetella pertussis. J Gen Microbiol* 1987; 133: 323–30.

42 McLafferty MA, Harcus DR, Hewlett EL. Nucleotide sequence and characterization of a repetitive DNA element from the genome of *Bordetella pertussis* with characteristics of an insertion sequence. *J Gen Microbiol* 1988; 134: 2297–306.

43 Park I, Saurin W, Ullmann A. A highly conserved 530 base-pair repeated DNA sequence specific for *Bordetella pertussis. FEMS Microbiol Lett* 1988; 52: 19–24.

44 Alsheikhly AR, Lofdahl S. Identification of a DNA fragment in the genome of *Bordetella pertussis* carrying repeated DNA sequences also present in other *Bordetella* species. *Microb Pathog* 1989; 6: 193–201.

45 Houard S, Hackel C, Herzog A, Bollen A. Specific identification of *Bordetella pertussis* by the polymerase chain reaction. *Res Microbiol* 1989; 140: 477–87.

46 Glare EM, Paton JC, Premier RR, Lawrence AJ, Nisbet IT. Analysis of a repetitive DNA sequence from *Bordetella pertussis* and its application to the diagnosis of pertussis using the polymerase chain reaction *J Clin Microbiol* 1990; 28: 1982–7.

47 Hata D, Kuze F, Mochizuki Y *et al.* Evaluation of DNA probe test for rapid diagnosis of *Mycoplasma pneumoniae* infections. *J Pediatr* 1990; 116: 273–6.

48 Kleemola SR, Karjalainen JE, Raty RK. Rapid diagnosis of *Mycoplasma pneumoniae* infection: clinical evaluation of a commercial probe test. *J Infect Dis* 1990; 162: 70−5.

49 Van Eys GJ, Gravekamp C, Gerritsen MJ *et al.* Detection of leptospires in urine by polymerase chain reaction. *J Clin Microbiol* 1989; 27: 2258−62.

50 Bessesen MT, Luo QA, Rotbart HA, Blaser MJ, Ellison RT, 3d detection of *Listeria monocytogenes* by using the polymerase chain reaction. *Appl Environ Microbiol* 1990; 56: 2930−2.

51 Wilson KH, Blitchington R, Shah P, McDonald G, Gilmore RD, Mallavia LP. Probe directed at a segment of *Rickettsia rickettsii* rRNA amplified with polymerase chain reaction. *J Clin Microbiol* 1989; 27: 2692−6.

52 Welch D, Lee CH, Larsen SH. Detection of plasmid DNA from all *Chlamydia trachomatis* serovars with a two-step polymerase chain reaction. *Appl Environ Microbiol* 1990; 56: 2494−8.

53 Dutilh B, Bebear C, Rodriguez P, Vekris A, Bonnet J, Garret M. Specific amplification of a DNA sequence common to all *Chlamydia trachomatis* serovars using the polymerase chain reaction. *Res Microbiol* 1989; 140: 7−16.

54 Engel JN, Pollack J, Malik F, Ganem D. Cloning and characterization of RNA polymerase core subunits of *Chlamydia trachomatis* by using the polymerase chain reaction. *J Bacteriol* 1990; 172: 5732−41.

55 Van den Berg FM, Zijlmans H, Langenberg W, Rauws E, Schipper M. Detection of *Campylobacter pylori* in stomach tissue by DNA *in situ* hybridisation. *J Clin Pathol* 1989; 42: 995−1000.

56 Kwok S, Higuchi R. Avoiding false positives with PCR. *Nature* 1989; 339: 237−8.

57 Porter-Jordan K, Garret CT. Source of contamination in polymerase chain reaction assay. *Lancet* 1990; 335: 1120.

58 Cone RW, Hobson AC, Huang MLW, Fairfax MR. Polymerase chain reaction decontamination: the wipe test. *Lancet* 1990; ii: 686−7.

59 Deich RA, Anilionis A, Fulginiti J *et al.* Antigenic conservation of the 15 000-dalton outer membrane lipoprotein PCP of *Haemophilus influenzae* and biologic activity of anti-PCP antisera. *Infect Immun* 1990; 58: 3388−93.

60 Larrick JW, Coloma MJ, del-Valle J, Fernandez ME, Fry KE. Immunoglobulin V regions of a bactericidal anti-*Neisseria meningitidis* outer membrane protein monoclonal antibody. *Scand J Immunol* 1990; 32: 121−8.

61 McCafferty J, Griffiths AD, Winter G, Chiswell DJ. Phage antibodies: filamentous phage displaying antibody variable domains. *Nature* 1990; 348: 552−4.

62 Suzuki Y, Orellana MA, Schreiber RD, Remington JS. Interferon-gamma: the major mediator of resistance against *Toxoplasma gondii. Science* 1988; 240: 516−18.

63 Pesanti EL. Interaction of cytokines and alveolar cells with *Pneumocystis carinii in vitro. J Infect Dis* 1991; 163: 611−6.

64 Jaffe HA, Buhl R, Mastrangeli A *et al.* Organ specific cytokine therapy: local activation of mononuclear phagocytes by delivery of an aerosol of recombinant interferon-gamma to the human lung. *J Clin Invest* 1991; 88: 297−302.

9 Molecular biology and respiratory disease

S. BERTEL SQUIRE, VINCENT C. EMERY
AND PAUL D. GRIFFITHS

Introduction

With the exception of adenovirus, viral respiratory syndromes in immuno-competent hosts are all associated with infection by RNA viruses (Table 9.1). The infections tend to be acute and although the symptoms are self-limiting, they are common and are associated with significant morbidity in the general population. For some groups of individuals, however, respiratory syndromes are more serious and, in some cases, may be life threatening. For example, a pneumonia associated with significant mortality, which may be solely viral or due to bacterial super-infection, may develop with influenza infections in elderly individuals or patients with chronic cardiorespiratory disease. Epidemics of acute respiratory disease due to adenovirus may occur in relatively closed communities, such as boarding schools and military camps. The morbidity and mortality associated with viral respiratory disease is greater in children than adults, leading to complications such as otitis media (e.g. following measles) and sinusitis (e.g. following influenza). Also some viruses, such as respiratory syncytial virus (RSV), may cause severe bronchiolitis and pneumonia in infants and small children.

By contrast with the viruses responsible for the majority of respiratory diseases in the normal population, the viruses associated with respiratory syndromes in immunocompromised hosts are all DNA viruses (Table 9.2). The infections are chronic so that recurrent infections (reactivations and reinfections) as well as primary infections can be associated with significant respiratory morbidity and mortality. For example, the mortality from cytomegalovirus (CMV) pneumonitis in bone marrow transplant recipients is 85% if treatment is not given [1].

Clinical management of the spectrum of virus-associated respiratory disease has evolved around strategies for prevention, specific diagnosis, understanding of disease processes and treatment. Molecular biological techniques apply to all of these areas although at present the potential of these techniques has not been fully realized in the clinical setting. This chapter aims to review the current state of molecular biological applications in the diagnosis and treatment of viral lung disease and highlight areas for future exploitation.

Table 9.1 Major viral causes of lower respiratory tract disease in immunocompetent hosts (all examples can also cause upper respiratory tract syndromes)

Genome	Children	Adults	Prevention	Treatment
RNA	RESPIRATORY SYNCYTIAL VIRUS		None	Nebulized ribavirin
RNA	PARAINFLUENZA VIRUSES	Parainfluenza viruses	None	None
RNA	MEASLES		Live vaccine	None
RNA	INFLUENZA	INFLUENZA VIRUSES	Killed vaccines (types A and B); amantidine/ rimantidine (type A)	Amantidine/rimantidine (type A)
RNA	Rhinoviruses	Rhinoviruses	None	Hot air
RNA	Coronaviruses		None	None
DNA	Adenoviruses	ADENOVIRUSES	Live vaccine (experimental)	None
DNA	Varicella zoster virus	Varicella zoster virus	Live vaccine (experimental)	Acyclovir

Relative importance of viruses in causing disease in the different patient groups is indicated by the use of capitals or lower case.

Table 9.2 Major causes of lower respiratory tract disease in immunocompromised hosts

Genome	Virus	Prevention	Treatment
DNA	CYTOMEGALOVIRUS	Screening of blood products: acyclovir, immunoglobulin, ganciclovir	Intravenous immunoglobulin plus ganciclovir
DNA	Herpes simplex virus	Acyclovir	Acyclovir
DNA	Varicella zoster virus	Live vaccine (experimental)	Acyclovir

Relative importance of viruses in causing disease in the different patient groups is indicated by the use of capitals or lower case.

Application to prevention of viral respiratory disease

Molecular biology has much to offer in the development of vaccines to respiratory viruses. This has been demonstrated by recent work on influenza where molecular techniques have allowed the detailed structure of the major immunogenic proteins of the virus to be defined. Thus, X-ray diffraction has been used to define the crystal structure of the surface proteins haemagglutinin and neuraminidase [2] and to define genetic variants which have mutated to escape antibody-mediated neutralization.

Haemagglutinin has been expressed in vaccinia virus to produce a vaccine which protects mice against influenza [3]. Likewise, cyclic peptides derived from haemagglutinin can be immunogenic and provide protection against infection [4]. Antibody levels can be enhanced if haemagglutinin or neuraminidase molecules are incorporated into liposomes [5].

Molecular techniques also have the potential to present authentic viral proteins to the immune system without selection by *in vitro* culture. For example, when clinical specimens are inoculated into embryonated hens' eggs and into mammalian cells, the eggs tend to select for variants with particular point mutations [6], presumably because these replicate better in eggs. It has been shown that the strains propagated in mammalian cells for vaccine production provide better protection against challenge in the ferret model than do the strains propagated in eggs [7].

Cell-mediated immune responses to internal structural proteins of influenza may also be protective; for example, nucleoprotein can induce T-helper responses [8]. The T-cell response against nucleoprotein is broader than the B-cell response against haemagglutinin so that immunization with one subtype of influenza A can provide cross-protection against others [3].

Finally, molecular reassortment of the segmented RNA genome of a human influenza strain has been performed with avian strains. The reassortants were tested in human volunteers and shown to be attenuated with respect to the parent human strain [9]. Such studies are potentially important because the haemagglutinin gene from any new pandemic human strain could potentially be reassorted into well-characterized recipient strains to produce high titre vaccine candidates rapidly.

Application to the diagnosis of viral respiratory disease

Traditional methods of detecting viruses associated with respiratory disease have relied upon detecting specific humoral host immune responses (i.e. serological assays) and characteristic cytopathic effects of virus replication in cell culture. Although simple to carry out, the detection of humoral immune responses is an indirect method giving information about infection of the host with a given virus, without necessarily giving information on the contribution of this infection to respiratory pathology. For diagnostic purposes, seroconversion should be clearly demonstrated, and this may not be possible either because there is pre-existing immunity or because, in immunocompromised hosts, humoral immune responses may be impaired. Finally, diagnostic information may not be available for several weeks which does not allow time for consideration of treatment options. If convalescent samples are required, only retrospective diagnoses can be made.

Cell culture followed by the demonstration of characteristic cytopathic effects (with or without visualization of characteristic virus particles by electron microscopy) has the advantage of direct detection of the virus in respiratory samples. However, these are laborious and time-consuming techniques and, again, may not give diagnostic information for several weeks. In some cases they prove impossible due to microbial contamination of specimens, non-infectious virus (for example, the presence of defective particles, inactivation or neutralization), difficulties with transport media and lack of susceptibility of the cultured cells to the viral agent.

With the development of monoclonal antibody technology, it has become possible to detect viral antigens either by enzyme immunoassays (EIAs) or immunofluorescence (IF) and these techniques have been used effectively in the development of rapid diagnostic tests. Viral antigens can either be detected directly on respiratory samples [10], or on infected cells in culture before full cytopathic effects have evolved [11]. The major disadvantage of these techniques has been the lack of sensitivity. They require the presence of sufficient viral replication in the tissue sampled either: (1) to lead to the expression of detectable quantities of viral antigens on the sample cells; or (2) to generate virus that is capable of infecting cultured cells.

It has therefore become an attractive proposition to pursue the

demonstration of viral nucleotide sequences in clinical samples for diagnosis. These techniques may in the future be more rapid and sensitive
than the techniques described above. In addition, they allow quantitation
of the viral nucleic acid which may have prognostic benefit.

Nucleic acid hybridization

Specific viral oligonucleotide probes can be used to anneal to viral RNA
or DNA either directly on biopsy sections or cytological preparations of
lung washings or respiratory secretions (*in situ* hybridization), or on
fragments of DNA produced by restriction endonuclease digestion followed by immobilization on suitable membranes (Southern blotting) or
alternatively on RNA samples transferred on to membranes (Northern
blotting). The probes used in such analyses are usually radioactively
labelled and visualized by autoradiography although, more recently, labels
such as biotin, fluorescein and digoxigenin have been used for probe
labelling. The aforementioned techniques have the advantage that they
can be used on fixed tissue specimens and they provide a permanent
record. *In situ* hybridization will allow localization of virus within tissues
and, sometimes, cell types. However, the technique requires samples to
be processed and fixed before cell lysis occurs and is unsuitable for
samples where the cellular morphology has not been reasonably well
preserved.

It is worth noting some of the disadvantages of these techniques. For
instance, false-positive results can arise from the hybridization of the
plasmid vector DNA (used to propagate the specific probes) to bacterial
DNA sequences in the sample. Appropriate controls have, therefore, to
be included in these assays. The choice of probe is important: it should
lie within a region that is abundantly transcribed in infected cells but is
relatively conserved among different strains of virus and should not
cross-hybridize with other viral or host nucleic acid sequences. Owing
to the presence of RNAases in clinical samples specialized fixation and
extraction procedures may have to be used to preserve RNA target
sequences, as has been demonstrated in the detection of rhinoviruses
[12].

In spite of these caveats the techniques involved can be carried out
within a day and may provide rapid diagnostic information.

Nucleic acid amplification techniques

Although the polymerase chain reaction (PCR) is the most well-known
nucleic acid amplification technology, the ligase chain reaction (LCR),
nucleic acid sequence-based amplification (NASBA) and the Q-β-replicase
methods will all find applications in diagnostic virology.

Specific DNA sequences from the DNA viruses can be amplified directly from respiratory samples by the PCR while complementary DNA (cDNA) sequences can be amplified from the RNA viruses following the use of reverse transcriptase. In either case the PCR provides an extremely sensitive method of detecting viruses in samples. However, the identification of viruses by this method requires some specific considerations. First, as with the hybridization techniques described above, primers used should be conserved within a species and should not cross-hybridize significantly with host or other viral DNA and RNA. Second, the target sequence for amplification is usually in the range 100−500 base pairs and third, the signal generated requires authentication by hybridization to an internal probe and/or reamplification with a nested set of oligonucleotide primers [13]. Strain-specific authentication may require more sophisticated analysis of the amplimers such as restriction enzyme digestion or direct DNA sequencing.

The exquisite sensitivity of the PCR and related techniques means that viral sequences may be detected in samples from asymptomatic patients or an apparently undiseased respiratory tract. Thus, while a positive PCR result will often diagnose infection, in some circumstances it may prove to be of little prognostic value in making decisions on clinical management. The availability of quantitative enzyme amplification methodologies should circumvent these problems. In addition, problems frequently arise with contamination from amplified material or plasmid DNA used as positive controls within the reaction. Thus stringent measures must be effected to overcome contamination, for example irradiation of the buffer components with ultraviolet [14]. At present these techniques have only been applied in the research laboratory; however, it is to be expected that within the next 5 years nucleic acid-based amplification techniques will take their place in the array of diagnostic tests.

Use of nucleotide hybridization and gene amplification in the diagnosis of specific viral infections associated with respiratory disease

Respiratory syncytial virus

RSV is a non-segmented, negative strand RNA virus and the major cause of bronchiolitis and pneumonia in infants and children. Most children are infected before reaching 2 years of age and recurrent infections are frequent. In infants, primary infection may be severe and require hospital care, while infections in children with congenital heart defects are frequently lethal. Reinfections in the elderly can also be associated with significant respiratory morbidity and mortality. In all of these patient groups, nosocomial acquisition can be very important and early positive diagnosis has become increasingly important to ensure maximum benefit from aerosol ribavirin therapy [15]. In a recent study a cDNA probe complementary to the RSV nucleocapsid protein gene was used to compare the sensitivity and specificity of hybridization with EIA and IF for the detection of RSV in nasopharyngeal aspirates [16]. Compared with IF, hybridization had a sensitivity of 49% and a specificity of 66%. Compared with EIA, hybridization had a sensitivity of 60% and a specificity of 92%. These disappointing results were obtained on frozen samples and the authors anticipated improved results with fresh clinical samples.

Adequate nasopharyngeal sampling for viral diagnosis requires the retrieval of significant numbers of exfoliated cells. The use of a human DNA probe to quantify the numbers of host cells obtained in nasopharyngeal samples has shown that nasopharyngeal aspiration is a superior sampling technique to nasopharyngeal swabbing for the diagnosis of RSV [17].

Influenza viruses

Influenza viruses are negative strand RNA viruses with segmented genomes and classified as orthomyxoviruses. Infections are typically associated with upper respiratory tract symptoms such as coryza and cough along with fever, myalgia and malaise. In addition, infection can lead to bronchitis and pneumonia in the elderly, infants and children. There has been a description of the detection of influenza virus in nasopharyngeal samples by hybridization, but no indication of specificity or sensitivity was given [18]. The use of molecular biology in the diagnosis of influenza infections has been overshadowed by its use in the development of vaccines and in structure−function studies on the neuraminidase and haemagglutinin proteins.

Adenoviruses

Adenoviruses are DNA viruses associated with several types of disease, particularly in children and young adults. As already described, in adults they can cause episodic outbreaks of pneumonia in relatively closed communities. As with other viruses, virus isolation and serology are the conventional approaches for viral diagnosis, but IF and immunoassays have contributed to rapid diagnosis, without, unfortunately, improving sensitivity [19]. The results of initial studies using DNA hybridization were confounded by false-positives due to cross-reaction of the sample with vector DNA sequences. These have been overcome by using a DNA sandwich hybridization assay with two different DNA probes. This assay has been used to screen children [20] and military recruits [21] but the sensitivity was no better than conventional radioimmunoassays. This lack of increased sensitivity was also found in a study of dot-blot hybridization using RNA transcripts as a means of avoiding the problem of vector DNA contamination [22]. These studies were carried out using radioactive labels, but similar results have been obtained using biotinylated DNA probes and fluorescein-labelled complementary RNA [23].

Herpes simplex virus

Herpes simplex virus (HSV) is a herpesvirus which is not usually associated with respiratory disease in immunocompetent hosts. However, there are reports of significant HSV pneumonia in bone marrow transplant recipients [24]. Hybridization techniques have been used for detection of HSV in cerebrospinal and vesicle fluid [22], but have not been evaluated fully in lung samples where conventional cell culture usually provides a diagnosis within 5 days.

Cytomegalovirus

CMV is also a member of the herpesvirus group, but unlike HSV is classically associated with severe disease in immunocompromised hosts. Respiratory disease associated with CMV differs among the various groups of immunocompromised patients such that human immunodeficiency virus infected patients do not appear to suffer from the life-threatening CMV pneumonia that affects recipients of allogeneic transplants [25, 26], especially bone marrow transplant recipients [1]. As recent therapeutic regimens using a combination of ganciclovir and intravenous immunoglobulin [27, 28] have started to improve mortality rates, rapid diagnostic tests for lung samples, notably bronchoalveolar lavage (BAL), have become increasingly important. The direct use of fluorescent-labelled monoclonal antibodies on lung samples and on cell cultures incubated with lung samples has dramatically improved the speed of detection of CMV over that achieved with conventional cell culture without compromising sensitivity and specificity [11].

A number of studies have used *in situ* hybridization to diagnose CMV pneumonitis [29−32]. In general, sensitivity was not improved, hence at present, the complicated methodology required for *in situ* hybridization on lung biopsies means that it is reserved for cases where conventional histology or culture are equivocal. Unfortunately, when hybridization has been applied to samples obtained by the less invasive technique of BAL it has not proved as sensitive as existing cell culture techniques combined with IF [33] although evaluation of new probes and labels is continuing [34].

PCR has been shown to be of equivalent [35] or increased [36] sensitivity when compared with hybridization techniques in detecting CMV in lung biopsy specimens from bone marrow transplant recipients with pneumonitis. However, it has not yet been evaluated in a prospective manner on BAL specimens.

Application to understanding pathogenesis of viral respiratory disease

As described earlier, *in situ* hybridization can provide information on the localization of virus within tissues, and even to cell types that can be distinguished by morphology and conventional histological staining [37]. However, in pathological studies in which it is important to discover what subsets of cell types are infected, double staining of cells with monoclonal antibodies against viral antigens and cell phenotypic markers is superior. In general, activated immune cells are easily identified using monoclonal antibodies; however, *in situ* hybridization can be used to localize cells producing messenger RNA (mRNA) for cytokines such as the tumour necrosis factor [38]. The advantage of *in situ* hybridization is that it can be applied to formalin-fixed, paraffin-embedded samples derived from a variety of sources, e.g. autopsy material. In general, monoclonal antibodies cannot be used on these types of tissue.

The sensitivity afforded by hybridization, and particularly by PCR, has led to screening of samples for viruses in diseases not usually associated with a viral aetiology as with adenoviruses in follicular bronchiectasis [39]. A variation on this theme has been to search for several different viruses in patients with lung conditions classically associated with one virus type such as in pneumonia in heart–lung transplant [32, 35] and bone marrow transplant [40] recipients.

Understanding the pathogenesis of viral infections often requires the identification of particular strains of a virus species either to follow their transmission and epidemiology in the general population, or to help in distinguishing reactivations of latent virus within a host, or reinfection with a new strain. Molecular biology has long been important in this process through the use of restriction enzyme analysis (REA) [41]. Probing these fragments with DNA and RNA probes has refined the technique from recognition of oligonucleotides according to length to recognition according to particular viral genes. In addition, REA requires considerable quantities of viral DNA or RNA which traditionally involved time-consuming cell culture and virus propagation. PCR now provides a means of amplifying viral DNA or RNA from clinical samples where it may only be present in small quantities [31]. In all of these situations, quantification of viruses by molecular techniques will provide important information on viral pathogenesis [30, 42].

Application to treatment of viral respiratory disease

Understanding pathogenetic mechanisms leads to advances in thera-peutics and molecular biology stands to contribute most to treatment of viral respiratory disease in this way. However, molecular techniques have been used to identify genes conferring resistance to treatment with rimantidine in influenza. When rimantidine was given to patients with influenza A and their family contacts and compared with families given placebo, it became clear that the rimantidine-treated group did not have a reduced incidence of either symptomatic or asymptomatic influenza infections [43]. It was shown that resistant strains of influenza A were responsible, and that resistance was conferred by mutations consisting of single amino acid changes in the M2 protein of the virus [43]. In addition to this type of study, molecular techniques may have some contribution to the assessment of antiviral agents in cell culture to replace time-consuming plaque-reduction assays [44].

Conclusions

The techniques of nucleic acid hybridization and gene amplification have been refined considerably in the last 5 years to tailor their use to the diagnosis of viral respiratory diseases. Despite the widespread use of molecular technology in research laboratories the application of these technologies in the diagnostic laboratory is still in its infancy. However, it is important to remember that in many cases these techniques have not yet been shown to be superior to traditional techniques or the techniques ushered in by the advent of monoclonal antibodies. This partly explains why such techniques are not yet in widespread clinical use. It is to be expected that, as more antiviral agents become available and the pressure for rapid, sensitive diagnostic tests increases, this situation is bound to change.

References

1 Meyers JD, Fluornoy N, Thomas ED. Risk factors for cytomegalovirus infections after human marrow transplantation. *J Infect Dis* 1986; 153: 478–88.
2 Air GM, Laver WG. The neuraminidase of influenza virus. *Proteins* 1989; 6: 341–56.
3 Endo A, Itamura S, Iinuma H *et al*. Homotypic and heterotypic protection against influenza virus infection in mice by recombinant vaccinia virus expressing the haemagglutinin or nucleoprotein of influenza virus. *J Gen Virol* 1991; 72: 699–703.
4 Muller S, Plaue S, Samama JP, Valette M, Briand JP, Van-Regenmortel MH. Antigenic properties and protective capacity of a cyclic peptide corresponding to site A of influenza virus haemagglutinin. *Vaccine* 1990; 8: 308–14.
5 Nerome K, Yoshioka Y, Ishida M *et al*. Development of a new type of influenza subunit vaccine made by muramyldipeptide-liposome: enhancement of humoral and cellular immune responses. *Vaccine* 1990; 8: 503–9.
6 Oxford JS, Newman R, Corcoran T *et al*. Direct isolation in eggs of influenza A (H1N1) and B viruses with haemagglutinins of different antigenic and amino acid composition. *J Gen Virol* 1991; 72: 185–9.
7 Katz JM, Webster RG. Efficacy of inactivated influenza A virus (H3N2) vaccines grown in mammalian cells or embryonated eggs. *J Infect Dis* 1989; 160: 191–8.
8 Tite JP, Hughes-Jenkins C, O'Callaghan D *et al*. Anti-viral immunity induced by

recombinant nucleoprotein of influenza A virus. II. Protection from influenza infection and mechanism of protection. *Immunology* 1990; 71: 202−7.

9 Clements ML, Sears SD, Christina K, Murphy BR, Snyder MH. Comparison of the virologic and immunologic responses of volunteers to live avian−human influenza A H3N2 reassortant virus vaccines derived from two different avian influenza virus donors. *J Clin Microbiol* 1989; 27: 219−22.

10 Hughes JH, Mann DR, Hamparian VV. Detection of respiratory syncytial virus in clinical specimens by viral culture, direct and indirect immunofluorescence, and enzyme immunoassay. *J Clin Microbiol* 1988; 26: 588−91.

11 Griffiths PD, Panjwani DD, Stirk PR *et al*. Rapid diagnosis of cytomegalovirus infection in immunocompromised patients by detection of early antigen fluorescent foci. *Lancet* 1984; ii: 1242−5.

12 Al-Nakib W, Stanway G, Forsyth M, Hughes PJ, Almond JW, Tyrrell DA. Detection of human rhinoviruses and their molecular relationship using cDNA probes. *J Med Virol* 1986; 20: 289−96.

13 Porter-Jordan K, Rosenberg EI, Keiser JF *et al*. Nested polymerase chain reaction assay for the detection of cytomegalovirus overcomes false positives caused by contamination with fragmented DNA. *J Med Virol* 1990; 30: 85−91.

14 Fox JC, Ait-Khaled M, Webster A, Emery VC. Eliminating PCR contamination: is UV irradiation the answer? *J Virol Methods* 1991; 33: 375−82.

15 Hall CB, McBride JT, Walsh EE *et al*. Aerosolised ribavirin treatment of infants with respiratory syncytial viral infection. A randomised double-blind study. *N Engl J Med* 1983; 308: 1443−7.

16 Van-Dyke RB, Murphy-Corb M. Detection of respiratory syncytial virus in naso-pharyngeal secretions by DNA−RNA hybridization. *J Clin Microbiol* 1989; 27: 1739−43.

17 Ahluwalia G, Embree J, McNicol P, Law B, Hammond GW. Comparison of nasopharyngeal aspirate and nasopharyngeal swab specimens for respiratory syn-cytial virus diagnosis by cell culture, indirect immunofluorescence assay, and enzyme-linked immunosorbent assay. *J Clin Microbiol* 1987; 25: 763−7.

18 Pljusnin AZ, Rozhdova SA, Nolandt OV, Bryandtseva EA, Kuznetsov OD, Noskov FS. Molecular hybridisation with DNA-probes as a laboratory diagnostic test for influenza viruses. *Virologie* 1987; 38: 111−14.

19 Harmon MW, Pawlik KM. Enzyme immunoassay for direct detection of influenza type A and adenovirus antigens in clinical specimens. *J Clin Microbiol* 1982; 15: 5−11.

20 Virtanen M, Palva A, Laaksonen M, Halonen P, Soderlund H, Ranki M. Novel test for rapid viral diagnosis: detection of adenovirus in nasopharyngeal mucus aspirates by means of nucleic acid sandwich hybridisation. *Lancet* 1983; i: 381−3.

21 Lehtomaki K, Julkunen I, Sandelin K *et al*. Rapid diagnosis of respiratory adenovirus infections in young adult men. *J Clin Microbiol* 1986; 24: 108−11.

22 Schuster V, Matz B, Wiegand H, Traub B, Neumann-Haefelin D. Detection of herpes simplex virus and adenovirus DNA by dot blot hybridization using *in vitro* synthesized RNA transcripts. *J Virol Methods* 1986; 13: 291−9.

23 Gomes SA, Nascimento JP, Siqueira MM, Krawczuk MM, Pereira HG, Russell WC. *In situ* hybridization with biotinylated DNA probes: a rapid diagnostic test for adenovirus upper respiratory infections. *J Virol Methods* 1985; 12: 105−10.

24 Ramsay PG, Fife KH, Hackman RC, Meyers JD, Corey L. Herpes simplex virus pneumonia. Clinical, virologic, and pathologic features in 20 patients. *Ann Intern Med* 1982; 97: 813−20.

25 Grundy JE, Shanley JD, Griffiths PD. Is cytomegalovirus pneumonitis in allogeneic transplant recipients an immunopathological condition? *Lancet* 1987; ii: 996−9.

26 Millar AB, Patou G, Miller RF *et al*. Cytomegalovirus in the lungs of patients with

AIDS: respiratory pathogen or passenger? *Am Rev Respir Dis* 1990; 141: 1474–7.

27 Emmanual D, Cunningham I, Jules-Elysee K *et al.* Cytomegalovirus pneumonia after bone marrow transplantation successfully treated with the combination of ganciclovir and high-dose intravenous immune globulin. *Ann Intern Med* 1988; 109: 777–82.

28 Reed EC, Bowden RA, Dandliker MSN, Lilleby KE, Meyers JD. Treatment of cytomegalovirus pneumonia with ganciclovir and intravenous cytomegalovirus immunoglobulin in patients with bone marrow transplants. *Ann Intern Med* 1988; 109: 783–8.

29 Myerson D, Hackman RC, Meyers JD. Diagnosis of cytomegaloviral pneumonia by *in situ* hybridization. *J Infect Dis* 1984; 150: 272–7.

30 Einsele H, Vallbracht A, Jahn G, Kandolf R, Muller CA. Hybridization techniques provide improved sensitivity for HCMV detection and allow quantitation of the virus in clinical samples. *J Virol Methods* 1989; 26: 91–104.

31 Churchill MA, Zaia JA, Forman SJ, Sheibani K, Azumi N, Blume KG. Quantitation of human cytomegalovirus DNA in lungs from bone marrow transplant recipients with interstitial pneumonia. *J Infect Dis* 1987; 155: 501–9.

32 Weiss LM, Movahed LA, Berry GJ, Billingham ME. *In situ* hybridization studies for viral nucleic acids in heart and lung allograft biopsies [see comments]. *Am J Clin Pathol* 1990; 93: 675–9.

33 Gleaves CA, Hursh DA, Rice DH, Meyers JD. Detection of cytomegalovirus from clinical specimens in centrifugation culture by *in situ* DNA hybridization and monoclonal antibody staining. *J Clin Microbiol* 1989; 27: 21–3.

34 McClintock JT, Thaker SR, Mosher M *et al.* Comparison of *in situ* hybridization and monoclonal antibodies for early detection of cytomegalovirus in cell culture. *J Clin Microbiol* 1989; 27: 1554–9.

35 Jiwa M, Steenbergen RD, Zwaan FE, Kluin PM, Raap AK, van-der-Ploeg M. Three sensitive methods for the detection of cytomegalovirus in lung tissue of patients with interstitial pneumonitis. *Am J Clin Pathol* 1990; 93: 491–4.

36 Einsele H, Steidle M, Vallbracht A, Saal JG, Ehninger G, Muller CA. Early occurrence of human cytomegalovirus infection after bone marrow transplantation as demonstrated by the polymerase chain reaction technique. *Blood* 1991; 77: 1104–10.

37 Dankner WM, McCutchan JA, Richman DD, Hirata K, Spector SA. Localization of human cytomegalovirus in peripheral blood leukocytes by *in situ* hybridization. *J Infect Dis* 1990; 161: 31–6.

38 Wakamiya N, Stone R, Takeyama H, Spriggs D, Kufe D. Detection of tumor necrosis factor gene expression at a cellular level in human acute myeloid leukaemias. *Leukaemia* 1989; 3: 51–6.

39 Hogg JC, Irving WL, Porter H, Evans M, Dunnill MS, Fleming K. *In situ* hybridization studies of adenoviral infections of the lung and their relationship to follicular bronchiectasis. *Am Rev Respir Dis* 1989; 139: 1531–5.

40 Carrigan DR, Drobyski WR, Russler SK, Tapper MA, Knox KK, Ash RC. Interstitial pneumonitis associated with human herpesvirus-6 infection after marrow transplantation. *Lancet* 1991; 338: 147–9.

41 Huang ES, Alford CA, Reynolds DW, Stagno S, Pass RF. Molecular epidemiology of cytomegalovirus infections in women and their infants. *N Engl J Med* 1980; 303; 958–62.

42 Saltzman RL, Quirk MR, Mariash CN, Jordan MC. Quantitation of cytomegalovirus DNA by blot hybridization in blood leukocytes of viremic patients. *J Virol Methods* 1990; 30: 67–77.

43 Hayden FG, Belshe RB, Clover RD, Hay AJ, Oakes MG, Soo W. Emergence and apparent transmission of rimantidine-resistant influenza A virus in families.

N Engl J Med 1989; 321: 1696−702.

44 Dankner WM, Scholl D, Stanat SC, Martin M, Sonke RL, Spector SA. Rapid antiviral DNA−DNA hybridization assay for human cytomegalovirus. *J Virol Methods* 1990; 28: 293−8.

10 Application to pathology

JAMES C. HOGG

Introduction

Pathologists have the privilege of examining human lung tissue that has been either resected during life or obtained at autopsy. This examination traditionally involves the macroscopic study of the gross specimen followed by microscopic examination of smaller samples selected from it. The histology of the lung is usually evaluated using a standard staining procedure such as haematoxylin and eosin (H&E) followed by special stains that are used to examine specific structural features of both normal and diseased lung. Relatively recently this traditional process has been enhanced by the introduction of new techniques that allow specific identification of molecules of DNA, RNA and protein. These powerful methods have improved the pathologist's ability to examine the structure of the normal lung, to investigate its growth and ageing and begin to understand the aetiology and pathogenesis of many of the disease processes which affect it.

This chapter will attempt to provide a brief review of the methods available to the pathologist to study the three basic levels of molecular organization (i.e. DNA, RNA and protein) in the lung. The value of these new techniques will be illustrated primarily by studies of the inflammatory response in smokers' lungs and recent studies of adenoviral infection in human lungs rather than by an extensive review of the literature.

The detection and localization of specific proteins in human lungs

The ability to demonstrate proteins and other complex molecules in tissue is based on an application of the principles that are involved in binding antibodies to antigens. The first step in detecting the target molecule of interest in a histological specimen is to apply an appropriate primary antibody to bind to it. Because this primary antibody–antigen complex is invisible, secondary steps are required to visualize the target with either the light or electron microscope. These secondary procedures all follow the general principle of linking the primary antigen–antibody complex to a visible detection system.

Antibodies are immunoglobulin molecules of approximately 150 000 kD molecular weight that consist of one pair of light chains each of 25 000 kD and one pair of heavy chains each of 50 000 kD bound together by disulphide bridges. The binding site or Fab fragment of the molecule is located on the terminal end of each light chain—heavy chain pair where the specificity of the binding site is determined by the amino acid sequences of the light and heavy chain. The sequences present at an antigen-binding site are referred to as the antibody's idiotype and are specific for each antigen. The end of the immunoglobulin molecule opposite the binding site shows less variation in amino acid sequence and is referred to as the constant region or Fc fragment.

Large molecules usually have several antigenic determinants or epitopes, each of which is dependent on a unique three-dimensional structure. The key to the second step procedures used to visualize the target molecule is the use of epitopes in the Fc fragment of the immuno-globulin molecule of one species to raise antibodies in a second. For example, the constant region of the murine immunoglobulin G (IgG) can be used to immunize a rabbit. Tracer molecules can then be attached to the rabbit antimurine IgG and linked to the protruding Fc fragment of the primary antibody—target antigen complex. The sensitivity of demon-strating the primary target has been greatly increased by a technique developed by Cordell et al. [1]. This is achieved by first adding the secondary antibody in great excess which allows some molecules to bind to the Fc fragment of the primary antibody with only one valency. A reagent [1] made by complexing a murine antibody against alkaline phosphatase to alkaline phosphatase (an alkaline phosphatase—anti-alkaline phosphatase or APAAP complex) is then added in excess. The free valency of the linkage antibody binds to the extended Fc fragment of the APAAP reagent joining the complex to the primary antibody. This brings a high concentration of alkaline phosphatase to the site of the primary antibody target molecule complex and provides a very sensitive technique for demonstrating the target antigen.

These immunocytochemical techniques have been widely used to characterize cells and tissues in nearly all the organs of the body in both health and disease [2]. With respect to the lung, they have been particu-larly useful in determining the cell types present in the inflammatory response in the airways of patients with asthma [3, 4] and of cigarette smokers with obstructive lung disease [5]. Plate 10.1 (facing p. 164) is an example from the recent work of Bosken et al. [5] where the CD8$^+$ T-suppressor cells (Plate 10.1a) demonstrated by the APAAP method are seen lined up along the base of the epithelium as well as scattered in small numbers throughout the airways wall. The monocyte line stained with the anti-CD68 antibody contains cells with variable morphologies that include large, smooth-edged alveolar macrophages within the air space as well as cells in the airways wall that have a dendritic appearance.

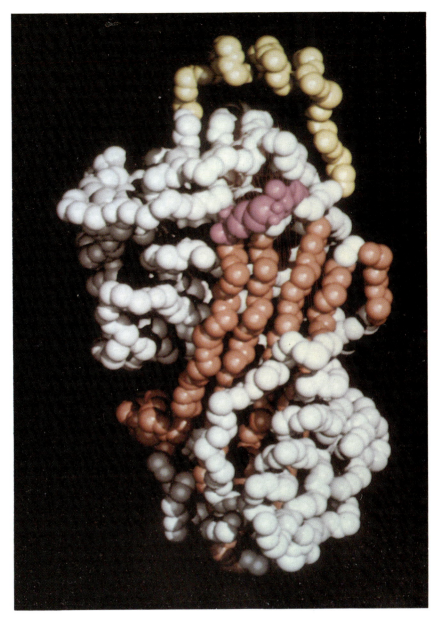

Plate 6.1 Ray tracing of α_1-antitrypsin modelled on ovalbumin. The reactive loop is shown in yellow, the β-pleated sheets in brown and the lysine (290)−glutamic acid (342) salt bridge in purple.

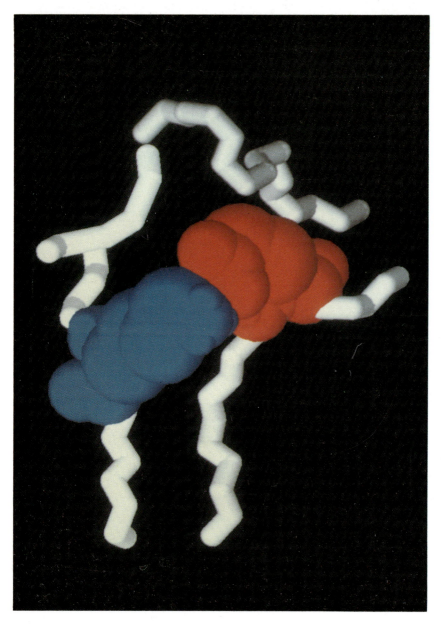

Plate 6.2 Licorice diagram of α_1-antitrypsin modelled on ovalbumin. The van der Waals forces of lysine (290) and glutamic acid (342) are shown in blue and red, respectively, to illustrate their ability to form a salt bridge.

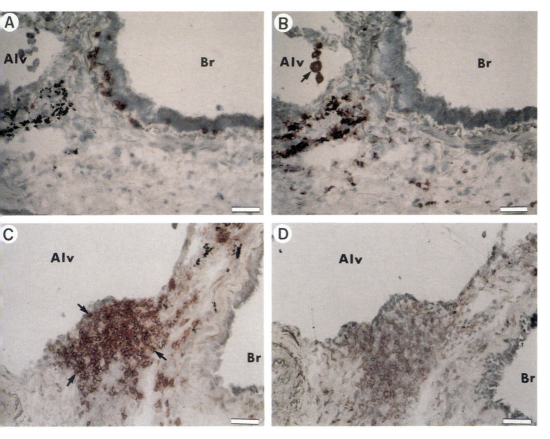

Plate 10.1 (A) Small airways treated with monoclonal antibody against CD8 where positive cells can be seen lining up against the basement membrane. (B) Same airways as in (A) stained with monoclonal antibody CD68, which reacts with cells of the monocytic line. This antibody stains alveolar macrophages (arrow) and tissue macrophages present in the airway wall. (C) Lymphoid nodule in the airway wall treated with a monoclonal antibody against CD19 which stains the surface of the β-lymphocytes. This shows that the lymphatic nodule is in the outer wall of the airways and bulges into the alveolar lumen and contains many β-cells. (D) The same airways as in (C) treated with antibody against CD4, which stains numerous T lymphocytes in the nodule and throughout the airway wall (Alv = alveolus; Br = bronchial lumen). (From Bosken *et al.* [5] with permission.)

Bosken *et al.* [5] also found that the mean polymorphonucleocyte (PMN) count (CD35$^+$ cells) in the airways wall was related to the total amount smoked (CD35$^+$ cells = 15.1 + 0.083* cigarette years; $r = 0.541$, $P < 0.02$) but there were no statistically significant differences in the number of PMNs in the airways of patients from either the obstructed or non-obstructed groups ($P = 0.071$). Although cigarette smokers with airways obstruction had more β-cells (CD19) in the adventitia of the small airways than patients with normal airways function, the total cell count was not affected by this increase in β-cells because they accounted for less than 15% of the total inflammatory cell population in the airways wall (Fig. 10.1). However, this increase in β-cells in the airways of smokers with obstructive lung disease is interesting because of the documented association between cigarette smoking, elevated levels of serum IgE and airways obstruction [6].

Bosken *et al.* [5] also found that the bronchial-associated lymphoid tissue (BALT) present in the airways of cigarette smokers differed in location from the classically described BALT in rodents [7−9]. The nodules in human lungs contained a core of densely packed CD19$^+$ β-cells and a moderate number of CD4$^+$ T-helper cells (Fig. 10.1c and d). Quantitative studies showed that the nodules consisted of 55% CD19 cells (range 42−70%), 23% CD4 cells (range 1−40%), 10% CD8 cells

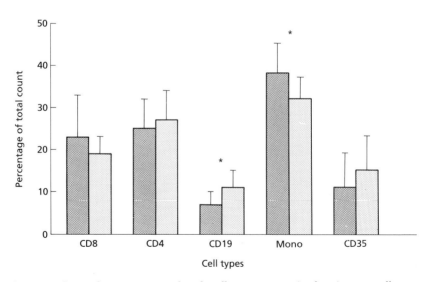

Fig. 10.1 Shows the percentage of each cell type present in the airways walls. Monocytes (CD68) were the most numerous followed by CD4 and CD8 lymphocytes. The β-cells (CD19) and PMNs (CD35) were observed less frequently. The airways from patients with airways obstruction contained a greater percentage of β-cells (CD19) ($P<0.05$) and a slightly lower percentage of monocytes ($P<0.05$) than airways from patients with normal function. The dark grey bars represent the control group; the light grey bars represent patients with airways obstruction (mean ± SEM). (From Bosken CH, Hards J, Catter K, Hogg JC. *Am Rev Respir Dis* 1992; 145: 911−17.)

(4−25%) and 12% macrophages (range 2−22%) with no differences between patients with airways obstruction and controls. In rodents the BALT lies in the submucosa, bulges into the bronchial lumen and is covered by a flattened epithelium lacking cilia. However, in humans Bosken *et al.* [5] reported the BALT to be more frequently found in the outer airways wall where it protruded into the adjacent air space rather than the bronchial lumen. The position of the lymphoid nodules in humans suggests that in cigarette smokers the uptake of antigen may occur in the lympho-epithelial structures located in the outer wall of the small airways. This site could be important in processing antigens present in the very small particulate or gas phase of cigarette smoke because these antigens would penetrate to the alveolar surface of the lung whereas larger particulates deposit in the central airways.

Pabst and Gehrke [9] have reported that BALT was not found in human lungs in the absence of a history of respiratory infection. This conclusion is based on an interspecies comparative study where no BALT was found in 34 human autopsies. Bosken *et al.* [5], however, found BALT in 65% of the lungs examined, but only in approximately one in five airways. This suggests that these lymphatic collections are easily missed if only a few airways are examined. Furthermore, the patients in Bosken *et al.*'s studies were all cigarette smokers while the smoking status of the patients described by Pabst [9] is uncertain. It is possible that cigarette smoking promotes the development of the lymphoid nodules by providing a chronic antigenic stimulus to the respiratory tract.

These and other studies show that the development of immunocyto-chemistry has made it possible to study the inflammatory reaction in the human lung in great detail. These techniques, plus the growing availability of antibodies to a wide variety of molecules that characterize tissues, cells, cytokines, hormones and other substances, have greatly enhanced the pathologist's ability to advance our knowledge of the lung in both health and disease.

The detection and localization of nucleic acid in human lungs

Specific nucleic acids present in cells can be detected and localized by hybridizing a complementary probe to them. Very sensitive methods are now available for detecting target DNA or RNA in tissue by first extracting it from the tissue, amplifying the target sequences using the polymerase chain reaction (PCR) [10] and performing standard Southern [11] or Northern [12] blotting procedures for DNA and RNA, respectively. The nucleic acid present on these filters can be semiquantitated by hybridizing a radiolabelled probe to the target sequence, performing autoradiography and quantitating the appropriate bands using densitometric techniques.

The target nucleic acid sequences can also be localized in tissue by using an *in situ* hybridization procedure but the sensitivity (approximately 10 copies per cell) is much less than the filter hybridization procedures which can detect single copies of nucleic acid targets. However, the recent combination of PCR with the *in situ* hybridization procedures [13] has made it possible to detect much lower copy numbers of the target sequence in the cells and tissue of interest.

The hybridization procedures are based on the fact that the two strands forming a nucleic acid duplex are held together by non-covalent forces that are easily disrupted by increasing temperature. The factors which determine the rate and strength of hybridization of one nucleic acid strand to another are critical to successful demonstration of DNA and RNA targets, both *in situ* in tissues and by filter hybridization techniques. Stringency refers to the degree to which hybridization reactions favour the dissociation of nucleic acid duplexes. Among the most important of the factors which determine stringency are: 1, the ionic strength of the hybridization solution; 2, the percentage of guanine−cytosine (GC) pairs; and 3, the length of the duplex molecule.

The ionic strength of the hybridization solution is important because nucleic acid duplexes become stabilized by increasing ionic strength due to the neutralization of the electrostatic repulsive forces between the negatively charged phosphate groups on opposing strands of the DNA duplex. The percentage of GC base pairs in the DNA molecule affects the strength of binding between strands because they contain three hydrogen bonds compared with the two between the adenine−thymine (AT) pairs. Therefore, duplexes with high GC content are more stable than those with a low number of GC pairs. The length of the probe is the third important factor determining hybrid stability because long complementary sequences contain more hydrogen bonds than short ones.

It follows from the above discussion that stringency can be increased by elevating temperature and decreasing salt concentration and by selecting a target sequence that is long and has a high GC content. The addition of formamide to hybridization mixtures further increases stringency because it destabilizes hydrogen bonds. Hybridization reactions performed at low stringencies allow non-specific interactions between less homologous DNA strands. A series of post-hybridization washes at increasing stringency are then frequently used to allow the imperfect hybrids to dissociate and increase the specificity of probe and target interaction.

The technique of *in situ* hybridization enables the precise localization and identification of individual cells containing a specific nucleic acid sequence. Although hybridization in solution occurs most rapidly with long probes of low complexity at high probe concentrations, these conditions do not always apply to *in situ* hybridization reactions in a straightforward manner. For example, in tissue, short probes may provide a better hybridization signal because access to the target DNA may be decreased by the limited diffusion of longer probes to the target site.

Most hybridization reactions are designed to allow the probe to be present in vast excess over the target. Under these conditions, the rate of hybrid formation follows pseudo-first-order kinetics and the time required for half the probe to hybridize to an immobilized DNA target depends primarily on the length of the probe and its concentration. Double-stranded probes create a situation where in addition to hybridization of the probe to the target, there is also re-annealing of the complementary probe strands to each other. This eliminates some of the probe from the desired hybridization reaction and slows the rate of hybrid formation between the probe and the target DNA. The inclusion of the anionic polymer, dextran sulphate, in the hybridization mixture promotes the aggregation of partially overlapping sequences of re-annealed probe molecules and effectively increases the concentration of a single-stranded probe near the target DNA.

Double-stranded complementary DNA probes can be used to detect RNA targets because one strand of the DNA can be made complementary to the RNA target. Alternatively, a DNA duplex can be inserted into a plasmid containing promoters on either side that allow the single strands of the inserted DNA to be copied from either end. A single strand produced by this procedure can then be used as a specific probe for RNA targets utilizing RNA–RNA hybridization. Alternatively, if one is aware of the sequence of the target messenger RNA (mRNA), oligonucleotide probes can be synthesized and purified for use in detecting specific mRNA.

The nucleic acid probes utilized for *in situ* hybridization can be visualized by labelling them with either radioactive or non-radioactive material. The advantage of using radioactive probes is that they can be used in conjunction with a photographic emulsion to obtain quantitative information on single cells by counting the silver grains produced as a result of radioactive decay. The disadvantage is the fact that these methods often require prolonged exposure periods that can be as long as 2 months when tritium is used. ^{35}S and ^{32}P labelling shortens this development time because the decay energy of these isotopes is greater. However, the down side of these higher energy probes is the loss of resolution because the track of the particle is longer.

The non-radioactive detection systems are very similar to those used to identify target molecules of protein and depend on the incorporation of either biotin or digoxigenin into the probe. When biotin is incorporated, it can be linked to an avidin–alkaline phosphatase complex which can then be used to localize the probe target hybrid. The incorporation of digoxigenin into the probe molecule allows it to be detected with a primary antibody against digoxigenin followed by one of the secondary detection systems used for protein detection.

The solution hybridization techniques provide exquisite sensitivity in detecting specific DNA and RNA targets extracted from tissue. When coupled with the PCR technology for amplifying target sequences, these techniques are capable of detecting single copies per cell. The sensitivity of the *in situ* techniques is currently much lower but may improve with the introduction of *in situ* PCR.

Figures 10.2 and 10.3 show examples of how *in situ* hybridization can be used to detect a lytic infection with adenovirus. Figure 10.2a shows a histological preparation of cultured Hep II cells that have been infected with the adenovirus and subjected to the *in situ* hybridization technique with an appropriate probe. The positivity of the experimental cells treated with a specific adenoviral DNA probe over the control cells treated with a non-specific probe is clearly evident.

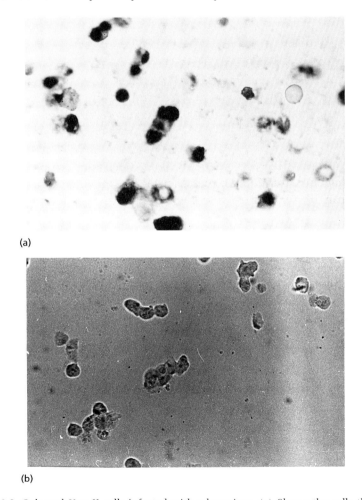

(a)

(b)

Fig. 10.2 Cultured Hep II cells infected with adenovirus. (a) Shows the cells that were treated with a specific probe for the adenovirus where the hybridization studies result in dark staining of the nuclei. (b) Shows the same uninfected cells treated with a non-specific probe where no hybridization resulted.

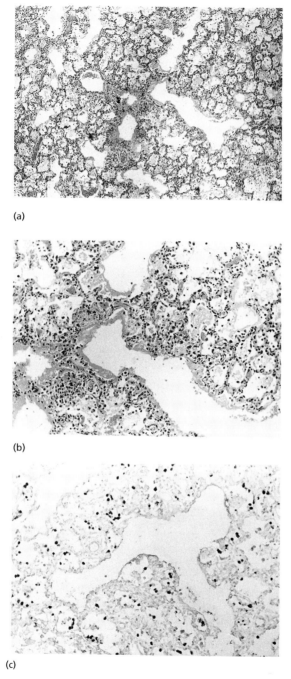

(a)

(b)

(c)

Fig. 10.3 (a) Low power view of a lung with haemorrhagic pulmonary oedema. (b) A higher magnification where the hyaline membrane can be appreciated in the airways. (c) Shows an *in situ* hybridization from the same region where many of the cells stained positively for the adenovirus. The *in situ* hybridization performed in this case was completed in a single working day and therefore provides a powerful diagnostic method for proving that the haemorrhagic pulmonary oedema was due to adenovirus infection.

Figure 10.3 shows a low power view of an H&E section of a lung showing haemorrhagic oedema with hyaline membrane formation (Fig. 10.3a and b). An *in situ* hybridization study of the same area (Fig. 10.3c) shows that this diffuse alveolar injury is caused by a lytic infection with adenovirus which affects many of the cells in the lung. These studies illustrate that DNA hybridization can provide an accurate rapid identification of a viral DNA in an acute infection.

Lytic viral infections, particularly with DNA viruses, are easy to detect with *in situ* hybridization and the method provides a technique for rapid, accurate diagnosis of acute viral lung disease. As antiviral drugs develop, the selection of therapeutic agents appropriate for specific viral pathogens will likely be based on this technique in the same way that sensitivity tests are used to select appropriate antibiotics for bacterial infection. As we are in an era where the current antiviral agents are probably at a level comparable with sulphonamides for bacterial infections, the perfection of both solution and *in situ* hybridization techniques may prove to be valuable in providing rapid, accurate diagnostic procedures needed to evaluate new antiviral agents.

In summary, the development of immunocytochemistry and nucleic acid hybridization technology has greatly enhanced our ability to study the lung in both health and disease. The extreme power of these molecular techniques has only begun to be exploited and they will undoubtedly provide new diagnostic methods as well as better methodology for scientists to ask questions about lung biology and pathology.

References

1 Cordell JL, Falini B, Erber WN *et al*. Immunoenzymatic labelling of monoclonal antibodies using immune complexes of alkaline phosphatase and monoclonal anti-alkaline phosphatase (APAAP complexes). *J Histochem Cytochem* 1984; 32: 219–29.

2 Taylor CR. Immunomicroscopy: a diagnostic tool for the surgical pathologist. In: Benington JL, consulting ed. *Major Problems in Pathology*, Vol. 19. Philadelphia: WB Saunders, 1986; pp. 10–362.

3 Beasley R, Roche WR, Roberts JA, Holgate ST. Cellular events in mild asthma before and after mild provocation. *Am Rev Respir Dis* 1989; 139: 806–17.

4 Holgate ST, Wilson JR, Howarth PH. New insights into airway inflammation by endobronchial biopsy. *Am Rev Respir Dis* 1992; 145: S2–6.

5 Bosken CH, Hards J, Gatter K, Hogg JC. Characterization of the inflammatory reaction in the peripheral airways of cigarette smokers using immunocytochemistry. *Am Rev Respir Dis* 1992; 145: 911–17.

6 Vollmer WM, Buist AS, Johnson LR, McCamant LE, Halonen M. Interactions of smoking and immunologic factors in relation to airways obstruction. *Chest* 1983; 84: 657–61.

7 Berman JS, Beer DJ, Theodore AC, Kornfeld H, Bernardo J, Center DM. Lymphocyte recruitment to the lung. *Am Rev Respir Dis* 1990; 142: 238–57.

8 Fournier M, Vai F, Derenne JP, Pariente H. Bronchial lymphoepithelial nodules in the rat. *Am Rev Respir Dis* 1977; 116: 685–94.

9 Pabst R, Gehrke I. Is the bronchus associated lymphoid tissue (BALT) an integral structure of the lung in normal mammals, including humans? *Am J Respir Cell Mol Biol* 1990; 3: 131−5.

10 Imprain CC, Saiki RK, Erlich HA, Teplitz RL. Analysis of DNA extracted from formalin-fixed paraffin-embedded tissue by enzymatic amplification and hybridization with sequence specific oligonucleotides. *Biochem Biophys Res Commun* 1987; 142: 710−6.

11 Ausubel FM, Brent R, Kingston RE *et al.* eds. *Current Protocols in Molecular Biology*, Vol. 1, Section 2.9. New York: Wiley & Son, 1987. Supplement 13, pp. 1−15.

12 Ausube FM, Brent R, Kingston RE *et al.* eds. *Current Protocols in Molecular Biology*, Vol. 1, Section 4.9.1−7. New York: Wiley & Son, 1987. Supplement 13.

13 Nuovo GJ, MacConnell P, Forde A, Delvenne P. Detection of human papillomavirus DNA in formalin-fixed tissues by *in situ* hybridization after amplification by polymerase chain reaction. *Am J Pathol* 1991; 139: 847−54.

11 Oncogenes, cancer and growth factors

EVA SZABO AND MICHAEL J. BIRRER

Introduction

Despite major technological advances in medical oncology in recent years, lung cancer continues to be one of the major causes of death world-wide. Although the introduction of multi-agent chemotherapy has made a real impact on survival in small cell lung cancer, it affords little advantage for the other more common types of lung cancer. In addition, the recognition of environmental causes such as cigarette smoke, asbestos and radon has not yet been translated into decreased mortality, and early detection efforts have only recently begun to uncover markers for mass screening. Thus, at present, the vast majority of lung cancer victims die of their disease.

Nevertheless, our understanding of lung carcinogenesis has made great strides over the past decade. Recent studies on human lung cancers have revealed a variety of molecular abnormalities in key target genes, which conspire to produce malignant transformation of the respiratory epithelium [1−3]. These abnormalities include chromosomal deletions and translocations, point mutations and gene amplification. The target genes can be classified into three basic groups:

1 Dominantly acting oncogenes whose altered expression or over-expression contributes to the malignant phenotype.

2 Recessive oncogenes, or tumour suppressor genes, whose inactivation or loss allows for deregulation of cell growth.

3 Genes coding for growth factors or their receptors, providing the malignant cell with a growth advantage over the surrounding normal cells, especially in cases where the malignant cell itself produces these growth factors (autocrine loops; Fig. 11.1).

The delineation of the molecular genetics of lung cancer has not only deepened our general understanding of the process of carcinogenesis, but has provided promising new therapeutic, early detection and, potentially, chemopreventative approaches to this disease.

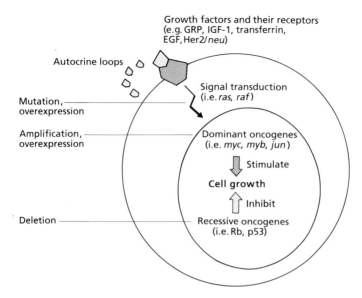

Fig. 11.1 Molecular mechanisms of lung carcinogenesis.

Genetic changes in lung cancer

Inherited predisposition

Although lung cancer is not classically thought of as a genetic disease, it has long been suspected that there exists a genetic component. A number of epidemiological studies have identified families with an excess of lung cancers [4–6], while first-degree relatives of lung cancer patients have a two- to fourfold risk of lung cancer [4, 6] as well as increased risk of other, non-smoking-related cancers [7]. A recent study of 337 families with lung cancer in Louisiana revealed the Mendelian inheritance of a two-allele autosomal locus with incomplete dominance influencing the age of onset of lung cancer [8]. With increasing smoking and advancing age, the relative contribution of this gene towards cancer diminishes. It is estimated that 0.27% of the population has the homozygous genotype while 9.9% of the population is heterozygous and, therefore, most people with lung cancer before the age of 70 years are gene carriers. Further evidence for an inherited predisposition to cancer is found with the observation that survivors of lung cancer have a significantly increased risk of a second malignancy, especially another lung cancer [9, 10]. While it is difficult to exclude the role of carcinogen exposure in these second cancers (particularly since a number of these cancers are potentially smoking related, such as respiratory tract, oral cavity, bladder and kidney), an excess of smoking-unrelated cancers (breast, female genital tract, liver) has also been reported [10].

While epidemiological studies support the existence of lung cancer susceptibility genes, it is not clear what role these genes may play in lung cancer. One possible connection is through an inherited predisposition to chronic obstructive pulmonary disease (COPD). In a study of 835 subjects with COPD attending an emphysema clinic, lung cancer incidence with a 4.3 year median follow-up was four to five times higher than in other comparable series of smokers or subjects with bronchitis [11]. In addition, smokers with known ventilatory obstruction have a significantly greater risk of cancer than those without obstruction [12]. It has been hypothesized that the chronic damage to lung tissue characterizing this lung process predisposes to subsequent neoplasia.

An additional suggested role for inherited genes in lung cancer is found with the debrisoquine metabolic phenotype [13]. Debrisoquine is an antihypertensive drug whose metabolism is under autosomal dominant control. Extensive metabolizers have a significantly increased risk of lung cancer compared with poor or intermediate metabolizers (odds ratio = 6.1; 95% confidence interval = 2.2−17.1). Whether this reflects a direct role for this enzymatic pathway in carcinogenesis, a related one in processing key carcinogens involved in the genesis of lung cancer or simply linkage to another more important gene is not clear.

Somatic mutations

Recent studies have shown that a large number of acquired (somatic) mutations occur in lung cancer. Cytogenetic analysis has revealed a wide range of chromosome aberrations, ranging from numerical abnormalities (hypodiploidy, hyperdiploidy, tetraploidy) to structural ones (translocations and deletions) [14]. While multiple abnormalities are frequently present within any one tumour, certain patterns, such as consistent deletions of 3p or 17p, have also emerged as common to all lung cancers.

The development of restriction fragment length polymorphism (RFLP) technology has greatly facilitated further characterization of these abnormalities and has confirmed that DNA from specific loci is lost in many cases. RFLP analysis is dependent on minor differences in DNA sequence occurring in different alleles of a gene, thus allowing detection of different sized fragments by restriction endonuclease digestion (Fig. 11.2). If two different alleles are present in normal tissue but only one allele is present in tumour tissue (referred to as loss of heterozygosity, LOH), then, clearly, one allele has been lost.

RFLP analysis has been applied extensively to all histological subtypes of lung cancer. Non-random LOH has been identified on at least 15 different chromosomes: chromosomes 1, 2, 3, 5, 6, 9, 10, 11, 12, 13, 14, 16, 17, 18 and 20 [14−16]. In addition, the frequency of LOH varies greatly according to chromosome, with chromosomes 3, 13 and 17 showing the most frequent and consistent deletions in lung cancer,

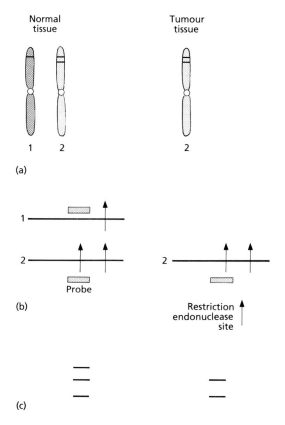

Fig. 11.2 RFLP analysis. (a) Chromosomes: tumour tissue frequently loses part of a chromosome or a whole chromosome. (b) DNA: minor differences in the DNA sequence of the two alleles result in differences in recognition sites for restriction endonucleases that cleave DNA at specific sequences resulting in RFLPs (see text and Chapter 1). Thus chromosome 1 harbours one such site while chromosome 2 has two such sites. (c) DNA is digested with the appropriate restriction endonuclease, separated on the basis of size by agarose gel electrophoresis, transferred to a nitrocellulose filter, and hybridized with a radiolabelled probe. In this example, the probe recognizes one large fragment of chromosome 1 and two smaller fragments of chromosome 2. Since tumour tissue has lost the corresponding portion of chromosome 1 or the whole chromosome, only the two smaller fragments are detected in the tumour tissue by hybridization with the probe. Thus loss of heterozygosity is confirmed at a molecular level.

thereby suggesting the presence of key target genes involved in the genesis of lung cancer.

Oncogenes

Oncogenes are a group of genes that have been identified as playing a key role in the process of carcinogenesis. Two distinct types have been characterized. Dominant oncogenes are genes whose increased expression or function contributes to neoplasia (i.e. genes with growth stimulatory characteristics). The recessive oncogenes, or tumour suppressor genes, characterized more recently are genes whose absence allows the neoplastic state to occur (i.e. genes possessing growth inhibitory characteristics). In the case of lung cancer, members of both groups have been shown to be important (Table 11.1), with multiple oncogenes usually involved in any one tumour.

Dominant oncogenes

With the development of polymerase chain reaction (PCR) technology allowing for the amplification of minute amounts of DNA from tumour specimens, the role of dominant oncogenes in various histological subtypes of lung cancer is beginning to be defined. The presence of activated dominant oncogenes in lung cancer has been estimated at anywhere from 13 to 86% of lung cancer specimens [17−19]. However, the specific contribution of each oncogene to the process of carcinogenesis has yet to be determined.

The dominant oncogene most extensively studied in lung cancer is *ras* [20−25]. The *ras* family consists of three members, N-, Ha- and Ki-*ras*, all of which code for a 21 kD protein with a putative role in signal transduction. These membrane-associated proteins exist in two functional states: the active GTP (guanine triphosphate)-bound form, and the inactive GDP (guanine diphosphate)-bound form. Conversion between the two involves an intrinsic GTPase activity that is stimulated by an associated GTPase activating protein (GAP). Mutations in codons 12, 13 and 61 lead to a constitutive activation of the Ras protein (i.e. loss of the GTPase-dependent activity) and, as a result, they perpetuate the growth stimulatory signal.

Analysis of non-small cell lung cancer has identified a mutation at codon 12 in the Ki-*ras* gene in approximately one-third of adenocarcinomas, mainly in smokers [22]. Slebos *et al.* [26] studied 69 patients with adenocarcinoma whose tumours could be completely removed by radical surgery (stages I−IIIa). Nineteen were positive for codon 12 mutations of the Ki-*ras* gene. The tumours harbouring an activated Ki-*ras* gene tended to be smaller but less well differentiated and, significantly, with a median follow-up of 36 months, they defined a subgroup with poor prognosis. Differences were seen in disease-free survival, overall survival and deaths due to cancer despite the fact that the tumours with *ras* mutations tended to fall into the earlier stage categories. Other histological subtypes of lung cancer appear not to be associated with activated *ras* genes and the Ha-*ras* and N-*ras* family members are rarely involved. Interestingly, deletion of Ha-*ras* is also associated with a poor prognosis [18], although it is not nearly as common an event and it is not clear whether it merely serves as a

Table 11.1 Dominant oncogenes and tumour suppressor genes in lung cancer

Gene	Histology	Mutation type	Frequency	Function	References
Dominant					
Ki-*ras*	NSCLC (adenocarcinoma)	PM	26–50%	Signal transduction	[20–25]
Ha-*ras*	NSCLC	D	9%	Signal transduction	[18]
c-*myc*	SCLC*	A;O	11–44%	Cell proliferation	[17, 18, 31–33]
	NSCLC	O	10%		
L-*myc*	SCLC	O	5–33%	Cell proliferation	[17, 33, 34]
	NSCLC	O	4%		
N-*myc*	SCLC	O	6–25%	Cell proliferation	[17, 31, 33]
Her2/*neu*	NSCLC	O	27–36%	?Growth factor receptor	[46, 47]
c-*myb*	SCLC	O	87%	Cell proliferation	[49]
c-*raf*-1	SCLC	O	Common	Signal transduction	[50]
	NSCLC	O	Common		
c-*jun*	SCLC	E	NA	Transcription factor	[51]
	NSCLC	E	NA		
Recessive					
Rb	SCLC	D;PM	+90%	Cell cycle regulation	[60–62]
p53	SCLC	D;PM;R	+50%	?Transcription factor	[69, 70]
	NSCLC	D;PM;R	+45%		
3p	SCLC	D	+90%	Putative tumour suppressor	[16, 82–87]
	NSCLC	D	25–50%	PTPG-signal transduction	[88]
				RAR-β-differentiation	[89]

A, amplification; D, deletion; E, expression; NA, not available; NSCLC, non-small cell lung cancer; O, overexpression; PM, point mutation; R, rearrangement; SCLC, small cell lung cancer.

marker being associated with a tumour suppressor gene located on chromosome 11, which is also lost.

The exact role of *ras* in the pathogenesis of lung cancer is not clear. Studies of carcinogen-induced tumours in mice with a high incidence of spontaneous lung tumours reveal a specific pattern of Ki-*ras* activation that is seen both in the adenomas as well as the carcinomas, suggesting that these mutations may be early events in the neoplastic process [27]. However, although blockage of Ki-*ras* with antisense oligonucleotides results in growth inhibition, cells remain viable and tumour growth in nude mice still occurs at high inoculums, albeit at a reduced rate [28]. In addition, insertion of the viral counterpart of the Ha-*ras* oncogene into a variant small cell lung cancer cell line induces features typical of large cell undifferentiated carcinoma, suggesting that *ras* may play a role in phenotype transitions and tumour progression [29]. Whatever the precise role may be in lung oncogenesis, the identification of *ras* mutations as a poor prognostic factor in lung cancer has clear and important clinical implications. Indeed, adjuvant therapy could be targeted specifically to patients with resectable but locally advanced tumours. In addition, mevalonate inhibitors are now available which could be used to interfere specifically with Ras membrane attachment and function [30].

A second group of dominant oncogenes abnormally expressed in lung cancer is the *myc* gene family. All three members of the family (c-, N- and L-*myc*) have been found to be overexpressed in lung cancers [31−33], with L-*myc* originally being identified on the basis of its high level expression in small cell lung cancer [34]. In particular, *myc* gene family amplification in small cell lung cancer has been identified in up to 11% of tumours from untreated patients and 28−44% of tumours from treated patients [35, 36]. The clinical significance of *myc* overexpression is suggested by the observation that patients who relapsed with tumours exhibiting *myc* amplification had a significantly shorter median survival than those relapsing without *myc* amplification (33 vs. 53 weeks) [35]. In addition, many small cell lung cancer cell lines and tumours have single copy overexpression of *myc* gene family members resulting in high levels of Myc protein. On the other hand, *myc* gene family amplification has not been found frequently in non-small cell lung cancer, although overexpression may still occur by mechanisms other than gene amplification.

Several mechanisms for deregulated *myc* expression in lung cancer have been identified. These include gene amplification and rearrangement, promoter activation and loss of transcriptional attenuation normally seen at the exon 1−intron 1 border in c-*myc* and L-*myc* [37]. Interestingly, in any one cell line or tumour, however, only one *myc* family member appears deregulated [32, 34].

The function of c-*myc* in normal cells has not been fully elucidated despite extensive characterization. Its protein product is a nuclear phosphoprotein containing both a leucine zipper and helix−loop−helix motif with DNA-binding capacity [38]. As such, c-*myc* has the structural requirements to function as a transcription factor and, indeed, has recently been found to regulate gene expression. In addition, c-*myc* appears to be intimately involved with cellular proliferation, perhaps as a 'competence' factor, since *myc* is expressed during cell growth while being down-regulated with terminal differentiation and cessation of cell growth. All *myc* family members can cooperate with an activated *ras* gene to transform primary rat embryo cells [39−41]. Small cell lung cancer cell lines overexpressing c-*myc* (variant cell lines) exhibit faster growth and higher cloning efficiency *in vitro* than cell lines that do not overexpress c-*myc* [42]. Indeed, a small cell carcinoma cell line overexpressing a transfected c-*myc* gene takes on the morphological and more aggressive growth characteristics of variant lines [43], suggesting that *myc* has a direct and potent effect on cell growth.

Recently, the product of the Her2/*neu* oncogene has been identified as a significant prognostic indicator in breast and ovarian cancer [44, 45]. Similar studies using both immunoprecipitation and immuno-histochemistry have shown that the Neu protein is present in approximately 30% of non-small cell lung cancers, particularly adenocarcinomas [46, 47]. It is also expressed in normal adult ciliated bronchiolar epithelium, albeit at lower levels. Activation of this oncogene occurs primarily through overexpression, and in at least one study, overexpression in adenocarcinomas of the lung was correlated with older age and a shortened median survival (83.7 vs. 188.5 weeks, $P = 0.01$) [46].

The Neu protein has homology to the epidermal growth factor receptor, encoding a 185 kD transmembrane glycoprotein [47]. Its carboxy terminus has features typical of an intracellular tyrosine kinase domain. Although its exact function remains unknown, its homology suggests that it is a growth factor receptor. In fact, in support of this suggestion, a potential ligand has recently been identified [48].

Other dominant oncogenes expressed in lung cancer include c-*myb*, c-*raf*-1 and c-*jun* [49−51]. c-*myb* appears to be expressed in most small cell lung cancer cell lines, while c-*raf*-1 appears to be expressed in all tumour cell types as well as normal lung. The c-*raf* proto-oncogene codes for a serine−threonine protein kinase involved in signal transduction. The nuclear proto-oncogene c-*jun* is also expressed in all histologies of lung cancer as well as in normal lung. c-*jun* is of particular interest because it encodes a component of the transcription factor AP-1, that appears to be at least one part of the molecular mechanism by which tumour promoters such as phorbol esters act [52]. As c-*jun* expression is easily stimulated by growth factors in both primary bronchial epithelium and some small cell lung cancer cell lines, it offers an attractive mediator for the 'promoting' effects of known growth factors for lung epithelial cells [53].

Tumour suppressor genes

The first tumour suppressor gene to be characterized was the retino-blastoma (Rb) gene located on chromosome 13q14 [54–56]. Its existence was predicted by Knudson in 1971 based on his observations of families with inherited retinoblastoma [57]. According to his hypothesis, in familial retinoblastoma, one defective allele is inherited through the germ line, while the second allele is inactivated by somatic mutation. Thus, in the familial form of the disease, every cell inherits one non-functional Rb gene and only one other mutation is necessary to inactivate this gene fully. This explains why multifocality, bilaterality and onset at an early age are hallmarks of the disease. On the other hand, in the sporadic form of the disease, two somatic mutations are necessary to inactivate the Rb gene product, and thus these tumours tend to be unilateral and occur at a later age than in the familial form. The Rb gene identified at chromosome locus 13q14 satisfies the requirements of this hypothesis since in every case examined, its normal protein product is not expressed in the tumour, while it is found in normal cells from the same individual [58]. In addition, reintroduction of the Rb gene into a retinoblastoma cell line at least partially reverses the neoplastic phenotype [59].

Examination of small cell lung cancer cytogenetics reveals a frequent loss of heterozygosity at 13q, with more detailed molecular analysis pin-pointing these abnormalities to the Rb locus [16, 60]. In a study by Harbour *et al.* [60], gross DNA abnormalities in the Rb gene were found in approximately 20% of small cell lung cancer cell lines (13% of primary tumours), while mRNA expression was absent in 60% of cell lines. More detailed analysis revealed that the Rb protein is absent or abnormal in greater than 90% of small cell lung cancer cell lines [61, 62]. On the other hand, 90% of non-small cell lung cancer cell lines express normal Rb mRNA.

Despite extensive characterization of the Rb protein as a nuclear phosphoprotein, its exact function in normal cells remains unclear [63]. Changes in its degree of phosphorylation have been correlated with the cell cycle, suggesting a direct role in this process [64]. In addition, the transforming proteins of DNA tumour viruses such as adenovirus E1A form specific complexes with Rb, suggesting that the resulting functional loss of Rb contributes to the cell growth deregulation associated with these transforming viruses [65].

Although attempts to introduce the Rb gene into small cell lung cancer cell lines have not yet been successful, the above findings suggest that the retinoblastoma gene functions as a tumour suppressor in small cell lung cancer in a similar fashion as in retinoblastoma. Indeed, the finding that relatives of patients with familial retinoblastoma have a 15-fold increase in lung cancer (mainly of the small cell variety) supports this concept further [66]. Finally, the recent reports of early onset of small cell lung cancer in patients with familial retinoblastoma suggest that the connection is not random [67].

A second tumour suppressor gene associated with lung cancer is the p53 oncogene. Originally characterized as a dominant oncogene, it has only recently been appreciated that p53 actually possesses tumour suppressor function [68]. It is located on chromosome region 17p13, and is a frequent target of allelic loss in both small cell and non-small cell lung cancers [16]. Molecular analysis by RNase protection assay or DNA sequencing has revealed that p53 is a frequent target of mutation in all types of lung cancer [69, 70]. In one study of 30 non-small cell lung cancer cell lines, 57% showed p53 DNA or mRNA abnormalities while another 17% expressed only very low levels of p53 mRNA. Abnormalities included homozygous deletions, abnormally sized mRNAs, splicing mutants and point mutations or small deletions in the open reading frame, resulting in amino acid sequence changes within a region of highly conserved evolution [71].

Of interest, p53 mutations tend to be clustered within the evolutionarily conserved amino acids in exons 5 to 8 and both the location and type of amino acid substitution vary according to tumour type [72]. In the case of non-small cell lung cancer, Chiba *et al.* [70] reported that 22 of 23 mutations were G to T transversions, in contrast to the G:C−A:T transitions seen in colon cancer [72]. In addition, there appears to be a clear strand bias in that the guanine residue tends to be located on the non-transcribed strand [72]. These findings support the hypothesis that these tumours are in part carcinogen induced with different carcinogens providing different mutational signatures.

The role of p53 in normal cells has not yet been clearly defined, although evidence suggests that it may function as a transcriptional activator. p53 is a nuclear phosphoprotein with the ability to bind DNA in a sequence-specific manner [73]. In addition, when fused with the DNA-binding domain of the yeast transcriptional activator GAL4, p53 can act as a potent transcriptional activator [74, 75]. Mutant p53, on the other hand, appears to have an altered transcriptional capacity. Mutant p53 proteins can cooperate with an activated *ras* gene to transform cells, while wild-type p53 suppresses this transformation [76, 77]. In addition, wild-type p53 transfected into human colon carcinoma cell lines suppresses neoplastic growth, whereas mutant p53 is unable to do so [78]. This evidence firmly establishes that p53 can function as a tumour suppressor gene on a molecular level. *In vivo* confirmation is shown in the fact that a germ line p53 abnormality has been found in the hereditary Li−Fraumeni syndrome, where affected individuals have a very high incidence of malignancies, especially lung, breast and bone cancers [79, 80] and that transgenic mice carrying a mutant p53 gene have a high incidence of cancer, particularly of the lung [81].

As mentioned previously, cytogenetic analysis of small cell lung cancer reveals non-random deletions in chromosome 3p in greater than 90% of cases, with the shortest region of overlap at 3p14-23 [82−84]. These findings have been confirmed and expanded by RFLP analysis, both in primary tumours and in cell lines [16, 84, 85]. Further, since lymphoblastoid cell lines from the same patients did not reveal the same chromosomal deletion, these mutations are tissue specific and must be somatically acquired [82]. In addition, a 3p deletion has been found in all histological subtypes of non-small cell lung cancer (albeit with lesser frequency) and in renal cell carcinomas (particularly the inherited forms) suggesting that it may play a more general role in the pathogenesis of cancer [86, 87].

The finding of the 3p deletion has led to a massive effort to identify the target gene, since its absence may play a role in the establishment or progression of the malignant phenotype in several tumour types. Recently, a candidate gene on 3p21 has been identified [88]. This gene codes for receptor protein tyrosine phosphatase-γ (PTPG), a transmembrane protein which may function in signal transduction. As phosphorylation of tyrosyl residues has been implicated in the control of cell growth and a number of oncogenes have been shown to possess tyrosine kinase ability, the notion that a tyrosine phosphatase (opposing the action of a tyrosine kinase) could function as a tumour suppressor gene is very attractive. One PTPG allele was shown to be deleted in five of 10 lung cancers and in three of five renal carcinoma cell lines, in keeping with its putative role as a tumour suppressor [88]. Confirmation of this role, however, will require the demonstration that the PTPG protein is absent or non-functional in these tumours (i.e. that the remaining allele is also mutated or inactive), and that restoration of intact PTPG protein reverses the neoplastic phenotype.

Another gene located on the short arm of chromosome 3 characterized recently is the retinoic acid receptor-β (RAR-β). As retinoic acid is required for normal differentiation of human bronchial epithelial cells, this gene or loss of its expression may well be involved in lung carcinogenesis. A recent study of lung cancer cell lines and primary lung tumours of all histological types showed alterations of RAR-β expression or inducibility in a large proportion of samples studied (50 and 30%, respectively) [89]. Further work is required to determine the exact role of this gene in the development of lung cancer.

Growth factors and their receptors

While the delineation of oncogene mutations in lung cancer provides support for the initiation and progression events of the multistage hypothesis of lung carcinogenesis, there exists a body of accumulating evidence that growth factors also play a crucial role in this process, perhaps as tumour promoters. This role may involve paracrine or autocrine mechanisms. The autocrine hypothesis states that a cell produces and secretes growth factors which interact with specific receptors on its membrane surface to produce deregulated cellular proliferation. To date, four growth factors which may function in an autocrine fashion in lung cancer have been characterized (Table 11.2).

The growth factor characterized best is gastrin-releasing peptide (GRP). Originally identified in amphibians as bombesin, mammalian GRP is detected in 70% of small cell lung cancer cell lines [90−92] but only rarely in non-small cell lung cancer cell lines [93]. Growth of small cell lung cancer cell lines is stimulated markedly by GRP in serum-free medium [94] and can in turn be inhibited by an anti-bombesin mono-clonal antibody [93] or synthetic bombesin receptor antagonists [95]. Furthermore, the growth of established tumours in nude mice is reduced markedly by the anti-bombesin antibody [94], which forms the basis for the present clinical trial using this antibody in patients with small cell lung cancer [96].

Transcription of the GRP gene results in three mRNA forms through alternative mRNA processing [97, 98], and subsequent post-translational modification (including amidation) is required for full biological activity of the peptide [99, 100]. GRP functions by binding to high affinity receptors to activate intracellular signalling pathways that lead to intra-cellular calcium mobilization, phosphatidyl inositol turnover and acti-vation of protein kinase C [100, 101]. In addition, there is constitutive activation of a tyrosine kinase that phosphorylates a 115 kD protein associated with the GRP receptor complex [102]. Responsiveness to GRP appears to be correlated with both GRP and L-*myc* expression [103]. Responsive cell lines tend to express L-*myc*, while non-responsive lines express little or no GRP and overexpress c-*myc* or N-*myc*, suggesting that these *myc* family members may have allowed the cell to escape this growth factor dependence.

GRP is mitogenic for normal bronchial epithelium [104], and bom-besin-like immunoreactivity has been detected in human foetal lung [105], suggesting a physiological role in normal lung development. A mitogenic peptide normally present during development might function

Table 11.2 Autocrine growth factors in lung cancer

Factor	Histology	References
Gastrin-releasing peptide	SCLC	[90−92]
Transferrin	SCLC	[107, 108]
Insulin-like growth factor-1	SCLC, NSCLC	[109, 110]
Epidermal growth factor	NSCLC	[111, 112]

NSCLC, non-small cell lung cancer; SCLC, small cell lung cancer.

as a tumour promoter during the early stages of the carcinogenic process. GRP could expand a cell population by autocrine and/or paracrine stimulation, allowing the accumulation of genetic lesions that would ultimately lead to neoplastic transformation. In this context, the finding of GRP immunoreactivity in bronchial lavage fluid in smokers offers further evidence for an early 'promotional' role in carcinogenesis and a possible candidate for identification of patients at high risk for subsequent cancers [106].

Much less is known about other autocrine growth loops. Small cell lung cancer cell lines able to grow in serum-free medium have been shown to produce transferrin, and conditioned medium from these cells can support the growth of other transferrin-sensitive cell lines [107, 108]. Furthermore, anti-transferrin receptor antibodies inhibit the growth of these cell lines, as do gallium salts interfering with iron uptake. Similarly, insulin-like growth factor-1 (IGF-1) has also been demonstrated to stimulate the growth of small cell lung cancer cell lines, while an IGF-1 precursor is detectable by Western blot analysis and a monoclonal antibody to the IGF-1 receptor interferes with cell growth [109]. IGF-1 precursor molecules and high affinity IGF-1 receptors have also been identified in non-small cell lung cancer cell lines [110].

Non-small cell lung cancer cell lines, on the other hand, have been shown to express epidermal growth factor (EGF) receptors in up to 80% of cases, while small cell lung cancers do not [111, 112]. This correlation is particularly strong for the squamous cell subtype, with increased expression in stage III tumours as opposed to stages I and II [112]. Significantly, these changes have also been noted in the normal bronchial epithelium of patients with a first or second primary lung tumour, suggesting that they may be early changes during carcinogenesis [113].

The application of molecular genetics to the diagnosis and treatment of lung cancer

The recent discoveries in the molecular genetics of lung cancer have provided us not only with a better understanding of the process of lung carcinogenesis, but also with a wealth of new approaches for treatment, early detection and potential chemoprevention of lung cancer. Already attempts are being made to use monoclonal antibodies against growth factors in advanced cancers, as well as to screen for early, possibly preneoplastic changes in sputum and bronchial lavage fluids. Stratification according to prognosis in non-small cell lung cancer on the basis of the presence of an activated Ki-*ras* gene can serve as a model to predict which patients need adjuvant treatment after surgery, perhaps with mevalonate inhibitors that interfere specifically with *ras* function. The identification of patients with early preneoplastic lesions by screening sputum samples or bronchial biopsies for genetic abnormalities such as p53 mutations may allow for early intervention and potentially curative therapy. Finally, an understanding of the early biochemical and molecular events during the development of lung cancer may allow for the production of rational chemoprevention approaches. The complexity of the molecular changes in lung cancer affords both a challenge and a hope for the development of new methodologies that will be more efficacious in the prevention and treatment of this disease than those currently available.

References

1 Bishop JM. The molecular genetics of cancer. *Science* 1986; 235: 305–311.
2 Birrer MJ, Minna JD. Molecular genetics of lung cancer. *Semin Oncol* 1988; 15: 226–35.
3 Birrer MJ, Minna JD. Genetic changes in the pathogenesis of lung cancer. *Annu Rev Med* 1989; 40: 305–17.
4 Tokuhata GK, Lilienfeld AM. Familial aggregation of lung cancer in humans. *J Natl Cancer Inst* 1963; 30: 289–312.
5 Goffman TE, Hassinger DD, Mulvihill JJ. Familial respiratory tract cancer: opportunities for research and prevention. *J Am Med Assoc* 1982; 247: 1020–3.
6 Ooi WL, Elston RC, Chen VW, Bailey-Wilson JE, Rothschild H. Increased familial risk for lung cancer. *J Natl Cancer Inst* 1986; 76: 217–22.
7 Lynch HT, Kimberling WJ, Markvicka SE *et al*. Genetics and smoking-associated cancers. A study of 485 families. *Cancer* 1986; 57: 1640–6.
8 Sellers TA, Bailey-Wilson JE, Elston RC *et al*. Evidence for Mendelian inheritance in the pathogenesis of lung cancer. *J Natl Cancer Inst* 1990; 82: 1272–9.
9 Boice JD Jr, Fraumeni JF Jr. Second cancer following cancer of the respiratory system in Connecticut, 1935–1982. *Natl Cancer Inst Monogr* 1985; 68: 83–98.
10 Olsen JH. Second cancer following cancer of the respiratory system in Denmark, 1943–1980. *Natl Cancer Inst Monogr* 1985; 68: 309–24.
11 Davis A. Bronchogenic carcinoma in chronic obstructive pulmonary disease. *J Am Med Assoc* 1976; 235: 621–2.
12 Tockman MS, Anthonisen NR, Wright EC, Donithan MG. Airway obstruction and the risk for lung cancer. *Ann Intern Med* 1987; 106: 512–18.
13 Caporaso NE, Tucker MA, Hoover RN *et al*. Lung cancer and the debrisoquine metabolic phenotype. *J Natl Cancer Inst* 1990; 82: 1264–72.
14 Whang-Peng J. 3p deletions and small cell lung carcinoma. *Mayo Clinic Proc* 1989; 64: 256–60.
15 Shiraishi M, Morinaga S, Noguchi M, Shimorato Y, Sekiya T. Loss of genes on the short arm of chromosome 11 in human lung carcinomas. *Jpn J Cancer Res (Gann)* 1987; 78: 1302–8.
16 Yokota J, Wada M, Shimosato Y, Terada M, Sugimura T. Loss of heterozygosity on chromosomes 3, 13, and 17 in small-cell carcinoma and on chromosome 3 in adenocarcinoma of the lung. *Proc Natl Acad Sci USA* 1987; 84: 9252–6.
17 Shiraishi M, Noguchi M, Shimosato Y, Sekiya T. Amplification of protooncogenes in surgical specimens of human lung carcinomas. *Cancer Res* 1989; 49: 6474–9.
18 Hajj C, Akoum R, Bradley E, Paquin F, Ayoub J. DNA alterations at protooncogene loci and their clinical significance in operable non-small cell lung cancer. *Cancer* 1990; 66: 733–9.
19 Reynolds SH, Anna CK, Brown KC *et al*. Activated protooncogenes in human lung tumors from smokers. *Proc Natl Acad Sci USA* 1991; 88: 1085–9.

20 Kurzrock R, Gallick GE, Gutterman JU. Differential expression of p21^{ras} gene products among histologic subtypes of fresh primary human lung tumors. *Cancer Res* 1986; 46: 1530−4.

21 Rodenhuis S, vande Wetering ML, Mooi WJ, Evers SG, van Zandwijk N, Bos JL. Mutational activation of the K-*ras* oncogene: a possible pathogenetic factor in adenocarcinoma of the lung. *N Engl J Med* 1987; 317: 929−35.

22 Rodenhuis S, Slebos RJC, Boot AJM *et al*. Incidence and possible clinical significance of K-*ras* oncogene activation in adenocarcinoma of the human lung. *Cancer Res* 1988; 48: 5738−41.

23 Bos JL. *ras* oncogenes in human cancer: a review. *Cancer Res* 1989; 49: 4682−9.

24 DeBiasi F, DelSal G, Horan Hand P. Evidence of enhancement of the *ras* oncogene protein product (p21) in a spectrum of human tumors. *Int J Cancer* 1989; 43: 431−5.

25 Kobayashi T, Tsuda T, Noguchi M *et al*. Association of point mutation in c-Ki-*ras* oncogene in lung adenocarcinoma with particular reference to cytologic subtypes. *Cancer* 1990; 66: 289−94.

26 Slebos RJC, Kibbelaar RE, Dalesio O *et al*. K-*ras* oncogene activation as a prognostic marker in adenocarcinoma of the lung. *N Engl J Med* 1990; 323: 561−5.

27 You M, Candrian U, Maronpot RR, Stoner GD, Anderson MW. Activation of the Ki-*ras* protooncogene in spontaneously occurring and chemically induced lung tumors of the strain A mouse. *Proc Natl Acad Sci USA* 1989; 86: 3070−4.

28 Mukhopadhyay T, Tainsky M, Cavender AC, Roth JA. Specific inhibition of K-*ras* expression and tumorigenicity of lung cancer cells by antisense RNA. *Cancer Res* 1991; 51: 1744−8.

29 Mabry M, Nakagawa T, Nelkin BD *et al*. v-Ha-*ras* oncogene insertion: a model for tumor progression of human small cell lung cancer. *Proc Natl Acad Sci USA* 1988; 85: 6523−7.

30 Schafer WR, Kim R, Sterne R, Thorner J, Kim S-H, Rine J. Genetic and pharmacologic suppression of oncogenic mutations in *ras* genes of yeast and humans. *Science* 1989; 245: 379−85.

31 Wong AJ, Ruppert JM, Eggleston J, Hamilton SR, Baylin SB, Vogelstein B. Gene amplification of c-*myc* and N-*myc* in small cell carcinoma of the lung. *Science* 1986; 233: 461−4.

32 Kiefer PE, Bepler G, Kubasch M, Havemann K. Amplification and expression of protooncogenes in human small cell lung cancer cell lines. *Cancer Res* 1987; 47: 6236−42.

33 Yokota J, Wada M, Yoshida T *et al*. Heterogeneity of lung cancer cells with respect to the amplification and rearrangement of *myc* family oncogenes. *Oncogene* 1988; 2: 607−11.

34 Nau MM, Brooks BJ, Battey J *et al*. L-*myc*, a new *myc*-related gene amplified and expressed in human small cell lung cancer. *Nature* 1985; 318: 69−73.

35 Johnson BE, Ihde DC, Makuch RW *et al. myc* family oncogene amplification in tumor cell lines established from small cell lung cancer patients and its relationship to clinical status and course. *J Clin Invest* 1987; 79: 1629−34.

36 Brennan J, O'Connor T, Makuch RW *et al. myc* family DNA amplification in 107 tumors and tumor cell lines from patients with small cell lung cancer treated with different combination chemotherapy regimens. *Cancer Res* 1991; 51: 1708−12.

37 Krystal G, Birrer M, Way J *et al*. Multiple mechanisms for transcriptional regulation of the *myc* gene family in small-cell lung cancer. *Mol Cell Biol* 1988; 8: 3373−81.

38 Luscher B, Eisenman RN. New light on *myc* and *myb*. Part I. *myc. Genes Dev* 1990; 4: 2025−35.

39 Land H, Parada LF, Weinberg RA. Tumorigenic conversion of primary embryo fibroblasts requires at least two cooperating oncogenes. *Nature* 1983; 304: 596−602.

40 Yancopoulos GP, Nisen PD, Tesfaye A, Kohl NE, Goldfarb MP, Alt FW. N-*myc* can cooperate with *ras* to transform normal cells in culture. *Proc Natl Acad Sci USA* 1985; 82: 5455−9.

41 Birrer MJ, Segal S, DeGreve J, Kaye F, Sausville EA, Minna JD. L-*myc* cooperates with *ras* to transform primary rat embryo fibroblasts. *Mol Cell Biol* 1988; 8: 2573−668.

42 Gazdar AF, Carney DN, Nau MM, Minna JD. Characterization of variant subclasses of cell lines derived from small cell lung cancer having distinctive biochemical, morphological, and growth properties. *Cancer Res* 1985; 45: 2924−30.

43 Johnson BE, Battey J, Linnoila I *et al*. Changes in the phenotype of human small cell lung cancer cell lines following transfection and expression of the c-*myc* proto-oncogene. *J Clin Invest* 1986; 78: 525−32.

44 Slamon DJ, Clark GM, Wong SC, Levin WJ, Ullrich A, McGuire WL. Human breast cancer: correlation of relapse and survival with amplification of the HER 2/*neu* oncogene. *Science* 1987; 235: 177−82.

45 Wright C, Angus B, Nicholson S *et al*. Expression of the c-erbB-2 oncoprotein: a prognostic indicator in human breast cancer. *Cancer Res* 1989; 49: 2087−90.

46 Kern JA, Schwartz DA, Nordberg JE *et al*. p185^{neu} expression in human lung adenocarcinomas predicts shortened survival. *Cancer Res* 1990; 50: 5184−91.

47 Weiner DB, Nordberg J, Robinson R *et al*. Expression of the *neu* gene-encoded protein (p185^{neu}) in human non-small cell carcinomas of the lung. *Cancer Res* 1990; 50: 421−425.

48 Lupu R, Colomer R, Zugmaier G *et al*. Direct interaction of a ligand for the erbB2 oncogene product with the EGF receptor and p185erbB2. *Science* 1990; 249: 1552−5.

49 Griffin CA, Baylin SB. Expression of the c-*myb* oncogene in human small cell lung carcinoma. *Cancer Res* 1985; 45: 272−5.

50 Rapp U, Huleihel M, Pawson T *et al*. Role of *raf* oncogenes in lung carcinogenesis. *Lung Cancer* 1988; 4: 162−7.

51 Schutte J, Nau MM, Birrer M, Thomas F, Gazdar A, Minna J. Constitutive expression of multiple mRNA forms of the c-*jun* oncogene in human lung cancer cell lines. *Proc Am Assoc Cancer Res* 1988; 29: 455.

52 Bohmann D, Bos TJ, Admon A, Nishimura T, Vogt PK, Tjian R. Human proto-oncogene c-*jun* encodes a DNA binding protein with structural and functional properties of transcription factor AP-1. *Science* 1987; 238: 1386−92.

53 Birrer MJ, Alani R, Cuttita F *et al*. Early events in the neoplastic transformation of respiratory epithelium. *J Natl Cancer Inst* 1992; 13: 31−7.

54 Friend SH, Bernards R, Rogelj S *et al*. A human DNA segment with properties of the gene that predisposes to retinoblastoma and osteosarcoma. *Nature* 1986; 323: 643−6.

55 Fung Y-KT, Murphree AL, T'Ang A, Qian J, Hinricks SH, Benedict WF. Structural evidence for the authenticity of the human retinoblastoma gene. *Science* 1987; 236: 1657−61.

56 Lee W-H, Bookstein R, Hong F, Young L-J, Shew J-Y, Lee E Y-HP. Human retinoblastoma susceptibility gene: cloning, identification, and sequence. *Science* 1987; 235: 1394−9.

57 Knudson AG. Mutation and cancer: statistical study of retinoblastoma. *Proc Natl Acad Sci USA* 1971; 68: 820−3.

58 Horowitz JM, Park S-H, Bogenmann E *et al*. Frequent inactivation of the retinoblastoma anti-oncogene is restricted to a subset of human tumor cells. *Proc Natl*

Acad Sci USA 1990; 87: 2775−9.

59 Huang H-JSH, Yee J-K, Shew J-Y *et al*. Suppression of the neoplastic phenotype by replacement of the RB gene in human cancer cells. *Science* 1988; 242: 1563−6.

60 Harbour JW, Lai S-L, Whang-Peng J, Gazdar AF, Minna JD, Kaye FJ. Abnormalities in structure and expression of the human retinoblastoma gene in SCLC. *Science* 1988; 241: 353−7.

61 Yokota J, Akiyama T, Fung Y-KT *et al*. Altered expression of the retinoblastoma (RB) gene in small-cell carcinoma of the lung. *Oncogene* 1988; 3: 471−5.

62 Hensel CH, Hsieh CL, Gazdar AF *et al*. Altered structure and expression of the human retinoblastoma susceptibility gene in small cell lung cancer. *Cancer Res* 1990; 50: 3067−72.

63 Lee W-H, Shew J-Y, Hong FD *et al*. The retinoblastoma susceptibility gene encodes a nuclear phosphoprotein associated with DNA binding activity. *Nature* 1987; 329: 642−5.

64 Furukawa Y, DeCaprio JA, Freedman A *et al*. Expression and state of phosphorylation of the retinoblastoma susceptibility gene product in cycling and noncycling human hematopoietic cells. *Proc Natl Acad Sci USA* 1990; 87: 2770−4.

65 Green MR. When the products of oncogenes and anti-oncogenes meet. *Cell* 1989; 56: 1−3.

66 Sanders BM, Jay M, Draper GJ, Roberts EM. Non-ocular cancer in relatives of retinoblastoma patients. *Br J Cancer* 1989; 60: 358−65.

67 Leonard RCF, MacKay T, Brown A, Gregor A, Crompton GK, Smyth JF. Small-cell lung cancer after retinoblastoma. *Lancet* 1988; ii: 1503.

68 Mowat M, Cheng A, Kimura N, Bernstein A, Benchimol S. Rearrangements of the cellular p53 gene in erythroleukaemic cells transformed by Friend virus. *Nature* 1985; 314: 633−6.

69 Takahashi T, Nau MM, Chiba I *et al*. p53: a frequent target for genetic abnormalities in lung cancer. *Science* 1989; 246: 491−4.

70 Chiba I, Takahashi T, Nau MM *et al*. Mutations in the p53 gene are frequent in primary, resected non-small cell lung cancer. *Oncogene* 1990; 5: 1603−10.

71 Takahashi T, D'Amico D, Chiba I, Buchhagen DL, Minna JD. Identification of intronic point mutations as an alternative mechanism for p53 inactivation in lung cancer. *J Clin Invest* 1990; 86: 363−9.

72 Hollstein M, Sidransky D, Vogelstein B, Harris CC. p53 mutations in human cancers. *Science* 1991; 253: 49−53.

73 Kern SE, Kinzler KW, Bruskin A *et al*. Identification of p53 as a sequence-specific DNA-binding protein. *Science* 1991; 252: 1708−11.

74 Fields S, Jang SK. Presence of a potent transcription activating sequence in the p53 protein. *Science* 1990; 249: 1046−9.

75 Raycroft L, Wu H, Lozano G. Transcriptional activation by wild-type but not transforming mutants of the p53 anti-oncogene. *Science* 1990; 249: 1049−51.

76 Eliyahu D, Michalovitz D, Eliyahu S, Pinhasi-Kimhi O, Oren M. Wild-type p53 can inhibit oncogene-mediated focus formation. *Proc Natl Acad Sci USA* 1989; 86: 8763−7.

77 Finlay CA, Hinds PW, Levine AJ. The p53 proto-oncogene can act as a suppressor of transformation. *Cell* 1989; 57: 1083−93.

78 Baker SJ, Markowitz S, Fearon ER, Willson JKV, Vogelstein B. Suppression of human colorectal carcinoma cell growth by wild-type p53. *Science* 1990; 249: 912−15.

79 Malkin D, Li FP, Strong LC *et al*. Germ line p53 mutations in a familial syndrome of breast cancer, sarcomas, and other neoplasms. *Science* 1990; 250: 1233−8.

80 Srivastava S, Zou Z, Pirollo K, Blattner W, Chang EH. Germ-line transmission of a mutated p53 gene in a cancer-prone family with Li−Fraumeni syndrome. *Nature* 1990; 348: 747−9.

81 Lavigueur A, Maltby V, Mock D, Rossant J, Pawson T, Bernstein A. High incidence of lung, bone, and lymphoid tumors in transgenic mice overexpressing mutant alleles of the p53 oncogene. *Mol Cell Biol* 1989; 9: 3982−91.

82 Whang-Peng J, Kao-Shan CS, Lee EC *et al.* Specific chromosome defect associated with human small cell lung cancer: deletion 3p (14−23). *Science* 1982; 215: 181−2.

83 Falor WH, Ward-Skinner R, Wegryn S. A 3p deletion in small cell lung cancer. *Cancer Genet Cytogenet* 1985; 16: 175−7.

84 Buys CHCM, Osinga J, van der Veen AY *et al.* Genome analysis of small cell lung cancer (SCLC) and clinical significance. *Eur J Respir Dis* 1987; 149 (Suppl): 29−36.

85 Johnson BE, Sakaguchi AY, Gazdar AF *et al.* Restriction fragment length polymorphism studies show consistent loss of chromosome 3p alleles in small cell lung cancer patients' tumors. *J Clin Invest* 1988; 82: 502−7.

86 Kok K, Osinga J, Carritt B *et al.* Deletion of a DNA sequence at the chromosomal region 3p21 in all major types of lung cancer. *Nature* 1987; 330: 578−81.

87 Zbar B, Brauch H, Talmadge C, Linehan M. Loss of alleles of loci on the short arm of chromosome 3 in renal cell carcinoma. *Nature* 1987; 327: 721−4.

88 LaForgia S, Morse B, Levy J *et al.* Receptor protein−tyrosine phosphatase-γ is a candidate tumor suppressor gene at human chromosome region 3p21. *Proc Natl Acad Sci USA* 1991; 88: 5036−40.

89 Gebert JF, Moghal N, Frangioni JV, Sugarbaker DJ, Neel BG. High frequency of retinoic acid receptor-β abnormalities in human lung cancer. *Oncogene* 1991; 6: 1859−68.

90 Moody TW, Pert CB, Gazdar AF, Carney DN, Minna JD. High levels of intracellular bombesin characterize human small-cell lung carcinoma. *Science* 1981; 214: 1246−8.

91 Erisman MD, Linnoila RI, Hernandez O, DiAugustine RP, Lazarus LH. Human lung small-cell carcinoma contains bombesin. *Proc Natl Acad Sci USA* 1982; 79: 2379−83.

92 Hamid Q, Addis B, Springall D *et al.* Expression of the C-terminal peptide of human probombesin in 361 lung endocrine tumours, a reliable marker and possible prognostic indicator for small cell carcinoma. *Virchows Arch* 1987; 411: 185−92.

93 Cuttita F, Carney DN, Mulshine J *et al.* Bombesin-like peptides can function as autocrine growth factors in human small-cell lung cancer. *Nature* 1988; 316: 823−6.

94 Carney DN, Cuttita F, Moody TW, Minna JD. Selective stimulation of small cell lung cancer clonal growth by bombesin and gastrin-releasing peptide. *Cancer Res* 1987; 47: 821−5.

95 Trepel JB, Moyer JD, Cuttita F *et al.* A novel bombesin receptor antagonist inhibits autocrine signals in a small cell lung carcinoma cell line. *Biochem Biophys Res Commun* 1988; 156: 1383−9.

96 Mulshine JL, Avis I, Treston AM *et al.* Clinical use of a monoclonal antibody to bombesin-like peptide in patients with lung cancer. *Ann N Y Acad Sci* 1988; 547: 360−72.

97 Spindel ER, Chin WW, Price J, Rees LH, Besser GM, Habener J. Cloning and characterization of cDNAs encoding human gastrin-releasing peptide. *Proc Natl Acad Sci USA* 1984; 81: 5699−703.

98 Sausville EA, Lebacq-Verheyden AM, Spindel ER, Cuttita F, Gazdar AF, Battey

J. Expression of the gastrin-releasing peptide gene in human small cell lung cancer: evidence for alternative processing resulting in three distinct mRNAs. *J Biol Chem* 1986; 261: 2451−7.

99 Moody TW, Carney DN, Cuttita F, Quattrocchi K, Minna JD. High affinity receptors for bombesin/GRP-like peptides on human small cell lung cancer. *Life Sci* 1985; 37: 105−13.

100 Lebacq-Verheyden A, Kasprzyk P, Raum M, Coelingh KVW, Lebacq J, Battey J. Posttranslational processing of endogenous and of baculovirus-expressed human gastrin-releasing peptide precursor. *Mol Cell Biol* 1988; 8: 3129−35.

101 Heikkila R, Trepel JB, Cuttita F, Neckers LH, Sausville EA. Bombesin-related peptides induce calcium mobilization in a subset of human small cell lung cancer cell lines. *J Biol Chem* 1987; 262: 16456−60.

102 Gaudino G, Cirillo D, Naldini L, Rossino P, Comoglio PM. Activation of the protein−tyrosine kinase associated with the bombesin receptor complex in small cell lung carcinomas. *Proc Natl Acad Sci USA* 1988; 85: 2166−70.

103 Trepel J, Moyer J, Heikkila R, Neckers L, Sausville E. Relationship of bombesin responsiveness to *myc* gene family expression in small cell lung cancer cell lines. *Clin Res* 1987; 35: 528A.

104 Willey J, Lechner J, Harris C. Bombesin and the C-terminal tetradecapeptide of gastrin-releasing peptide are growth factors for normal human bronchial epithelial cells. *Exp Cell Res* 1984; 153: 245−8.

105 Yamaguchi K, Abe K, Kameya T *et al.* Production and molecular size heterogeneity of immunoreactive gastrin-releasing peptide in fetal and adult lungs and primary lung tumors. *Cancer Res* 1983; 43: 3932−9.

106 Aguayo S, Kane M, Schwarz M *et al.* Bombesin like immunoreactivity in broncho-alveolar lavage from smokers and interstitial lung disease. *Clin Res* 1987; 35: 530A.

107 Nakanishi Y, Cuttita F, Kasprzyk PG *et al.* Growth factor effects on small cell lung cancer cells using a colorimetric assay: can a transferrin-like factor mediate autocrine growth? *Exp Cell Biol* 1988; 56: 74−85.

108 Vostrejs M, Moran PL, Seligman PA. Transferrin synthesis by small cell lung cancer cells acts as an autocrine regulator of cellular proliferation. *J Clin Invest* 1988; 82: 331−9.

109 Nakanishi Y, Mulshine JL, Kasprzyk PG *et al.* Insulin-like growth factor-1 can mediate autocrine proliferation of human small cell lung cancer cell lines *in vitro. J Clin Invest* 1988; 82: 354−9.

110 Natale RB, Cuttita F, Nakanishi Y, Minna J, Gazdar A, Mulshine J. IGF-1 can stimulate proliferation of non-small cell lung cancer cell lines *in vitro. Proc Am Soc Clin Oncol* 1988; 7: 197.

111 Hendler FJ, Ozanne BW. Human squamous cell lung cancers express increased epidermal growth factor receptors. *J Clin Invest* 1984; 74: 647−51.

112 Veale D, Ashcroft T, Marsh C, Gibson GJ, Harris AL. Epidermal growth factor receptors in non-small cell lung cancer. *Br J Cancer* 1987; 55: 513−16.

113 Sozzi G, Miozzo M, Tagliabue E *et al.* Cytogenetic abnormalities and overexpression of receptors for growth factors in normal bronchial epithelium and tumor samples of lung cancer patients. *Cancer Res* 1991; 51: 400−4.

12 Molecular biology of lung receptors

PETER J. BARNES

Introduction

Receptors play a critical role in regulation of cellular responsiveness and have traditionally been investigated by pharmacological studies of functional responses or by direct binding studies with radioligands. Recently, many receptors have been cloned, opening up new insights into receptor structure and function, and providing new opportunities to study receptor regulation in pulmonary cells and in lung disease [1]. In the future it may also lead to new and more specific therapeutic approaches. This chapter discusses some of the areas in which molecular biological approaches have been used to investigate receptor structure and function, although at present there have been few applications of these new techniques to lung disease. It is clear that the tools provided by molecular biology are extremely powerful and will allow questions which were previously unanswerable to be addressed.

Receptor cloning

The genes for many receptors have now been cloned and expressed. These receptors include: neurotransmitter, mediator and cytokine receptors, all of which may be relevant to pulmonary physiology and disease. The gene sequence coding for a particular receptor (complementary DNA, cDNA) may be identified by extraction of total RNA or messenger RNA (mRNA) from a tissue known to express the receptor of interest in high density using reverse transcriptase. The single strand of cDNA is then made double stranded using DNA polymerase and the cDNAs corresponding to all the species of mRNA originally present are each inserted into a plasmid vector for amplification in a non-pathogenetic strain of *Escherichia coli*. cDNA clones coding for receptors may then be identified using labelled synthetic probes which contain part of the predicted DNA sequence. Usually, short sequences of the receptor protein which may be known or predicted are used to synthesize short oligonucleotide probes of 20–30 bases, which are labelled. A cocktail of such probes may then be used to screen a cDNA library.

Once the receptor cDNA is identified it can be amplified, so that large numbers of exact copies can be made. This yields enough pure cDNA to allow determination of the nucleotide sequence, leading to prediction of the amino acid sequence of the receptor protein. Since receptor proteins are usually present in very low abundance in most cells, it has not previously been possible to determine their precise amino acid sequence; the application of molecular biology techniques has therefore been an enormous advance.

Because there are structural similarities between receptors, such as G-protein-linked receptors, it is possible to use a cDNA probe from one receptor to identify subtypes of the same receptor and other receptors in the same supergene family. For example, screening of a cDNA library with a cross-hybridizing probe for a β_2-adrenoceptor led to the discovery of the serotonin (5-HT$_{1A}$) receptor [2].

Since many receptors are only expressed at very low levels in most tissues it may be difficult to obtain a sufficient quantity of the receptor for the initial sequencing necessary to prepare a probe. More recently, the polymerase chain reaction (PCR) has been used to amplify enormously the number of mRNA copies in a cell in order to make a series of probes, which can then be used to screen a DNA library [3].

The receptor cDNA can also be inserted into an immortal cell line, resulting in its expression and thus providing a source of the receptor, so that it is possible to characterize the gene product pharmacologically. The cDNA may be directly microinjected into the large *Xenopus* toad oocyte, or transfected into a cultured mammalian cell which does not normally express the receptor, using a plasmid expression vector which, after suitable manipulation, inserts the cDNA into the cultured cell genome. Cultured Chinese hamster ovary (CHO) and B-82 (a mouse L-cell line) cells have been found to be very useful in studying neurotransmitter receptors, since they lack these receptors but possess other elements, such as G-proteins and adenylyl cyclase and phospholipase C, so that aspects of receptor coupling can be investigated. The cultured cells express the single receptor coded by the inserted cDNA and this can be studied directly by radioligand binding and by measuring cellular responses, such as cyclic 3′,5′-adenosine monophosphate (cAMP) concentrations or phosphoinositide (PI) hydrolysis. Using a series of suitable agonists and antagonists it is then possible to characterize carefully the pure cloned receptor pharmacologically. Factors that influence the pure receptor can then be studied in detail without variations in metabolism and the interfering effects of other related receptors.

The value of receptor cloning

The cloning of receptors has led to many important advances in our understanding of receptor structure and function, and has provided important tools for investigating the role of receptors in disease. Cloning of receptors has been valuable in several ways.

1 Molecular cloning has revealed the primary sequence of receptor proteins which were impossible to determine because of the limited amounts of purified protein which could be prepared by conventional techniques.

2 The isolation of receptor cDNA makes it possible to study the pharmacology of the pure receptor if expressed in a cultured cell line which does not normally express the receptor of interest or related receptors. In most intact tissues several receptors may be expressed, and this can make interpretation of responses difficult, especially when several subtypes of receptor are expressed in the same cell.

3 Knowledge of the nucleotide sequence of a receptor makes it possible to delete specific stretches, thus leading to removal of particular lengths of the amino acid sequence in the receptor encoded by the mutant cDNA (deletion mutagenesis). This is important in elucidating the parts of the protein structure which are important for ligand binding, signal transduction or in receptor regulation. More specific information is provided by the deletion or substitution of single coding sequences, leading to the substitution of particular amino acids (site-directed mutagenesis).

4 The availability of large quantities of purified receptor by cloning techniques has allowed the generation of specific antibodies, which may then be used for localization of receptors. After deletion of part of the cDNA sequence, it is also possible to generate immunological probes to specific parts of the receptor sequence. The antibodies which bind to these sequences may then be used to determine the functional domains of the receptor, the structural requirements for receptor binding and the localization of transmembrane signalling elements [4]. Site-directed antireceptor antibodies have confirmed the studies of site-directed mutagenesis.

5 Cloning of one receptor has often led to the discovery of closely related subtypes of receptors which may or may not have been previously recognized by pharmacological techniques. Thus the discovery of m_1-, m_2- and m_3-muscarinic receptors, which have been distinguished by the development of selective antagonists, was followed by the discovery of two additional muscarinic receptor subtypes (m_4 and m_5), which cannot yet be identified pharmacologically [5, 6] and six subtypes of α-adrenoceptor [7]. Using subtype-specific antireceptor antibodies, generated from the cloned receptors, it has recently been possible to study the distribution of receptor subtypes in tissues; muscarinic m_4- and m_5-receptors can thus be studied in the absence of any known selective drugs [8].

6 The expression of a pure receptor in a cultured cell may be useful in rapid drug screening. Thus human β_2-receptors have been co-expressed in yeast cells with the α-subunit of G_s, which then activates the enzyme β-galactosidase, which has a pheromone-responsive (FUS1) gene promoter site. This allows activation of the galactosidase activity as a colorimetric response and provides a rapid and sensitive screening test for β_2-agonists [9]. It is also applicable to other cloned receptors.

Molecular structure of receptors

G-protein-coupled receptors

While neurotransmitter receptors vary widely in terms of specificity for agonists, molecular biological characterization has recently revealed some common structural features. This is perhaps understandable, since these receptors interact with a guanine nucleotide regulatory protein (G-protein). G-proteins may stimulate (G_s) or inhibit (G_i) adenylyl cyclase and thus increase or decrease the intracellular concentration of cAMP [10, 11], or they may stimulate G-proteins which activate phospholipase C (G_q or G_{plc}), resulting in PI hydrolysis leading to the formation of inositol 1,4,5-triphosphate, the intracellular messenger which releases calcium ions from internal stores [12].

More than 30 G-protein-linked receptors have now been cloned and their sequences determined [13, 14]. The first and most carefully characterized receptor in this category was rhodopsin in light-sensitive rods of the retina which is linked to a unique G-protein called transducin [15, 16], and this has served as a useful model for other receptors in this group which were cloned later. Analysis of the amino acid sequence of rhodopsin has revealed seven hydrophobic (lipophilic) stretches of 20−25 amino acids which are linked to hydrophilic regions of variable length. The most likely spatial arrangement of the receptor in the cell surface membrane is for the seven hydrophobic sections (each of which is in the form of an α-helix) to span the cell membrane. The intervening hydrophilic sections are exposed alternately intracellularly and extracellularly with the amino (N)-terminal exposed to the outside and the carboxy (C)-terminal within the cytoplasm (Fig. 12.1). The extracellular domains of rhodopsin recognize the specific ligand (retinal) and the intracellular domains interact with transducin.

Several other G-protein-linked receptors have now been cloned and sequenced. These include neurotransmitter receptors such as β_1- [17], β_2- [18, 19] and β_3-adrenoceptors [20], three α_1- and three α_2-adrenoceptors [7], m_1-m_5-muscarinic receptors [21, 22], A_1- and A_2-adenosine receptors [23], neuropeptide receptors such as three tachykinin receptors NK_1, NK_2, NK_3 [24−27] and a vasoactive intestinal polypeptide (VIP)-receptor [28]. Inflammatory mediator receptors, such as platelet-activating factor [29], thromboxane [30] and bradykinin B_2-receptors [31], which are also linked to G-proteins have also recently been cloned. All of these receptors share the common feature of seven similar hydrophobic membrane-spanning segments. There is also some sequence homology of the intracellular loops (which interact with various

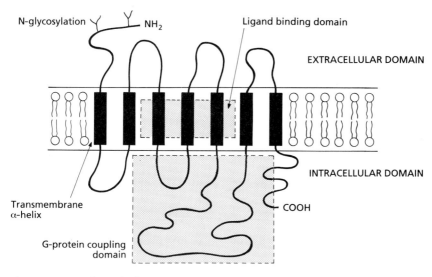

Fig. 12.1 Typical motif of G-protein-coupled surface receptors. The polypeptide chain is believed to be folded so that it crosses the membrane seven times. Extracellular loops may be glycosylated. Intracellular loops interact with the G-protein. The agonist appears to bind at a site deep in the membrane between transmembrane segments.

G-proteins) but less similarity in the extracellular domains. For example, there is a 50% homology between rat β_2-adrenergic and muscarinic m_2-receptors [32]. There is also close homology between the same receptor in different species. Thus there is 95% homology between rat and pig heart m_2-receptors [32]. These similarities demonstrate that G-receptor-linked receptors form part of a supergene family, which may have a common evolutionary origin [14].

Members of the G-protein receptor supergene family are generally 400−500 amino acids in length and the receptor cDNA sequence consists of 2000−4000 nucleotide bases (2−4 kilobases or kb). There is usually a striking lack of introns in the coding sequence of these receptors, compared with genes for other proteins. The molecular weight of the cloned receptors predicted from the cDNA sequence is 40 000−60 000 daltons (40−60 kD), which is usually less than the molecular mass of the wild receptors when assessed by sodium dodecylsulphate−polyacrylamide gel electrophoresis. This discrepancy is due to glycosylation of the native receptor. For example, β_2-receptors contain two sites for glycosylation on asparagine (Asn/N) residues near the amino terminus, and it is estimated that N-glycosylation accounts for 25−30% of the molecular mass of the native receptor. The functional significance of glycosylation is not yet clear [33]; it does not affect receptor affinity for ligand or coupling to G-proteins but may be important for the trafficking of the receptor through the cell during down-regulation, or for keeping the receptor correctly oriented in the lipid bilayer.

Steroid receptors

Steroids interact with intracellular (cytosolic) receptors rather than surface receptors. There is a family of steroid receptors that recognizes different endogenous steroids such as glucocorticosteroids, mineralocorticoids, androgens and oestrogens. Indeed, steroid receptors belong to a gene superfamily that also includes thyroid hormone and vitamin D receptors [34]. Several steroid receptors have now been cloned and their structures have been shown to differ [35, 36]. However, there is some homology between these receptors since they all interact with nuclear DNA, where they act as modulators of the transcription of specific genes [37]. For instance, corticosteroids switch on the transcription of the 37 kD protein, lipocortin, which may inhibit phospholipase A_2 [38], although it is likely that lipocortin is only one of several proteins induced by steroids. Only a limited number of genes appear to respond to steroids. Glucocorticosteroid receptors (GR) are normally present in the cytosol in an inactive form bound to two molecules of a 90 kD heat shock protein (HSP 90), which cover the DNA-binding domain. Binding of a steroid to its receptor results in the dissociation of HSP 90 and the occupied receptor then undergoes a conformational change that allows it to bind to DNA [39].

The DNA-binding domain of steroid receptors is rich in cysteine (Cys) residues. Formation of a complex with zinc is able to fold the peptide chain into a finger-shaped conformation and the zinc is either coordinated by two Cys and two histidine (His) or by four Cys residues. GRs have two 'zinc fingers' consisting of loops of about 15 residues with four Cys residues, which are held in place by a zinc atom and appear to be essential for recognition of specific DNA sequences — the so-called glucocorticoid response elements (GREs; Fig. 12.2). GREs have the consensus sequence GGTAnnnTGTTCT [40]. Dimers of GR occupied by steroid bind to the GRE on the DNA double helix and either increase

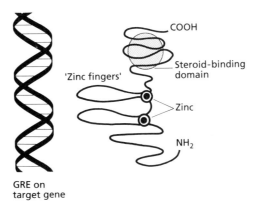

Fig. 12.2 Glucocorticosteroid receptor. There are two 'zinc fingers' which interact with specific glucocorticoid response elements (GREs) on target genes.

(+GRE) or decrease (nGRE) the rate of transcription by influencing the promoter sequence in the target gene. Indeed repression of target genes may be the most important aspect of steroid action in inflammatory diseases such as asthma, since steroids may inhibit the transcription of many cytokines, which are involved in the chronic inflammatory response [41].

By understanding the interactions between steroid receptors and DNA it may be possible to develop synthetic agents in the future that could mimic these responses. The steroid receptor–DNA interactions may be tissue-specific and this opens up the possibility for the development of more selective steroid-like agents for therapeutic use, thereby reducing the potential hazards of systemic therapy.

Cytokine receptors

Cytokines are a diverse collection of peptides, including interleukins (IL), growth factors and colony-stimulating factors, which play an important role in chronic inflammatory and immune pulmonary diseases [42]. The effects of cytokines are mediated via specific surface receptors, several of which have now been cloned [43]. Little is known about the intracellular mechanisms involved in cytokine signalling, although increasing evidence suggests that stimulation of various protein kinases leads to the activation of transcription factors, which regulate the expression of various target genes [44]. Some cytokine receptors (e.g. epidermal growth factor receptors) have intrinsic tyrosine kinase activity, leading to phosphorylation of cytosolic substrates that results in altered gene transcription. Many of the cloned cytokine receptors have a primary structure which is quite different from the seven transmembrane-spanning

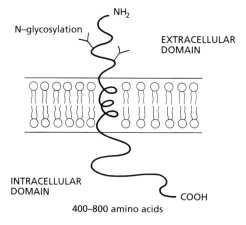

Fig. 12.3 Typical structure of a cytokine receptor, with a single membrane-spanning segment. The extracellular domain may be glycosylated and the intracellular domain may lead to the activation of transcription factors, or may have intrinsic protein tyrosine kinase activity.

segments associated with G-protein-linked receptors (Fig. 12.3). Thus the receptor for tumour necrosis factor (TNF)-α is a 55 kD peptide, which has recently been cloned and appears to have a single transmembrane-spanning helical segment, an extracellular domain which binds TNF-α and an intracellular domain [45]. The intracellular domain leads to activation of transcription factors such as nuclear factor kappa B (NF$_\kappa$B) and activator protein-1 (AP-1). The structure of the receptor is analogous to the nerve growth factor receptor. A second receptor for TNF-α has also been cloned, but differs markedly in sequence, and may be linked to different intracellular pathways [45].

Molecular cloning has now revealed that although cytokines may be structurally diverse, their receptors may be grouped into various families which share structural homology. One family of receptors includes the receptors for IL-1 and platelet-derived growth factor; these receptors belong to the immunoglobulin superfamily, which includes T-cell antigen receptors and certain cell-surface adhesion molecules [46]. Another cytokine receptor superfamily, the haematopoietin receptor superfamily, includes receptors for IL-2, IL-3, IL-4, IL-5, IL-6, IL-7, interferons and granulocyte—macrophage colony-stimulating factor (GM-CSF) [47, 48]. Prolactin, growth factor and erythropoietin receptors are also included in this family. The receptor proteins are oriented with an extracellular N-terminal domain and a single hydrophobic transmembrane-spanning segment. There is striking homology in the extracellular ligand-binding domain with four conserved Cys residues. There is very close homology between the receptors for IL-3, IL-5 and GM-CSF, all of which stimulate growth of eosinophils. Molecular cloning has demonstrated that each of these receptors consists of an α- and β-chain and share a common β-chain [49—51]. This explains why they have overlapping biological activities.

The IL-8 superfamily of cytokines appears to bind to receptors which are linked to G-proteins and their receptors have the seven transmembrane-spanning motifs typical of such receptors [52].

Receptor subtypes

The existence of receptor subtypes is often first indicated by differences in the potency of a series of agonists in different tissues. This could be due to differing proportions of coexistent receptor subtypes, or may indicate the existence of a novel receptor subtype. Molecular biology can resolve these possibilities, since molecular techniques can clearly discriminate between different subtypes of receptor and show that they are encoded by different genes. Thus, the human β_1-receptor is clearly different from the β_2-receptor in its amino acid sequence, with only 54% homology [53], and the neurokinin-1 (NK$_1$) receptor which is selectively activated by substance P has a 48% homology with the NK$_2$-

receptor, which is activated by the related tachykinin neurokinin A [25]. A third tachykinin receptor, NK_3-receptor, which is selectively activated by neurokinin B has also been cloned [26]. Molecular biology techniques have thus confirmed the evidence for the existence of receptor subtypes obtained by classical pharmacological techniques, using the rank order of potency of different agonists and antagonists.

Using cross-hybridization in which a known receptor cDNA sequence is hybridized with a genomic library it has also been possible to detect previously unknown subtypes of a receptor. For example, an atypical β-receptor, which does not clearly fit into the β_1- or β_2-receptor subtypes, has been suspected in adipose tissue and recently a 'β_3'-receptor has been identified, cloned, sequenced and expressed [20]. The β_3-receptor is clearly different from either β_1- or β_2-receptors (about 50% amino acid sequence homology). β_3-Receptors appear to be important in regulation of metabolic rate and have not yet been detected in lung homogenates. Without the techniques of molecular biology this receptor would probably still remain undiscovered.

Molecular biology has been particularly useful in advancing our understanding of muscarinic receptors. Five distinct muscarinic receptors have been cloned from rat and human tissues [5, 6]. The m_1-, m_2- and m_3-receptors correspond to the m_1-, m_2- and m_3-receptors identified pharmacologically, whereas m_4- and m_5-receptors are previously unrecognized pharmacological subtypes which occur predominantly in the brain, and for which no selective drugs have yet been developed. Interestingly, m_4-receptors have been demonstrated in rabbit lung using antibodies against the cloned m_4-receptor [8], and their presence has been confirmed by cDNA probes for the m_4-receptor [54]. These m_4-receptors are localized to vascular smooth muscle and alveolar walls [55], but have not been observed in lungs of other species, including humans. Other related, but as yet uncharacterized, genes could represent additional subtypes and up to nine subtypes have been predicted in the rat [6]. The reason for so many different subtypes of a receptor which recognize a single agonist is still not certain, but it seems likely that they are linked to different intracellular pathways and that the regulation of the intracellular portion of the amino acid sequence may be unique to each subtype. The m_1-, m_3- and m_5-receptors stimulate PI hydrolysis through a pertussis-insensitive G-protein, whereas m_2- and m_4-receptors inhibit adenylyl cyclase via G_i [56]. The picture is complicated further by the fact that, at higher agonist concentrations, m_2- and m_4-receptors can also stimulate PI hydrolysis [57]. It is possible that the difference in protein structure may reflect regulation at a transcriptional level from DNA through different promoters, leading to variations in tissue or developmental expression, or to differences at a post-translational level, allowing regulation by intracellular mechanisms such as phosphorylation at critical sites on intracellular loops.

It seems very likely that several other subtypes of known receptors will be identified in the future using the technique of cross-hybridization. This is likely to have important implications for the development of more selective receptor agonists and antagonists. The potential clinical importance of muscarinic receptor subtypes in airways is already apparent [58] and the recognition of different receptor subtypes has prompted the search for m_3-selective antagonists to treat airways obstruction. Similarly, for α-receptors additional subtypes have been identified by molecular cloning techniques. Thus, there appear to be at least three α_1- and three α_2-receptors [7].

Molecular approaches may be particularly valuable in the study of peptide receptors, where selective agonists and antagonists have until recently been difficult to develop. If the existence of distinct receptors is demonstrated (which has not been possible by conventional pharmaco-logical techniques), this may lead to the development of selective agonists and antagonists. For platelet-activating factor (PAF) there is some func-tional evidence for more than one subtype of receptor [59, 60]. The recent cloning of a PAF receptor from guinea-pig lung [29] opens up the possibility of finding subtypes of receptor in different cell types. The potential diversity of receptors is obviously an important consideration when designing agonists and antagonists for the treatment of lung diseases, but the coexistence of receptor subtypes raises the possibility that more selective drugs may be developed in the future.

Site-directed mutagenesis

Once the cDNA sequence for receptors is known it is possible to substitute single nucleotide bases at different positions in the sequence and thus produce a mutant receptor with predetermined alterations in its amino acid sequence. This is carried out by substituting the codon for one amino acid with that for another in a synthetic oligonucleotide, and creating a mutant gene which, when expressed, produces a receptor with minor specific changes. The technique of site-directed mutagenesis has proved to be invaluable in elucidating receptor structure and function [61, 62]. Replacement of the Cys residues at positions 106 and 184 in the second and third extracellular domain in the hamster lung β_2-receptor shows that they are important in maintaining the correct tertiary structure (three-dimensional shape) of the receptor in the cell membrane by the formation of a disulphide link between the two loops. Substitution of either of these Cys residues with isoleucine (Ile) impairs β-receptor ligand-binding affinity [63]. Similarly, substitution of either of the adjacent Cys residues at positions 190 and 191 on the third cytoplasmic loop of the human β_2-receptor markedly reduces binding affinity and coupling to adenylyl cyclase [64]. It is interesting that the Cys residues on the second and third extracellular loops are highly conserved among receptors and suggests that they may be important in stabilizing their three-dimensional structure.

Two of the most intriguing questions are the location of the ligand-binding site and the means by which an agonist changes the receptor so that it can interact with the appropriate G-protein. The ligand-binding domain of the β-receptor has been carefully characterized by selective deletion of sections of the gene encoding hydrophilic and hydrophobic domains of the receptor protein, expressing the mutant receptor genes in mammalian cell lines, and determining the binding and functional characteristics of the mutant receptor. These elegant studies have demonstrated that regions which form junctions between the transmembrane hydrophobic segments and the extramembranous loops result in altered protein folding. Curiously, most of the extracellular portions of the receptor can be deleted without affecting binding, which implicates regions within the hydrophobic membrane portion as being critical for binding [65]. Site-directed mutagenesis of single amino acids of the β_2-receptor has indicated that substitution of neutral amino acids for aspartate (Asp) residues in the second and third transmembrane segments affects agonist-binding affinity, but does not affect G_s activation. The importance of Asp residues may relate to the fact that they are believed to bind to the protonated group of catecholamines [61, 62, 66]. Interestingly, equivalent Asp residues are conserved in all other adrenergic receptors which all bind ligands with a charged amine group.

To explain how adrenergic receptors are selective for catecholamines, however, differences from G-protein-linked receptors which recognize different agonists must be examined. Site-directed mutagenesis of serine (Ser) residues, which may form a hydrogen bond with the catechol ring, suggests that Ser residues in the fifth transmembrane helix are important. These studies indicate that a ligand-binding pocket may fit between the third and sixth transmembrane helices [61]. Using the fluorescent β-blocker carazolol which binds with high affinity to the β_2-receptor it has been possible with fluorescence spectroscopy to demonstrate in quenching experiments that the ligand-binding site is buried deep (at least 11 Å) within the receptor [67].

The reason why β_2-receptors prefer adrenaline (which is more bulky) is not completely understood. Recent studies with chimeric receptors, which are a combination of the sequence of β_1- and β_2-receptors, indicate that the sequences of amino acids in transmembrane helices 4 and 5 are critical and probably determine the shape of the binding pocket [68].

The intracellular loops located on the inner surface of the plasma membrane interact with G-proteins. Deletion mutagenesis studies, in which stretches of the amino acid sequence are removed, indicate that the third intracellular loop is critical for interaction between β_2-receptors and G_s [69]. This loop contains a sequence of amino acids, which includes charged amino acids in the form of an α-helix. A similar sequence is found in all G-protein-linked receptors and the third cytoplasmic loop is also present in muscarinic receptors [6, 56]. The specificity for the particular G-protein (G_s, G_i, G_p or G_{plc}) is probably determined by the remaining intracellular loops.

Quantification and localization of receptor transcription

Transcription of the genes coding for receptors leads to the formation of specific mRNA which leaves the nucleus and localizes to ribosomes where amino acids are assembled in sequence to form the receptor protein. Total RNA, which includes mRNAs, can be extracted from tissues and specific receptor mRNA can then be identified by hybridization with a radiolabelled cDNA probe, which contains the unique receptor coding sequence. This probe may be the full receptor sequence or a unique oligonucleotide may be synthesized and end labelled.

Using Northern blot analysis the RNA is run on a size separation gel, and then hybridized with the labelled cDNA (or cRNA) probe to reveal whether there is a labelled band which corresponds to the receptor mRNA. Specific mRNA represents only a small percentage of total RNA and it may be difficult to detect, especially when the amounts are low (which is usually the case for receptor-specific mRNA). It may therefore be necessary to carry out a poly(A)$^+$ purification step.

Using this approach the distribution of muscarinic receptor subtype mRNAs has been determined in different tissues and indicates that both m_2- and m_3-receptors are found in porcine and rat tracheal smooth muscle [70] and in cultured human airways smooth muscle cells (Fig. 12.4) [71]. β_2-Receptor mRNA has also been detected in human and rat lung [72] and in guinea-pig lung mast cells [73]. The amount of radioactivity in the labelled band can be quantified by laser densitometry to give a semiquantitative estimate of the amount of mRNA present. This makes it possible to assess changes in gene transcription of a particular receptor. Results are usually expressed in comparison with those of a 'housekeeping' gene which shows consistent expression (e.g. β-actin or t-RNA synthase), or with the amount of RNA in the 18S ribosomal band, in order to overcome the variability in RNA purification.

As many receptors are present in relatively low abundance (compared with other proteins) there may be few mRNA copies present in a particular cell. Using the PCR it may be possible to amplify selectively the number of copies in order to detect the mRNA for a particular receptor subtype [3]. This technique is of potential relevance to the investigation of the role of receptors in lung disease, since it may be possible to detect and study receptor mRNA when only a small amount of tissue is available (e.g. from a bronchial or lung biopsy, from lavaged cells or from bronchial brushings). The major problem, however, is quantification since PCR

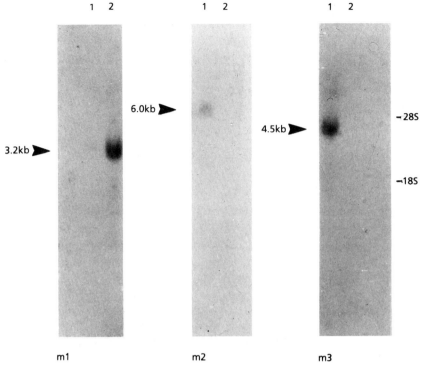

Fig. 12.4 Northern blot showing the presence of muscarinic receptor subtype specific mRNAs in cultured human airways smooth muscle cells (lane 1) and human peripheral lung (lane 2). Radiolabelled oligonucleotide probes against human m_1-, m_2- and m_3-muscarinic receptors were used. m_1-Receptor mRNA was identified in peripheral lung, whereas m_2- and m_3- receptor mRNA was localized to smooth muscle cells. Neither m_4- nor m_5-receptor mRNA was identified in either preparation.

will demonstrate only the presence of a particular receptor, and since most receptors are constitutively expressed this may not be useful. Development of quantitative PCR techniques may overcome these problems in the future [74].

In situ hybridization is capable of determining the distribution of receptor-specific mRNA in tissue sections. Since the amount of mRNA for receptors is present in only low concentrations a sensitive technique must be used. The use of cRNA probes (riboprobes), which are complementary to mRNA and therefore hybridize with the specific mRNA in the cell with greater affinity than the relevant cDNA probe, is probably the best technique. Autoradiography reveals the tissue distribution of receptor mRNA, and therefore the sites of gene expression of the receptor. With a full-length or long cDNA, and thus cRNA, sequence it is possible to label the probe at many sites, and then to increase the amount of radioactivity of the probe, so that there is a stronger signal.

Using this approach it has been possible to demonstrate the distribution

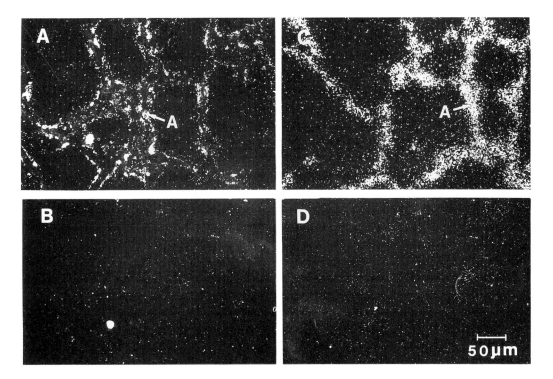

Fig. 12.5 *In situ* hybridization showing the distribution of β_2-receptor mRNA in sections of human peripheral lung, demonstrating positive hybridization in the alveolar wall (A). A radiolabelled partial cRNA probe to the human β_2-receptor was used. (B) Shows non-specific labelling using a sense sequence probe in the same way. (C) Shows the corresponding autoradiographic labelling of β_2-receptors in the alveolar wall (A) using $[^{125}I]$iodocyanopindolol in the presence of a β_1-selective antagonist. (D) Shows non-specific binding in the presence of excess β-agonist. From Hamid QA, Mak JC, Sheppard MN, Corrin B, Venter JC, Barnes PJ. *Eur J Pharmacol (Mol Pharmacol)* 1991; 206: 133–8.

of β_2-receptor-binding sites in lung tissue (Figs 12.5 & 12.6) [72]. The localization of receptor mRNA corresponds to the distribution of β_2-receptors as expected, but there are discrepancies between the relative density of mRNA and of receptors in certain cells. Thus, in airways smooth muscle there is a very high density of β-receptor mRNA, whereas the density of the β-receptors is relatively low; this suggests either that the rate of receptor synthesis is high, and there is a rapid turnover of receptors, or that the stability of mRNA is high. This may explain why it is difficult to down-regulate β-receptors in airways smooth muscle, and therefore to demonstrate tachyphylaxis to the bronchodilator action of β-agonists. By contrast, in the alveolar walls there is a low level of mRNA but a very high receptor density, which may indicate a low receptor turnover, and this would be consistent with the fact that down-regulation is readily produced in lung parenchyma. Using probes to muscarinic receptor subtypes it has been possible to demonstrate the

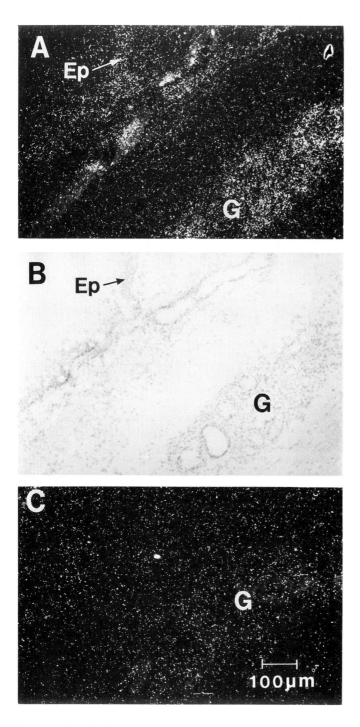

Fig. 12.6 (A) *In situ* hybridization showing the distribution of β₂-receptor mRNA in a human airways showing localization to airways epithelium (Ep) and submucosal gland (G). (B) Shows the tissue appearance and (C), non-specific hybridization.

sites of gene expression of different subtypes in human lung [71]. m_3-Receptors are expressed in airways smooth muscle and submucosal glands, as expected from the autoradiographic mapping of receptor expression [75]. m_3-Receptors are also strongly expressed in epithelial cells, which have few binding sites, indicating that there may be a rapid degradation of mRNA in these cells. m_1-Receptor mRNA is also localized to glands and to the alveolar wall, as predicted by the receptor mapping. Neither m_4- nor m_5-mRNA is detected in Northern analysis or by *in situ* hybridization. However, in rabbit lung there is evidence for m_4-receptor mRNA [54], which is localized to vascular smooth muscle and alveolar walls [55].

Similar approaches have also been adopted with steroid receptors, and glucocorticoid receptor mRNA has been localized in brain tissue [76]. Using a cDNA probe to the human glucocorticoid receptor-specific mRNA has been identified in human lung and is localized to endothelial cells and epithelial cells, but also to airways smooth muscle [77].

Regulation of receptor transcription

Perhaps one of the most interesting applications of molecular biology to receptor pharmacology will be in understanding further how receptors may be regulated in health and disease, although few such studies have so far been reported.

Desensitization

Tachyphylaxis or desensitization occurs with most receptors when exposed to an agonist. This phenomenon has been studied in some detail with β_2-receptors and involves several processes [53, 78]. In the short term desensitization involves phosphorylation which uncouples the receptor from G_s, via the action of an enzyme called β-adrenergic receptor-specific kinase (βARK) [79]. The site of this phosphorylation appears to be on the serine/threonine (Ser/Thr) rich region of the third intracellular loop and the C-terminal tail, since their replacement reduces the rate of desensitization [78, 80]. Longer term mechanisms include down-regulation of surface receptor number, a process which involves internalization of the receptor and its subsequent degradation. In a cultured hamster cell line, down-regulation of β_2-receptors results in a rapid decline in the steady-state level of β_2-receptor mRNA [81, 82]. This suggests that down-regulation is achieved, in part, either by inhibiting the genetic transcription of receptors or by increased post-transcriptional processing of the mRNA in the cell. Using actinomycin D to inhibit transcription it has been found that β_2-receptor mRNA stability is markedly reduced in these cells after exposure to β-agonists. Furthermore, by isolating nuclei and performing a nuclear run-on transcription assay it is apparent that β-agonist exposure does not directly alter receptor gene transcription [82]. Whether this also applies to β_2-receptors in various lung cells has not been reported.

Steroid modulation

Certain G-protein-linked receptors are also influenced by corticosteroids. Thus, rat pulmonary β-receptors are increased in density by pretreatment with corticosteroids [83] and corticosteroids increase the expression of β-receptors in rabbit foetal lung [84]. Steroids also prevent the desensitization and down-regulation of β-receptors on human leucocytes [85, 86]. Corticosteroids increase the steady-state level of β_2-receptor mRNA in cultured hamster smooth muscle cells, thus indicating that steroids may increase β-receptor density by increasing the rate of gene transcription [82, 87]. The increase in mRNA occurs rapidly (within 1 h), preceding the increase in β-receptors, and then declines to a steady-state level about twice normal. The mechanism by which steroids interact with the β-receptor gene is not yet understood, but the cloned β-receptor gene contains three potential GREs, which have the sequence [61]. In human lung and cultured airways smooth muscle cells steroids cause an increase in β_2-receptor mRNA, which appears to be due to increased gene transcription [88].

Steroids may also regulate their own receptors. Incubation of various cells with corticosteroids may result in a down-regulation of steroid receptors [89]. This appears to be due to a decrease in gene transcription of the receptors and the steroid receptor gene itself has GREs. In human lung the inhibition of receptor transcription is marked, with almost complete inhibition of transcription after incubation with a high concentration of dexamethasone (1 µmol l^{-1}) for 24 h [72]. This may have important implications for long-term management of airways disease by high doses of inhaled steroids, since this may lead to reduced steroid responsiveness, which may be an explanation of the apparent progression of asthma in some patients.

Ontogeny

Another area in which the molecular biology of receptors may be relevant is in the development of receptors, and the factors which determine expression of particular receptor genes during development.

Disease

There are several pulmonary diseases in which altered expression of receptors may be relevant to understanding their pathophysiology. Molecular biology offers a new perspective in investigating these abnormalities of receptor expression by providing insights into whether the abnormality arises through altered transcription of the receptor gene, or in post-transcriptional or post-translational processing.

There is debate about whether β-receptors function abnormally in asthmatic airways. Airways from patients who have died from asthma attacks show impaired relaxation to β-agonists *in vitro* [90]. Autoradiographic mapping studies in such patients have demonstrated a surprising increase in β-receptor density in airways smooth muscle, indicating that the reduced responsiveness to β-agonists is not likely to be due to loss of receptors, but more likely to be due to uncoupling of the receptors [91]. The unexpected increase in β-receptor number may be due to increased transcription of receptors in the absence of a negative feedback signal from intracellular cAMP via a cAMP responsive element (CRE).

Transcriptional control

Receptor genes, like any other genes, may be regulated by transcription factors, which may be activated within the cell under certain conditions, leading to increased or decreased receptor gene transcription, which may in turn alter the expression of receptors at the cell surface. Little is known about the transcription factors which regulate receptors, but these may be relevant to diseases, such as chronic inflammation. The transcription factor AP-1 is made up of the products of the early immediate genes c-*fos* and c-*jun* together with related proteins. Both c-*fos* and c-*jun* genes may be activated via protein kinase C, resulting in the formation of Fos and Jun nucleoproteins within the cell nucleus. AP-1 complexes are then formed, which interact with AP-1 regulatory sites on certain genes, leading to increased or decreased gene transcription. For example, the gene coding for the NK_1-receptor has an AP-1 site, which leads to increased gene transcription and a GRE which conversely results in decreased transcription [92]. Chronic cell stimulation, via activation of protein kinase C, may therefore lead to an increase in NK_1-receptor gene expression, which could lead to increased neurogenic inflammation. An increase in NK_1-receptors has been reported in the colon of patients with inflammatory bowel disease [93], and an increased NK_1-receptor gene expression is present in asthmatic airways [94]. By contrast corticosteroids reduce NK_1-specific mRNA in human lung [94]. Many other transcription factors have been described, including products of genes related to c-*fos* and c-*jun* (the leucine zipper supergene family). Thus Jun-B and FRA proteins form a transcription factor which appears to activate genes via a CRE [95]. $NF_\kappa B$ is also an important transcription factor, which may be activated in cells in response to cytokines such as TNF-α independently of protein kinase C activation [96].

Corticosteroids may exert their anti-inflammatory effect in chronic inflammatory diseases such as asthma by interacting with transcription factors [37]. GREs may be located on the same genes which may be activated by AP-1. An additional mechanism of control has recently been identified which involves a direct interaction between Jun and Fos proteins and the steroid receptor, resulting in reduced effects of AP-1 [97, 98]. Thus in human lung the stimulated increase in AP-1 may be inhibited by prior exposure to corticosteroids. Conversely increased formation of AP-1, perhaps by chronic exposure of cells to cytokines, may lead to a reduced density of cytosolic steroid receptors, resulting in reduced anti-inflammatory effects of steroids (Fig. 12.7).

Conclusions

The potential impact of molecular biology on the understanding of the structure and function of receptors is enormous. Use of these novel

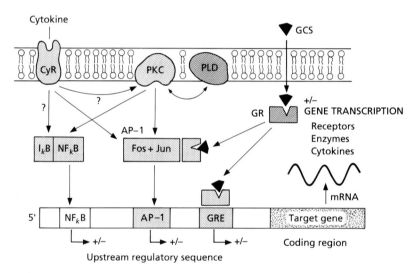

Fig. 12.7 The effect of cytokines and glucocorticosteroids on gene transcription. Cytokines interact with surface receptors (CyR) which leads to changes in receptor gene transcription by activating transcription factors, such as AP-1 and NF_kB. This may involve activation of protein kinase C (PKC) via diacylglycerol generated from activation of phosphoinositidase C (PIC). PKC in turn may activate phospholipase D (PLD) which generates more diacylglycerol to perpetuate activation of PKC. NF_kB is activated by phosphorylation of an inhibitory protein I_kB. AP-1 is made up of at least two protein products of the proto-oncogenes c-*fos* and c-*jun* (Fos and Jun, respectively). The transcription factors bind to particular sequences on the upstream regulatory element of target genes, leading to changes in transcription of the receptor gene. Corticosteroids (GCS) may counteract the effect of cytokines in gene transcription in at least two ways. First, the steroid binds to a cytosolic glucocorticoid receptor (GR), which then binds to the AP-1 complex preventing its effect on gene transcription. Second, the activated GR binds to a GRE on the same gene, which has the opposite effect on gene transcription from that of the activated transcription factors.

techniques should provide insight into the structure of the neuro-transmitter, inflammatory mediator and steroid receptors relevant to various lung diseases, and will give further understanding of abnormalities that may occur in disease. In the future this new knowledge should lead to advances in therapy, since understanding receptor structure and function will aid the development of new agonists or antagonists (which may be particularly valuable in the case of peptide receptors) and may also lead to novel drugs that interact with the transcription or post-translational processing of receptors.

References

1 Barnes PJ. Molecular biology of receptors: implications for lung disease. *Thorax* 1990; 45: 482−8.
2 Fargin A, Raymond JR, Lohse MJ, Kobilka BK, Caron MG, Lefkowitz RJ. The genomic clone G-21 which resembles a beta-adrenergic receptor sequence encodes the 5-HT1A receptor. *Nature* 1988; 335: 358−60.
3 Watson SP, James W. PCR and the cloning of receptor subtype genes. *Trends Pharmacol Sci* 1989; 10: 346−8.
4 Bahouth SW, Wang H-Y, Malbon CC. Immunological approaches for probing receptor structure and function. *Trends Pharmacol Sci* 1991; 12: 338−43.
5 Hulme EC, Birdsall NJM, Buckley NJ. Muscarinic receptor subtypes. *Annu Rev Pharmacol* 1990; 30: 633−73.
6 Bonner TI. New subtypes of muscarinic acetylcholine receptors. *Trends Pharmacol Sci* 1989; 10 (Suppl): 11−15.
7 Harrison JK, Pearson WR, Lynch KR. Molecular characterization of α_1- and α_2-adrenoceptors. *Trends Pharmacol Sci* 1991; 12: 62−7.
8 Dorje F, Levey AI, Brann MR. Immunological detection of muscarinic receptor subtype proteins (m1−m5) in rabbit peripheral tissues. *Mol Pharmacol* 1991; 40: 459−62.
9 King K, Dohlman HG, Thorner J, Caron MG, Lefkowitz RJ. Control of yeast mating signal transduction by a mammalian β_2-adrenergic receptor and $G_{s\alpha}$ subunit. *Science* 1990; 250: 121−3.
10 Gilman AG. G proteins: transducers of receptor-generated signals. *Annu Rev Biochem* 1987; 56: 615−49.
11 Bourne HR, Sanders DA, McCormick F. The GTPase superfamily: conserved structure and molecular mechanism. *Nature* 1991; 349: 117−27.
12 Berridge MJ, Irvine RF. Inositol phosphates and cell signalling. *Nature* 1989; 341: 197−205.
13 Dohlman HG, Caron MG, Lefkowitz RJ. A family of receptors coupled to guanine nucleotide regulatory proteins. *Biochemistry* 1987; 26: 2656−64.
14 Venter JC, Fraser CM, Kerlavage AR, Buck MA. Molecular biology of adrenergic and muscarinic cholinergic receptors: a perspective. *Biochem Pharmacol* 1989; 38: 1197−208.
15 Nathans J, Hogness DS. Isolation and nucleotide sequence of the gene encoding human rhodopsin. *Proc Natl Acad Sci USA* 1984; 87: 4851−5.
16 Martin RL, Wood C, Baehr W, Applesbury ML. Visual pigment homologies revealed by DNA hybridization. *Science* 1986; 232: 1266−9.
17 Frielle T, Collins S, Daniel KW, Caron MG, Lefkowitz RJ, Kobilka BK. Cloning of the cDNA for the β_1-adrenergic receptor. *Proc Natl Acad Sci USA* 1987; 84: 7920−4.

18 Dixon RAF, Kobilka B, Strader C *et al.* Cloning of the gene and cDNA for mammalian β-adrenergic receptor and homology with rhodopsin. *Nature* 1986; 321: 75−9.

19 Chung F-Z, Lentes K-U, Gocayne J *et al.* Cloning and sequence analysis of the human brain β-adrenergic receptor. *FEBS Lett* 1987; 211: 200−6.

20 Emorine LJ, Marullo S, Briend-Sutren M-M *et al.* Molecular characterization of the human β₃-adrenergic receptor. *Science* 1989; 245: 1118−21.

21 Bonner TI, Buckley NJ, Young AC, Brann MR. Identification of a family of muscarinic acetylcholine receptor genes. *Science* 1987; 237: 527−32.

22 Bonner TI, Young AC, Brann MR, Buckley NJ. Cloning and expression of the human and rat M₅ muscarinic acetylcholine receptor genes. *Neuron* 1988; 1: 403−10.

23 Linden J, Tucker AL, Lynch RR. Molecular cloning of adenosine A₁ and A₂ receptors. *Trends Pharmacol Sci* 1991; 12: 326−8.

24 Masu Y, Nakayama K, Tamaki H, Harada Y, Kuno M, Nakanishi S. cDNA cloning of bovine substance K receptor through oocyte expression system. *Nature* 1987; 329: 836−8.

25 Yokota Y, Sasai Y, Tanaka K *et al.* Molecular characterization of a functional cDNA for rat substance P receptor. *J Biol Chem* 1989; 264: 17649−52.

26 Shigemoto R, Yokota Y, Tsuchida K, Nakanishi S. Cloning and expression of a rat neuromedin K receptor cDNA. *J Biol Chem* 1990; 265: 623−8.

27 Gerard NP, Eddy RL, Shows TB, Gerard C. The human neurokinin A (substance K) receptor. *J Biol Chem* 1990; 265: 20455−62.

28 Speedharan SP, Robichen A, Peterson KE, Goetzl EJ. Cloning and expression of the human vasoactive intestinal peptide receptor. *Proc Natl Acad Sci USA* 1991; 88: 4986−90.

29 Honda Z, Nakamura M, Miki I *et al.* Cloning by functional expression of guinea pig lung platelet activating factor (PAF) receptor. *Nature* 1991; 349: 342−6.

30 Hirata M, Hayashi Y, Ushikubi F *et al.* Cloning and expression of cDNA for a human thromboxane A₂ receptor. *Nature* 1991; 349: 617−20.

31 McEachern AE, Bhakta S, Shelton ER *et al.* Expression cloning of a rat B₂-bradykinin receptor. *Proc Natl Acad Sci USA* 1991; 88: 7724−8.

32 Gokayne J, Robinson DA, Fitzgerald MG *et al.* Primary structure of rat cardiac β-adrenergic and muscarinic receptors obtained by automated DNA sequence analysis: further evidence for a multigene family. *Proc Natl Acad Sci USA* 1987; 89: 8296−300.

33 George ST, Ruoho AE, Malbon CC. N-Glycosylation in expression and function of β-adrenergic receptors. *J Biochem* 1986; 261: 16559−64.

34 Evans RM. The steroid and thyroid hormone receptor superfamily. *Science* 1988; 247: 889−95.

35 Miesfeld RL, Okret S, Wikstrom A-C, Wrange O, Gustafson J-Å, Yamamoto KR. Characterization of a steroid hormone receptor gene and mRNA in wild-type and mutant cells. *Nature* 1984; 312: 779−82.

36 Thompson BC. The structure of the human glucocorticoid receptor and its gene. *J Steroid Biochem* 1987; 27: 105−8.

37 Beato M. Gene regulation by steroid hormones. *Cell* 1989; 56: 335−44.

38 Flower RJ. Lipocortin and the mechanism of action of the glucocorticoids. *Br J Pharmacol* 1988; 94: 987−1015.

39 Munck A, Mendel DB, Smith LI, Orti E. Glucocorticoid receptors and actions. *Am Rev Respir Dis* 1991; 141: S2−10.

40 Miesfeld RL. Molecular genetics of corticosteroid action. *Am Rev Respir Dis* 1990; 141: S11−17.

41 Guyre PM, Girard MT, Morganelli PM, Manginiello PD. Glucocorticoid effects

on the production and action of immune cytokines. *J Steroid Biochem* 1988; 30: 89−93.

42 Kelley J. Cytokines of the lung. *Am Rev Respir Dis* 1990; 141: 765−88.

43 Shepherd VL. Cytokine receptors in lung. *Am J Respir Cell Mol Biol* 1991; 5: 403−10.

44 Muegge K, Durum SK. Cytokines and transcription factors. *Cytokine* 1990; 2: 1−8.

45 Sprang SR. The divergent receptors for TNF. *Trends Biochem Sci* 1990; 15: 366−8.

46 Williams AF, Barclay AN. The immunoglobulin superfamily − domains for cell surface recognition. *Annu Rev Immunol* 1988; 6: 381−405.

47 Cosman D, Lyman SD, Idzerda RL *et al*. A new cytokine receptor superfamily. *Trends Biochem Sci* 1990; 15: 265−70.

48 Bazan JF. Structural design and molecular evolution of a cytokine receptor superfamily. *Proc Natl Acad Sci USA* 1990; 87: 6934−8.

49 Tavernier J, Devos R, Cornelis S *et al*. A human high affinity interleukin-5 receptor (IL5R) is composed of an IL5-specific α chain and β chain with the receptor for GM-CSF. *Cell* 1991; 66: 1175−84.

50 Kitamura T, Sata N, Arai K, Miyajima A. Expression cloning of the human IL-3 receptor cDNA reveals a shared β subunit for the human IL-3 and GM-CSF receptors. *Cell* 1991; 66: 1165−74.

51 Gearing DP, King JA, Gough NM, Nicola NA. Expression cloning of a receptor for human granulocyte−macrophage colony stimulating factor. *EMBO J* 1989; 8: 3667−9.

52 Holmes WE, Lee J, Kuang W-J, Rice GC, Wood WI. Structure and functional expression of a human interleukin-8 receptor. *Science* 1991; 253: 1278−80.

53 Lefkowitz RJ, Caron MG. Adrenergic receptors. Models for the study of receptors coupled to guanine nucleotide regulatory proteins. *J Biol Chem* 1988; 263: 4993−6.

54 Lazareno S, Buckley NJ, Roberts FF. Characterization of muscarinic M_4 binding sites in rabbit lung, chicken heart and NG 108-15 cells. *Mol Pharmacol* 1990; 38: 805−15.

55 Mak JCW, Haldad EB, Buckley NJ, Barnes PJ. Visualization of muscarinic M_4 MRNA and M_4-receptor subtypes in rabbit lung. *Life Sci* 1993; 53: 1501−8.

56 Kurtenbach E, Curtis CAM, Pedder EK, Aiken A, Harris ACM, Hulme EC. Muscarinic acetylcholine receptors. *J Biol Chem* 1990; 265: 13702−8.

57 Ashkenazi A, Winslow JW, Peralta EG *et al*. A M_2-muscarinic receptor coupled to both adenylate cyclase and phosphoinositide turnover. *Science* 1987; 238: 672−5.

58 Barnes PJ. Muscarinic receptor subtypes in airways. *Life Sci* 1993; 52: 521−8.

59 Kroegel C, Yukawa T, Westwick J, Barnes PJ. Evidence for two platelet activating receptors on eosinophils: dissociation between PAF induced intracellular calcium mobilization, degranulation and superoxide anion generation. *Biochem Biophys Res Commun* 1989; 162: 511−21.

60 Dent G, Ukena D, Barnes PJ. PAF receptors. In: Barnes PJ, Page CP, Henson PM, eds. *PAF and Human Disease*. Oxford: Blackwell Scientific Publications, 1989; 68−81.

61 Strader CD, Sigal IS, Dixon RAF. Structural basis of β-adrenergic receptor function. *FASEB J* 1989; 3: 1825−32.

62 Fraser CM. Site-directed mutagenesis of β-adrenergic receptors. *J Biol Chem* 1989; 264: 9266−70.

63 Strader CD, Sigal IS, Candelore MR, Rands E, Hill WS, Dixon RAF. Conserved aspartic acid residues 79 and 113 of the β-adrenergic receptor have different roles in receptor function. *J Biol Chem* 1988; 263: 10267−71.

64 Fraser CM, Chung F-Z, Wang C-D, Venter JC. Site-directed mutagenesis of human

β-adrenergic receptors: substitution of aspartic acid-130 by asparagine produces a receptor with high-affinity agonist binding that is uncoupled for adenylate cyclase. *Proc Natl Acad Sci USA* 1988; 85: 5478–82.

65 Dixon RAF, Sigal IS, Rands E *et al*. Ligand binding to the β-adrenergic receptor involves its rhodopsin-like core. *Nature* 1987; 326: 73–7.

66 Chung F-Z, Wang C-D, Potter PC, Venter JC, Fraser CM. Site-directed mutagenesis and continuous expression of human β-adrenergic receptors. *J Biol Chem* 1988; 263: 4052–5.

67 Tota MR, Strader CD. Characterization of the binding domain of the β-adrenergic receptor with the fluorescent antagonist carazolol. *J Biol Chem* 1990; 265: 16891–7.

68 Kobilka BK, Kobilka TS, Daniel K, Regan JW, Caron MG, Lefkowitz RJ. Chimeric α_2- and β_2-adrenergic receptors: delineation of domains involved in effector coupling and ligand specificity. *Science* 1988; 240: 1310–16.

69 O'Dowd BF, Hnatowich M, Regan JW, Leader WM, Caron MG, Lefkowitz RJ. Site-directed mutagenesis of the cytoplasmic domains of the human β_2-adrenergic receptor. *J Biol Chem* 1988; 263: 15985–92.

70 Maeda A, Kubo T, Mishina M, Numa S. Tissue distribution of mRNAs encoding muscarinic acetylcholine receptor subtypes. *FEBS Lett* 1988; 239: 339–42.

71 Mak JCW, Baraniuk JN, Barnes PJ. Localization of messenger RNAs for muscarinic receptor subtypes in human lung. *Am J Respir Cell Mol Biol* 1992; 7: 344–8.

72 Hamid QA, Mak JC, Sheppard MN, Corrin B, Venter JC, Barnes PJ. Localization of β_2-adrenoceptor messenger RNA in human and rat lung using *in situ* hybridization: correlation with receptor autoradiography. *Eur J Pharmacol (Mol Pharmacol Section)* 1991; 206: 133–8.

73 Arbabian M, Graziano FM, Jicinsky J, Hadcock J, Malbon C, Ruoho A. Photoaffinity labeling of the guinea pig pulmonary mast cell beta receptor. *Am J Respir Cell Mol Biol* 1989; 1: 351–9.

74 Gilliand G, Perrin S, Blankhard K, Bunn MF. Analysis of cytokine mRNA and DNA: detection and quantification by competitive polymerase chain reaction. *Proc Natl Acad Sci USA* 1990; 87: 2725–9.

75 Mak JCW, Barnes PJ. Autoradiographic visualization of muscarinic receptor subtypes in human and guinea pig lung. *Am Rev Respir Dis* 1990; 141: 1559–68.

76 Aronsson M, Fuxe K, Dong Y, Agnati LF, Okret S, Gustafsson J-A. Localization of glucocorticoid receptor mRNA in the male rat brain by *in situ* hybridization. *Proc Natl Acad Sci USA* 1988; 85: 9331–5.

77 Adcock IM, Bronnegard M, Barnes PJ. Glucocorticoid receptor mRNA localization and expression in human lung. *Am Rev Respir Dis* 1991; 143: A628.

78 Bouvier M, Collins S, O'Dowd BF *et al*. Two distinct pathways for cAMP-mediated down-regulation of the β_2-adrenergic receptor. *J Biol Chem* 1989; 264: 16786–92.

79 Collins S, Caron MG, Lefkowitz RJ. From ligand binding to gene expression: new insights into the regulation of G-protein coupled receptors. *Trends Biochem Sci* 1992; 17: 37–9.

80 Bouvier MW, Hausdorff A, DeBlasi A *et al*. Removal of phosphorylation sites from the β-adrenergic receptor delays the onset of agonist-promoted desensitization. *Nature* 1988; 333: 370–3.

81 Hadcock JR, Williams DL, Malbon CC. Physiological regulation at the level of mRNA: analysis of steady state levels of specific mRNAs by DNA-excess solution hybridization. *Am J Physiol* 1989; 256: C457–65.

82 Hadcock JR, Wang HY, Malbon CC. Agonist-induced destabilization of β-adrenergic receptor mRNA: attenuation of glucocorticoid-induced up-regulation of β-adrenergic receptors. *J Biol Chem* 1989; 264: 19928–33.

83 Mano K, Akbarzadeh A, Townley RG. Effect of hydrocortisone on beta-adrenergic receptors in lung membranes. *Life Sci* 1979; 25: 1925–30.

84 Barnes PJ, Jacobs MM, Roberts JM. Glucocorticoids preferably increase fetal alveolar beta-receptors: autoradiographic evidence. *Pediatr Res* 1984; 18: 1191–4.

85 Davis AO, Lefkowitz RJ. Regulation of beta-adrenergic receptors by steroid hormones. *Annu Rev Physiol* 1984; 46: 119–30.

86 Davis AO, Lefkowitz RJ. Corticosteroid-induced differential regulation of beta-adrenergic receptors in circulating human polymorphonuclear leucocytes and mononuclear leucocytes. *J Clin Endocrinol Metab* 1980; 51: 599–605.

87 Collins S, Caron MG, Lefkowitz RJ. β-Adrenergic receptors in hamster smooth muscle cells are transcriptionally regulated by glucocorticoids. *J Biol Chem* 1988; 263: 9067–70.

88 Mak JCW, Adcock I, Barnes PJ. Dexamethasone increases β_2-adrenoceptor gene expression in human lung. *Am Rev Respir Dis* 1992; 45: 834.

89 Okret S, Dong Y, Brönnegård M, Gustafsson J-Å. Regulation of glucocorticoid receptor expression. *Biochimie* 1991; 73: 51–9.

90 Ihara H, Nakanishi S. Selective inhibition of expression of the substance P receptor mRNA in pancreatic acinar AR42J cells by glucocorticoids. *J Biol Chem* 1990; 36: 22441–5.

91 Bai TR. Abnormalities in airway smooth muscle in fatal asthma: a comparison between trachea and bronchus. *Am Rev Respir Dis* 1991; 143: 441–3.

92 Bai TR, Mak JCW, Barnes PJ. A comparison of β-adrenergic receptors and *in vitro* relaxant responses to isoproterenol in asthmatic airway smooth muscle. *Am J Respir Cell Mol Biol* 1992; 6: 647–51.

93 Mantyh CR, Gates TS, Zimmerman RP *et al.* Receptor binding sites for substance P but not substance K or neuromedin K are expressed in high concentrations by arterioles, venules and lymph nodes in surgical specimens obtained from patients with ulcerative colitis and Crohns disease. *Proc Natl Acad Sci USA* 1988; 85: 3235–59.

94 Adcock IM, Peters MJ, Gelder CM *et al.* Increased tachykinin receptors gene expression in asthmatic lung and its modulation by steroids. *J Mol Endocrinol* 1993; 11: 1–7.

95 Hai T, Curran T. Cross-family dimerization of transcription factors Fos/Jun and ATS/CREB alters DNA binding specificity. *Proc Natl Acad Sci USA* 1991; 88: 1–5.

96 Hohmann HP, Brockhaus M, Baeuerle PA, Remy R, Kolbeck R, van Loon AP. Expression of the types A and B tumor necrosis factor (TNF) receptors is independently regulated, and both receptors mediate activation of the transcription factor NF-kappa B. TNF alpha is not needed for induction of a biological effect via TNF receptors. *J Biol Chem* 1990; 265: 22409–17.

97 Schüle R, Rangarajan P, Kliewer S *et al.* Functional antagonism between oncoprotein c-Jun and the glucocorticoid receptor. *Cell* 1990; 62: 1217–26.

98 Yang-Yen H-F, Chambard J-C, Sun Y-L *et al.* Transcriptional interference between c-Jun and the glucocorticoid receptor: neutral inhibition of DNA binding due to direct protein–protein interaction. *Cell* 1990; 62: 1205–15.

13 The regulation of collagen and elastin gene expression in normal lung and during pulmonary disease

PETER K. MAYS AND GEOFFREY J. LAURENT

Introduction

The mechanical properties of the lung are largely determined by an extracellular matrix which comprises a large and growing number of identified components (see Table 13.1). These components all perform important functions (see Table 13.1), but in this chapter we focus only on the collagens and elastin. The collagens and elastin are the most abundant proteins in the lung and their ordered distribution is vital to maintain the structural integrity of the tissue.

A considerable amount of information is now available on the regulation of gene expression for the collagens and elastin, although the pulmonary system has not been the focus of these studies. Here we review the gene expression and protein biochemistry of these molecules commenting on the mechanisms known to regulate their expression and detailing where possible specific examples from the pulmonary system. A full and detailed review of the molecular biology of these proteins is inappropriate in a book such as this, but to give readers access to the literature more detailed reviews and key original manuscripts will be cited. Furthermore, we will give sufficient background information to guide researchers as to the important questions concerning regulation of collagen and elastin production, and most importantly identify the roles these proteins play in the pathogenesis of a wide range of pulmonary diseases (including, fibrotic disorders, emphysema, pulmonary hypertension and acute respiratory distress syndrome), where changes in the regulation of metabolism of these proteins may be a key event in the pathogenesis of these disorders.

Collagen

Collagen is not one unique protein, but a family of closely related proteins, each with a different but homologous amino acid sequence. Currently, about 30 distinct collagen polypeptide chains have been identified and these interact to form at least 18 distinct collagen types, which are identified by roman numerals (Table 13.2) [1−3]. Collagen is synthesized as a larger precursor, procollagen. Common to all collagens is a

Table 13.1 Some components of the extracellular matrix

Component	Functions	Location	References
Collagens	Tissue architecture, cell–matrix interactions, matrix–matrix interactions	Ubiquitously distributed among tissues, including lung	This chapter
Elastin	Tissue architecture, provides tissue elasticity	In tissues requiring elasticity, e.g. lung, blood vessels, heart, skin	This chapter
Fibronectin	Cell–matrix interactions	Basement membranes, epithelium	[212]
Proteoglycans	Cell–matrix interactions, matrix–matrix interactions, regulate cell proliferation	Basement membranes, cartilaginous tissues, interstitial tissue	[213] [214]
Laminin	Basement membranes, role in cell migration	Basement membranes	[215]
Thrombospondin	Modulates cell–matrix interaction	Transiently expressed associated with remodelling matrix	[216]
Tenascin	Modulates cell–matrix interaction	Transiently expressed associated with remodelling matrix	[216]
SPARC* (osteonectin)	Modulates cell–matrix interaction	Transiently expressed associated with remodelling matrix	[216]
Entactin (nidogen)		Basement membrane	[217]
Integrins	Cell surface proteins mediating cell adhesion	Ubiquitous	[218, 219]
Fibrillin	Microfibrillar component	Found in tissues requiring elasticity	[220]

* SPARC = secreted protein acidic and rich in cysteine.

triple-helical domain composed of three α-chains, with either the same or different amino acid composition. α-Chains are identified by arabic numerals, therefore proα1(I) is the procollagen α1-chain of collagen I. These α-chains characteristically have a high proportion of glycine, proline and hydroxyproline present in a repeating triplet Gly–X–Y, where

Table 13.2 Family of collagens

Type	α-Chains	Gene symbol	Chromosomal localization	Protein structure	Tissue distribution and function
I	α1(I) α2(I)	COL1A1 COL1A2	17q21.3–q22.05 7q21.3–q22.1	Fibril, 300 nm triple-helix	Interstitial, alveolar wall, blood vessels. Pulmonary architecture
II	α1(II)	COL2A1	12q13.1–q13.3	Fibril, 300 nm triple-helix	Cartilage in trachea Cartilage architecture
III	α1(III)	COL3A1	2q31–q32.3	Fibril, 300 nm triple-helix	Interstitial, alveolar wall, blood vessels. Pulmonary architecture.
IV	α1(IV) α2(IV) α3(IV) α4(IV) α5(IV) α6(IV)	COL4A1 COL4A2 COL4A3 COL4A4 COL4A5 COL4A6	13q34 13q34 2q36–q37 2q36–q37 Xq22–q23 Xq22–q23	Three-dimensional network	Basement membrane (α5 – glomerular basement membrane)
V	α1(V) α2(V) α3(V)	COL5A1 COL5A2 COL5A3	9q34.2–q34.3 2q14–q32	Fibril, 300 nm triple-helix	Interstitial, alveolar wall, blood vessels
VI	α1(VI) α2(VI) α3(VI)	COL6A1 COL6A2 COL6A3	21q22.3 21q22.3 2q37	Microfibrillar elements	Interstitial, alveolar wall, blood vessels
VII	α1(VII)	COL7A1	3p21	420 nm triple-helical domain	Dermis

VIII	α1(VIII)	COL8A1	3q12–q13.1	Filamentous lattice	Descemet's membrane, sclera, cornea, stroma
	α2(VIII)	COL8A2	1p32.3–p34.3		
IX	α1(IX)	COL9A1	6q12–q14	FACIT	Cartilage, associates with collagen II
	α2(IX)	COL9A2			
	α3(IX)	COL9A3			
X	α1(X)	COL10A1	6q21–q22.3	Filamentous lattice	Cartilage
XI	α1(XI)	COL11A1	1p21	Fibril, 300 nm triple-helix	Cartilage
	α2(XI)	COL11A2	6p21		
	α3(XI)	COL12A1	12q13.1–q13.3		
XII	α1(XII)	COL12A1	6q12–q14	FACIT	Interstitial
XIII	α1(XIII)	COL13A1	10q22	FACIT	
XIV	α1(XIV)	COL14A1		FACIT	Interstitial
XV	α1(XV)	COL15A1	9q21–q22	FACIT	
XVI	α1(XVI)	COL16A1	1p34–p35	FACIT	
XVII	α1(XVII)	COL17A1	10q24.3		Hemidesmosomal, cutaneous basement membrane
XVIII	α1(XVIII)	COL18A1		FACIT	

FACIT = fibril-associated collagens with interrupted triple-helices. See text for additional details and references.

approximately every third X is proline and every third Y is hydroxyproline [4]. Three of these α-chains fold together to form a stable triple-helix with a coiled-coil conformation. Essentially each polypeptide α-chain forms a left-handed helix in which every third residue is in the centre of a right-handed triple-helix. Sterically the glycyl residues must be at the centre of the triple-helix (Fig. 13.1) [1]; it is this requirement that gives collagen its unique structure and properties and dictates collagen's susceptibility to perturbations in its amino acid sequence. The repeating amino acid triplet, Gly−X−Y, is unique to collagenous proteins; however, other proteins contain this recurring triplet, but they are not classified as collagens (Table 13.3). By definition, in a collagen the repeating triplet domains must occupy a sizeable proportion of the molecule, and these molecules must form supramolecular aggregates whose primary function is to provide an extracellular matrix within a tissue [5].

The collagen family

At present there are 18 characterized collagen types with both a gene and protein product identified, and there are also a number of less well-characterized collagens [6, 7]. Each collagen has a specific role based on its biochemical, physical and packing properties.

Collagens I, II, III, V and XI are the major interstitial fibrillar collagens, which provide a scaffold for the tissue. These are comprised of three α-chains of approximately 95 kD molecular weight which are synthesized as a precursor, with C- and N-terminal globular extensions, of molecular weight 145 kD (Fig. 13.2). Collagen I is comprised of two α1(I) chains and one α2(I) chain. The triple-helical domain is ~300 nm in length and may be viewed as a rod (Fig. 13.2).

Collagens interact through specific intermolecular bonds to form fibrils which have a striated pattern due to their packing (Fig. 13.1) [8].

Table 13.3 Non-collagens containing 'Gly−X−Y' collagenous-like sequences

Protein	Reference
Acetylcholinesterase	[221]
Conglutinin	[222]
C1q component of complement	[223]
Mannose-binding protein	[224]
Surfactant apolipoprotein-A	[225]
Surfactant apolipoprotein-D	[226]

The Gly−X−Y collagenous sequences in these molecules are believed to be involved in cell recognition and cellular binding. In addition to these molecules, elastin is the only other hydroxyproline-containing protein; however, in elastin the hydroxyproline is not in a Gly−X−Y triplet [227].

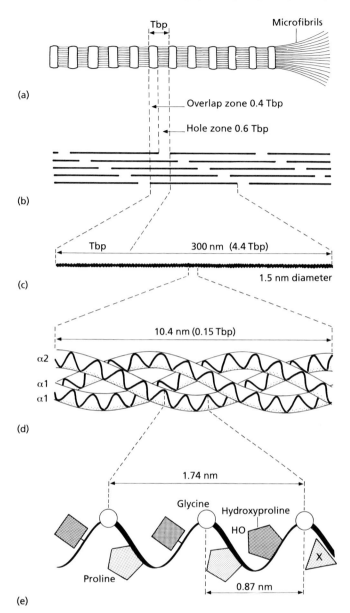

Fig. 13.1 Diagram showing the molecular packing of collagen I. (a) Shows the structure of striated collagen fibrils with the typical banding pattern (Tbp). (b) Illustrates the packing of collagen molecules in a microfibril. (c) Shows a single collagen molecule. (d) Shows a right-handed triple-helix in a collagen molecule. (e) Is a representation of the amino acid sequence in an α-chain. For further details on the molecular packing of collagen, see Piez KA. In: Piez KA, Reddi AH, eds. *Extracellular Matrix Biochemistry*. New York: Elsevier, 1984: 1−39. From Prockop DJ, Guzman NA. *Hosp Pract* 1977; 42: 61−8.

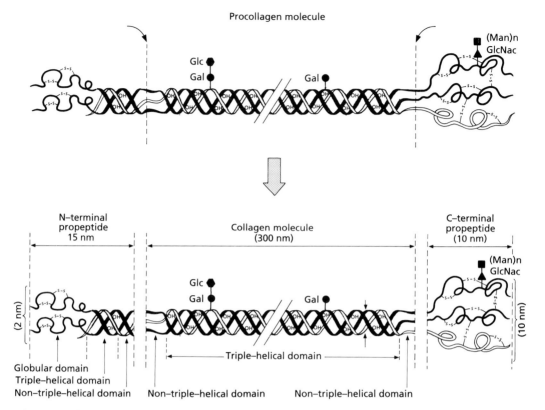

Fig. 13.2 Schematic diagram of the structure of the procollagen I molecule. The molecule is composed of two α1(I) chains (—) and one α2(I) chain (=). The central portion of the procollagen molecule is the triple-helical domain, which along with the short telopeptides, is deposited in the extracellular matrix as collagen following excision of the N- and C-propeptides. Gal, galactose; Glc, glucose; Man, mannose; GlcNac, N-acetylglucosamine; S–S, disulphide bonds. From Prockop DJ, Kivirikko KI, Tuderman L, Guzman NA. *N Engl J Med* 1979; 301: 13–23.

The fibrillar collagens often form heterofibres with interactions between collagens I and III [9, 10], collagens I and V [11] in interstitial tissues, and collagens II and IX in cartilaginous tissue [12]. These associations may be important in determining fibril diameter, and thus may define the functional properties of the fibril.

Collagen IV forms a mesh-like structure in the basement membrane which allows an intimate interaction with laminin, nidogen and heparin sulphate [13]. There are at least six different collagen IV α-chains (Table 13.2), which are distributed in a tissue-specific manner.

Collagens IX, XII and XIV share distinct physical and biochemical properties and have been described as 'fibril-associated collagens with interrupted triple-helices' by Shaw and Olsen [14]. These collagens are non-fibrillar and may act as bridges or links between components in the extracellular matrix. Collagen IX is generally associated with cartilaginous tissues, whereas collagens XII and XIV are often associated with the interstitial collagens. More recently, collagens XV, XVI and XVIII have been identified and are classified as members of the FACIT group of molecules.

Collagens VIII and X are similar in both gene structure and biochemistry; they are both expressed in highly specialized tissues; collagen VIII in Descemet's membrane and collagen X is only produced by hypertrophic chondrocytes. They both have a triple-helical segment of about 450−460 amino acids, with a number of imperfections in the Gly−X−Y sequences, and they both have relatively small C- and N-propeptide extensions.

Collagen VI is a non-fibrillar collagen, associated with microfibrils where it forms a headed filamentous structure. Collagen VII has a very long (420 nm), discontinuous triple-helical region with large globular extensions at each terminus, and is found principally in the dermis. At present the exact molecular structure of collagen XIII is unknown. Collagen XVII is a hemidesmosomal protein located in the cutaneous basement membrane.

The major collagens present in the interstitium of the lung are collagens I, III, V and VI, while collagens II, IX, XI are present in cartilaginous structures associated with the airways. Collagens I and III are the most abundant and in adult human lung they are present in a 2:1 ratio of I:III [15]. It is unclear whether alterations in this ratio occur during either development or ageing. However, in the rat lung the proportion of collagens I and III alters from a 2:1 ratio at birth to a 1:1 ratio at 1 year of age, due to increased deposition of collagen III [16]. The precise roles of these collagens are unknown; however, it has been hypothesized that collagen I confers tensile strength and rigidity to tissues, whereas collagen III bestows compliance [16, 17].

Collagen gene structure

Each procollagen α-chain is coded for by one gene. These genes are widely dispersed throughout the genome (see Table 13.2). Procollagen genes are characterized by a high GC-content, due to the recurring Gly−X−Y triplet within the collagenous triple-helical domains. This repetitive nucleotide sequence is an easily identifiable marker which has facilitated the cloning of novel procollagen genes. A considerable amount of information has been obtained on the structure and organization of procollagen genes, as well as the regulatory *cis*-elements and the *trans*-acting factors which direct procollagen gene transcription. Several recent reviews cover this field in greater depth [18−21].

Procollagens I, II and III share a highly conserved gene structure (see Table 13.4), with approximately 50 exons interspersed with introns of greatly varying sizes [19]. The 3′ untranslated regions in procollagen

Table 13.4 Genomic organization of the genes for procollagens I, II and III

Gene	Size of gene (kb)	Size of mRNA (kb)	Number of exons
Proα1(I)	18	4.8, 5.8	51
Proα2(I)	38	4.2, 4.4, 4.5, 4.9, 5.0	52
Proα1(II)	30	5.0	53
Proα1(III)	44	4.8, 5.4	52

Data from [19, 21, 228].

messenger RNAs (mRNAs) are relatively long, e.g. proα1(I), 1300 base pairs (bp); proα1(III), 870 bp (for details, see ref. 19), and these regions may be involved in coordinate regulation of gene expression as well as determining mRNA stability [22]. The variable use of different poly(A) sites in the 3′ untranslated region in procollagen genes gives rise to multiple-sized mRNA products (see Table 13.4). The triple-helical regions of collagens I, II and III are coded by 44 exons [20]. These 44 exons have a conserved 54-bp structure, representing six complete in-frame 9-bp repeats of the recurring codons for the Gly−X−Y triplet, which is proposed to represent a primordial gene [23]. Although fibrillar collagens share this basic 54-bp structure, other collagen genes are more divergent and do not always adhere to this pattern; for example, in collagen X the triple-helical domain is coded for by one large exon [24].

In general the different collagens arise from separate genes; however, divergency in protein structure may also arise from alternative splicing of primary pre-mRNA transcripts. There are a number of reports of

Table 13.5 Alternative splicing of procollagen genes

Gene	Description	References
Proα2(I)	Utilizes an alternative transcription start site in chick chondrocytes *in vitro*	[229]
Proα1(II)	Exon 2 alternatively spliced in humans and chicks	[230, 231]
Proα2(VI)	Generates divergence in C-terminal coding region and 3′ non-coding region of human collagen VI	[232, 233]
Proα1(IX)	Two alternatively spliced transcripts are observed in chicks	[234]
Proα1(XII)	Short form collagen XII generated by internally splicing 1164 bp	[235]
Proα1(XIII)	Two exons in collagenous region are alternatively spliced	[236]

alternative mRNA splicing for procollagen transcripts (Table 13.5); how-ever, the functional significance of these transcripts and their products has not been determined. A recent report has proposed that alternatively spliced products may direct cell-specific expression [25].

In some procollagen genes the upstream promoter sequences which are involved in the regulation of transcription have been determined [19, 26]. Collagens I and III share some common features such as a 'TATA' box and a 'CCAAT' box. Experiments utilizing chimeric constructs of chloramphenicol transferase fused to procollagen promoters in trans-genic mice have indicated that 2000–2500 bp of 5' upstream sequences are necessary to allow full tissue- and developmental-specific expression of procollagen I [27]. This has also been confirmed using a human proα1(I) collagen minigene in transgenic mice [28]. Within this 2000-bp 5' sequence a large number of regulatory *cis*-elements, to which *trans*-acting factors may bind, have been identified [19]. As the genes encoding the other procollagens have been isolated and characterized it is clear that many of them have different promoter regions, for instance proα1(II) has no 'CCAAT' box and proα1(IV) and proα2(IV) genes are arranged back-to-back [29] and share a common 'TATA'-less promoter [30]. A common feature of the fibrillar procollagen genes is that they contain so-called enhancer sequences within their first intron [31]. It is controversial whether these sequences are of importance [28, 32], but it has been postulated that they determine both tissue- and developmental-specific expression.

Within procollagen genes there are a number of well-characterized polymorphisms [19]. Many of these may now be characterized by a polymerase chain reaction (PCR)-based strategy, thereby allowing rapid and accurate determination which increases their usefulness in haplo-typing individuals [33, 34]. In addition, in the gene for procollagen III, two variable number tandem repeats (or minisatellites) have been deter-mined, and these should prove to be extremely useful in linkage analyses [35, 36].

Collagen biosynthesis

The principal steps of collagen biosynthesis are outlined below and have been described in more detail in several recent reviews [3, 37]. Collagens are synthesized in the lung predominantly by fibroblasts, although other cell types are also capable of synthesizing collagens including: type II pneumocytes, epithelial and endothelial cells.

Collagen DNA is transcribed in the nucleus and the primary RNA transcript is spliced to mRNA and translocated to the cytoplasm where translation occurs. The translated product, termed preprocollagen, has a small hydrophobic signal peptide at the N-terminal end which is proteolytically cleaved coincident with transport into the rough endoplasmic reticulum. Cleavage of this signal peptide produces a single procollagen α-chain, which after post-translational modification interacts with two other α-chains to form a triple-helical procollagen molecule within the endoplasmic reticulum [38]. One α-chain of a fibrillar procollagen molecule consists of about 1400 amino acids, of which about 1000 amino acids occur in Gly−X−Y repeats which form the triple-helical region (Table 13.6). At each end of the triple-helical region of the molecule there are short non-triple-helical telopeptides containing lysine residues which are involved in cross-link formation and fibrillogenesis. The N- and C-terminal propeptides are predominantly devoid of triple-helical regions, although the N-terminal propeptide of proα1(I) contains a short highly conserved Gly−X−Y triple-helical region, as do several other N-propeptides (Fig. 13.2). The intact C-propeptides on procollagen orientate the three α-chains in the correct conformation to form the triple-helix [39]. The cleaved N- and C-propeptides enter the circulation, where they have been measured as indices of collagen metabolism [40].

The intact procollagen α-chain undergoes a number of co-translational and post-translational modifications [38]; these include hydroxylation of proline and lysine in the Y position to 4-hydroxyproline and hydroxy-lysine, respectively. These reactions are carried out by specific disulphide isomerases, prolyl 4-hydroxylase and lysyl hydroxylase, and their genes have been cloned and characterized [41, 42]. Hydroxylation of proline is initiated during polypeptide elongation and proceeds until virtually all Y position prolines are hydroxylated. 4-Hydroxyproline is essential for the stability of the triple-helix and may determine the rate of triple-helix formation [43]. Underhydroxylated procollagen is highly unstable, susceptible to degradation [44] and is unable to form stable triple-helices [45]. The hydroxylysine residues in the procollagen are glycosylated by galactyl-transferase and glucosyl-transferase. Hydroxylysines in the triple-helical region participate in cross-link formation by interacting with

Table 13.6 Comparison of the number of amino acids of the various regions in collagens I and III

	Number of amino acid residues		
Region of the molecule	Proα1(I)	Proα2(I)	Proα1(III)
Signal peptide	22	22	24
N-Propeptide	139	57	129
N-Telopeptide	17	11	14
Triple-helical region	1014	1014	1029
C-Telopeptide	26	15	25
C-Propeptide	246	247	246

Data obtained from [237−241].

lysine residues in the telopeptides to generate the characteristic quarter-stagger pattern of collagen fibrils [46].

On completion of these post-translational modifications, triple-helix formation occurs through a nucleation centre in the C-propeptides, which is followed by the formation of inter- and intra-chain disulphide bonds in the C-propeptide which initiates triple-helix formation [47]. Once procollagen attains a triple-helical structure it is transported to the Golgi apparatus, packaged into vacuoles and secreted.

Procollagen molecules are susceptible to rapid degradation during biosynthesis [48]. This degradation may be a schocastic process which occurs in either the endoplasmic reticulum or Golgi apparatus [49]. Alternatively, it may represent defective procollagens being degraded in the lysosome [50]. The process occurs *in vivo* and between 30 and 80% of newly synthesized collagen is degraded within 30 min of synthesis in the lungs of experimental animals [51]. This pathway has been proposed to modulate net collagen production [52, 53].

Procollagen molecules are secreted with intact propeptides which are cleaved coincident with or after secretion by specific N- and C-proteinases [54, 55]. The N- and C-propeptides may both have a role in feedback control of procollagen synthesis [56, 57]. Both the rate and extent of cleavage of the N-propeptide may determine the fibril diameter [46]. The individual triple-helical collagen molecules interact probably at the involuted fibroblast plasma membrane to initiate fibrillogenesis [58, 59]. A nucleation centre of four molecules is sufficient for fibril growth and fibrils grow from this nucleation centre in a pointed fashion [60]. The fibrils are initially held together by electrostatic interactions; but as they mature they are stabilized by reducible covalent bonds which become more stable with time [61, 62].

Collagen degradation

The native collagen molecule and the polymerized fibrils it forms are relatively stable to proteolytic degradation. A specific group of metallo-proteinases have been identified which are capable of degrading extra-cellular collagens. These enzymes, listed in Table 13.7, are synthesized predominantly in fibroblasts as well as by phagocytic cells (e.g. neutrophils, macrophages). These enzymes are often secreted as inactive or latent precursors which are activated by proteolysis [63, 64]. Furthermore, both in serum and in the extracellular space there are numerous inhibitors of this class of metalloproteinases, including α_2-macroglobulin and tissue inhibitor of metalloproteinases [65], and therefore under steady-state conditions these degradative enzymes may not be active. Interstitial collagenase cleaves the triple-helical region of collagen three-quarters of the way along the molecule from the N-terminal end, producing two fragments TC_A (the larger fragment) and TC_B (the smaller fragment).

Table 13.7 Metalloproteinases capable of degrading extracellular matrix substrates

Metalloproteinase class	Matrix substrate
Interstitial collagenase (MMP1)	Collagens I, II, III, VII, X
Neutrophil collagenase (MMP8)	Collagens I, II, III
72-kD gelatinase (72-kD type IV gelatinase) (MMP2)	Collagens IV, V, VII, X Fibronectin Elastin
92-kD gelatinase (92-kD type IV gelatinase) (MMP9)	Collagens IV, V
Stromelysin-1 (MMP3)	Proteoglycan link protein Fibronectin, laminin Collagens III, IV, V, IX Procollagen peptides
Stromelysin-2 (MMP10)	Collagens III, IV, V Fibronectin
Matrilysin (Uterine metalloproteinase) (MMP7)	Proteoglycan Fibronectin

Adapted and abridged from [63, 64].

These two fragments are highly unstable, they denature at body temperature and are susceptible to proteolysis [66]. In highly cross-linked collagen matrices the neutrophil enzymes, elastase and cathepsin G, are believed to play a role in solubilizing irreducible cross-links and thereby enabling proteolysis by collagenase [65]. However, it is controversial whether the mature cross-linked extracellular matrix is degraded under normal pathological conditions [51].

An alternative degradative pathway has been proposed based on morphological evidence where fibroblasts internalize collagens (and most likely peptidyl fragments too) by phagocytosis [67]. Once internalized these peptides are degraded by thiol proteases, notably cathepsins B and N, in the lysosome [68].

Regulation of collagen gene expression

The regulation of collagen gene expression may occur at a number of sites (Table 13.8), the most important of which are reviewed below.

Transcriptional regulation

Collagens are synthesized in a cell-, tissue- and developmental-specific manner, which is most likely controlled at the level of transcription, by activating or inactivating particular genes. Currently the regulatory *cis*-acting elements and their counterpart *trans*-acting factors which deter-

Table 13.8 Points during collagen gene expression and biosynthesis at which regulation may occur

mRNA transcription and splicing
mRNA degradation (stability)
mRNA translation
Post-translational modifications
Intracellular degradation of newly synthesized collagen
Extracellular degradation prior to deposition in the matrix
Extracellular degradation of cross-linked matrix

mine the developmental expression of procollagens have not been identified. However, these regulatory *cis*-elements are believed to be present in the promoter, the first exon and the first intron. Using transgenic mice, it has been shown that a segment of DNA within the first intron of human proα1(I) may be necessary for correct expression in both lung and skeletal muscle [69], although currently no specific DNA sequences responsible for this process have been identified.

The macromolecular organization of chromatin around actively transcribed genes is different to that associated with inactive genes, thereby making the DNA more susceptible to digestion by DNAase1 or S1 nuclease [70]. Barsh *et al.* [71] investigated the sensitivity of the human proα1(I) gene to DNAase digestion and established the presence of a number of hypersensitive sites over 70 kilobases (kb) of DNA. In the mov13 mouse, where the proα1(I) gene is transcriptionally inactivated by the insertion of a Moloncy leukaemia virus in the first intron of proα1(I), there are detectable differences in the DNAase hypersensitive sites, suggesting that these sites may be important in determining procollagen gene expression [72]. Methylation of DNA at the cytosine of CpG dinucleotides is also believed to inactivate genes [73]. In procollagens, DNA methylation at these sites has been determined to correlate inversely with gene expression during normal development in mice [74], in the mov13 mouse [75] and in transiently transfected cell lines [76].

The C- and N-propeptides from procollagen have been shown to down-regulate collagen synthesis by a feedback mechanism [56, 57]. It is presently unclear at which step in the regulatory pathway these propeptides may act or even if they are of any importance *in vivo*, but it has been proposed that they may act by blocking DNA transcription, decreasing the half-life of procollagen mRNA or altering the rate of mRNA translation [77−79].

The rate of procollagen synthesis will be primarily determined by the steady-state levels of mRNA. Steady-state mRNA levels are determined by a dynamic equilibrium between the rate of synthesis of mRNA (i.e. rate of (DNA) transcription, splicing, etc.) and mRNA degradation. Various growth factors and other agents have been shown to affect collagen production in cultured cells (Table 13.9). Most of these factors

Table 13.9 Agents which may regulate collagen production *in vitro*

Agent	Effect on mRNA steady-state level	Procollagen synthesis	Intracellular degradation	Cell type	Reference
Ascorbate	Increase $proα1(I)$	Increase	—	Human skin fibroblasts	[242]
ECGF	Decrease $proα1(I)$	Decrease	—	Human smooth muscle cells	[243]
EGF-1	Decrease $proα1(I)$	Decrease	—	Human skin fibroblasts Rat lung epithelial cells	[244] [245]
bFGF	—	Increase	—	Bovine vascular endothelial cells	[246]
Fibrinogen fragments	Decrease $proα1(I)$	Decrease	—	Human skin fibroblasts	[247]
Glucocorticoids	Decrease $proα1(I)$	Decrease	—	Chick skin fibroblasts	[248]
Heparin	Decrease $proα1(I)$	Decrease	—	Human smooth muscle cells	[243]
Insulin	Increase $proα1(I)$ Increase $proα1(III)$	Increase	—	Human lung fibroblasts	[249]
IGF-1	Increase $proα1(I)$ Increase $proα1(III)$	Increase	—	Human lung fibroblasts	[249]
IL-1α	Increase $proα1(I)$ Increase $proα1(III)$	Decrease Decrease	—	Human skin fibroblasts	[84]
IL-1β	Increase $proα1(I)$ Increase $proα1(III)$	Decrease Decrease	—	Human skin fibroblasts	[84]
Interferon-α	—	Decrease	—	Human skin fibroblasts	[250]
Interferon-γ	Decrease $proα1(I)$	Decrease	—	Human skin fibroblasts Human lung fibroblasts	[251] [252]

Factor				Cell type	Reference
Leukoregulin	—	Decrease	—	Human skin fibroblasts	[253]
MDCF	No effect	No effect	—	Human lung fibroblasts	[254]
Oestradiol	Increase proα1(I)	—	—	Rat calvarial	[255]
Parathyroid hormone	Decrease proα1(I)	Decrease	—	Rat calvarial cells	[256]
PDGF	No effect	No effect	—	Human lung fibroblasts / Smooth muscle cells	[257] / [31]
PGE_1	—	Decrease	Increase	Human lung fibroblasts	[258]
PGE_2	Decrease proα1(I)	Decrease	Increase	Human lung fibroblasts / Human lung fibroblasts / Human skin fibroblasts	[259] / [260] / [261]
PMA	Decrease proα1(I)	Decrease	—	Human lung fibroblasts	[80]
Retinoic acid	Decrease proα1(I) / Decrease proα2(I)	Decrease	—	Human skin fibroblasts	[262]
TGF-β1	Increase proα1(I)	Increase	Decrease	Human skin fibroblasts / Foetal rat fibroblasts	[86] / [87]
TNF-α	Decrease proα1(I)	Decrease	—	Human skin fibroblasts / Human fibroblasts	[84] / [263]
t-PA	Increase proα1(I)	Increase	—	Human skin fibroblasts	[247]
Vitamin D	Decrease proα1(I) / Decrease proα2(I)	Decrease	—	Rat osteosarcoma cells	[264]
	No effect	No effect	—	Rat periosteal fibroblasts	[262]

Dashes in the table indicate that no data were available. ECGF, endothelial cell growth factor; EGF, epidermal growth factor; bFGF, basic fibroblast growth factor; IGF-1, insulin-like growth factor; IL-1α, interleukin-1α; IL-1β, interleukin-1β; MDCF, macrophage-derived competence factor; mRNA, messenger RNA; PDGF, platelet-derived growth factor; PGE_1, prostaglandin E_1; PGE_2, prostaglandin E_2; PMA, phorbol 12-myristate 13-acetate; TGF-β, transforming growth factor-β; TNF-α, tumour necrosis factor-α; t-PA, tissue plasminogen activator.

have been shown to mediate at least part of their effect by altering the steady-state levels of mRNA for procollagens (Table 13.9). In many instances, the precise mechanism which brings about this alteration is unclear. It has been hypothesized that protein kinase C activity may be an important determinant of the rate of procollagen gene transcription [80]. The secondary messenger cyclic adenosine monophosphate (cAMP) may also be important given that prostaglandin E_2 works, at least in part, by altering cAMP levels. Interleukin-1 and tumour necrosis factor-α may also exert part of their effects by increasing production of prostaglandin E_2 via cyclooxygenase production [81]. Furthermore, it appears that a number of cytokines may interact to either augment or inhibit one another [82–84]. Thus, it is clear that, although the individual factors have specific effects which may be demonstrated *in vitro* (Table 13.9), it should be emphasized that in normal lung these factors will be interacting homeostatically with other agents. In addition, many of the factors exert their effects at more than one regulatory level (Table 13.8). For instance, transforming growth factor (TGF)-β acts by increasing both the rate of transcription of procollagen genes, which is mediated via a nuclear factor-1 consensus sequence in the proα1(I) promoter [85], and the mRNA stability [86], as well as decreasing the degradation of newly synthesized collagen thereby augmenting the increase in collagen production [87].

Post-transcriptional regulation

The rate of translation of procollagen mRNA is generally not considered to be the limiting step in collagen production. Once the polypeptidyl procollagen has been synthesized it is subject to extensive post-translational modifications. The most important is the formation of hydroxyproline from peptidyl proline by prolyl 4-hydroxylase, which has been proposed to be a rate-limiting step in collagen synthesis [88]. More recent evidence indicates that the steady-state levels of mRNA for the α-subunit of prolyl 4-hydroxylase and proα1(I) and proα2(I) chains are coordinately regulated [89], and that the α-subunit of prolyl 4-hydroxylase is the main regulatory determinant of prolyl 4-hydroxylase activity [90]. This evidence supports the hypothesis that prolyl 4-hydroxylase activity is a rate-limiting step for collagen synthesis. Currently, no information is available on the coordinate expression of the other genes coding for the enzymes involved in post-translational modifications.

Another major determinant of collagen production is the rate of intracellular degradation of newly synthesized collagen [91]. Figure 13.3 demonstrates the age-related changes in collagen metabolism in lungs of male rats and shows that rapid degradation, which corresponds to intracellular degradation, is an important determinant of collagen

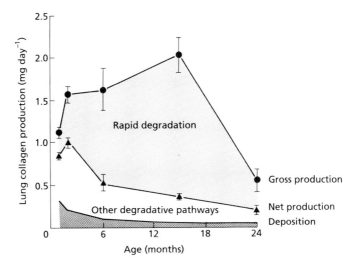

Fig. 13.3 Age-related changes in collagen metabolism. Collagen metabolism was measured using the flooding-dose method with [^{14}C]proline in male Lewis rats aged between 1 month and 2 years. 'Rapid degradation' corresponds to the degradation of newly synthesized collagen. From Mays PK, McAnulty RJ, Laurent GJ. *Am Rev Respir Dis* 1989; 140: 410–6.

production. Similarly, extracellular degradation of recently synthesized collagens, probably occurring during the early stages of fibrillogenesis, also determines the amount of deposition in the matrix. At present only a few studies have examined the effects of cytokines on the intracellular degradation of newly synthesized collagen (Table 13.9).

The final step in collagen production is deposition and stabilization into an extracellular matrix. This process is catalysed by the enzyme lysyl oxidase [92], which also performs the same function in stabilizing elastin in the extracellular matrix.

Proteolytic degradation of the mature cross-linked extracellular matrix is a process that is highly regulated and many cytokines affect the activity of these proteinases [63, 64].

Role of collagen in lung development and during ageing

Within pulmonary structures both collagen and elastin are critical for maintaining the correct functional architecture of the lung [93]. During lung ontogeny elastin has been proposed to play a key role during alveolarization [94]. Elastin is deposited to form a complete ring around the alveolar mouth opening, whereas collagen forms a mesh-like network in the alveolar duct wall between the mouth openings [93]. Collagen deposition proceeds as the lung grows and slows down with age, although synthesis continues throughout life (Fig. 13.3) [51]. This continual deposition results in an increasing lung collagen content. The physiological effect of this increased collagen content is unknown, but it may contribute to the decreased elastic recoil observed in the lung with age [95].

Pathologies associated with collagen

There are a number of diseases specifically associated with genetic mutations in procollagen genes (Table 13.10) [96−98].

Collagens are especially susceptible to alterations in their molecular structures which affect the ability of the procollagen α-chains to fold together into a stable triple-helix [99]. It is believed that as the mutated α-chains start to fold they form a defective triple-helix which is susceptible to degradation [100, 101], a process which has since been termed 'procollagen suicide' [102]. The molecular defects which, to date, have been characterized are deletions, insertions, single base substitutions replacing glycine in the Gly−X−Y triplet or substitutions giving rise to aberrant mRNA splicing [103]. Currently no defects have been found in the regulatory cis-elements, nor have there been mutations associated with specific pulmonary diseases.

The hypothesis of procollagen suicide has gained wide acceptance, and in many cases of osteogenesis imperfecta and Ehlers−Danlos syndrome type IV the principal manifestation of the disease may be attributed

Table 13.10 Diseases caused by mutations in procollagen genes

Disease	Mutated collagen gene(s)	Key reference
Alport's syndrome	Proα5(IV)	[265]
Dystrophic epidermolysis bullosa	Proα1(VII)	[266]
Ehlers−Danlos syndrome type IV	Proα1(III)	[267]
Ehlers−Danlos syndrome type VII	Proα1(I) Proα2(I)	[268]
Familial aortic aneurysms	Proα1(III)	[269]
Osteoarthritis	Proα1(II)	[270]
Osteogenesis imperfecta	Proα1(I) Proα2(I)	[271]
Osteoporosis	Proα2(I)	[272]
Skeletal dysplasias	Proα1(II)	[273]
Smooth muscle tumours	Proα5(IV) Proα6(IV)	[274]
Stickler syndrome	Proα1(II)	[275]

Further details and a full bibliography may be obtained from [103, 276, 277].

to decreased amounts of collagens I and III, respectively, in the tissues. The actual site of degradation of the defective molecules is unknown, and may occur either intracellularly or extracellularly, which may depend on the severity of the disruption of the triple-helical portion of the molecule. There are several well-characterized mutations in which pro-collagen suicide is not the mechanism responsible for the disease, since in a subset of mutations defective collagens are secreted from the cell and form extracellular matrices, which are functionally deficient [104].

Pulmonary complications in the diseases listed in Table 13.10 are rare and often these conditions are fatal in early life and therefore pulmonary disease may not be manifest. In one documented case an individual with Ehlers−Danlos syndrome type IV developed recurrent pneumothoraces [105]. Analysis of lung tissue obtained at biopsy revealed that collagen was more soluble than that from normal individuals, and that the proportion of collagens I:III was increased in the patient. Furthermore, cultured lung fibroblasts from the patient synthesized less collagen III than controls. Although no genetic mutations in procollagen genes have been associated with specific diseases affecting the lung, there are a number of pulmonary diseases which result in, or from, an imbalance in collagen metabolism. These diseases and the possible mechanism(s) giving rise to them will be briefly discussed here.

Pulmonary fibrosis

Fibrosis is the end point of a sequence of events involving inflammation, with associated oedema and cellular infiltration, epithelial and endothelial cell injury, resident cell proliferation and finally excessive deposition of connective tissue [106−108]. A number of diseases give rise to pulmonary fibrosis, including cryptogenic fibrosing alveolitis (idiopathic pulmonary fibrosis), adult respiratory distress syndrome, sarcoidosis, asbestosis and pneumoconiosis. In addition, fibrosis may be caused by the antineoplastic agent bleomycin and pulmonary x-irradiation. A number of experimental animal models have been utilized to study the development of acute pulmonary fibrosis [109]. These models, in general, have examined the respective roles of pulmonary inflammation [110], fibroblast proliferation [111] and deposition of connective tissue components [112] during the development of pulmonary fibrosis.

Since a large number of cytokines affect collagen metabolism (Table 13.9), a great deal of effort has focused on the potential roles these may play in the development of fibrosis [113−115]. During the development of pulmonary fibrosis the ability to induce both cell replication and collagen metabolism may be important. One of the most potent agents for inducing collagen production, so far examined, is TGF-β; however, the ability of TGF-β to induce cell proliferation varies depending on the cell type and the ability of the cell to synthesize and respond to platelet-derived growth factor (PDGF) [113]. TGF-β has been shown to be localized at sites of active extracellular matrix gene expression in humans with pulmonary fibrosis [116, 117] and in animal models of pulmonary fibrosis [118, 119]. Furthermore, PDGF has been implicated in the initial acute lung injury preceding pulmonary fibrosis in both humans [120, 121] and in animal models [122]. Other growth factors have also been pursued as candidates, including alveolar macrophage-derived growth (competence) factor [123, 124] and insulin-like growth factor (IGF)-I [125].

In pulmonary fibrosis in humans there is deposition of extracellular matrix within the expanded interstitium [126], and similarly in experimental models of pulmonary fibrosis there is also excessive deposition of collagen. An increased collagen synthesis rate and a decreased degradation of newly synthesized collagen are believed to be responsible for the increased collagen deposition during the development of pulmonary fibrosis in experimental animals. In humans with pulmonary fibrosis collagen III N-terminal propeptide levels are increased in both serum [128] and bronchoalveolar lavage fluid [129], indicating that collagen III is being actively synthesized. However, pulmonary fibroblasts cultured from patients with pulmonary fibrosis showed no marked differences in either their procollagen synthesis rate or in the ability of TGFb to upregulate their procollagen synthesis rate compared with normal pulmonary fibroblasts. These discrepant results may reflect alterations in the fibroblast phenotype when cultured *in vitro* or alternatively that the fibroblast is only activated in the interstitium of the lung.

It has been clear for some considerable time that pulmonary fibrosis may be a heritable disorder [132−136]. Linkage analysis has implicated immunoglobin-γ allotypes on chromosome 14 to familial pulmonary fibrosis [135]. In addition, biochemical data on α_1-antitrypsin deficiencies in individuals with familial pulmonary fibrosis also suggest involvement of a gene(s) on chromosome 14 [137, 138]. At present no linkage analyses have been performed directed towards either the cytokines which may be implicated in the pathogenesis of pulmonary fibrosis or to the extracellular matrix components deposited in the lung.

Emphysema

Collagen has not been generally implicated in the pathogenesis of emphysema. Emphysema is characterized by a destruction of functional elastic fibres in the interstitium of the lung, thereby giving rise to an increased compliance and decreased recoil [139]. However, it is known that collagen and elastin interact in maintaining the functional architecture of the lung [93]. Therefore, since in emphysema there is considerable degradation of the matrix, possibly mediated by elastases and oxidant damage, the role of collagen destruction in the pathogenesis of the disease ought to be re-evaluated. This may be especially important since neutrophil elastase may play a role in degrading cross-linked collagens and this enzyme has been implicated in the pathogenesis of emphysema [140, 141].

Pulmonary hypertension

This condition arises due to increased blood pressure within the pulmonary artery; one aetiological factor in the pathogenesis of this process is pulmonary fibrosis itself. Under sustained pulmonary hypertension excessive collagen and elastin deposition occurs within the wall of the vessel [142]. At present cellular infiltration, an inflammatory response and deposition of connective tissue have been demonstrated in animal models of pulmonary hypertension [143]. It is therefore conceivable that the molecular signals and pathways leading to increased connective tissue deposition in the hypertensive vessel may be similar to those which mediate excessive deposition in pulmonary fibrosis.

Other

Recently, the Goodpasture's syndrome, which is characterized by glomerulonephritis and pulmonary haemorrhage, has been shown to arise from auto-antibodies to endogenous α3(IV) collagen [144, 145]. Furthermore in Goodpasture's syndrome, in the alveolar basement membrane there is active involvement of the IV auto-antibody collagen [146].

Elastin

Elastin is present in all tissues requiring compliance and extensibility. It is a protein only found in vertebrates and therefore is phylogenetically younger than collagen [147]. Elastin is an integral component of the elastic fibres of the pulmonary extracellular matrix, comprising approximately 2.5% of the dry weight of the lung. The other major components of the elastic fibres are microfibrils; these are glycoproteins which self-assemble into microfibrils approximately 10−12 nm in diameter [148]. Elastin is present in the lung as an amorphous polymer, which unlike collagen has no ordered quaternary structure. It is synthesized as a soluble monomer, termed tropoelastin, which is deposited on a microfibril network and then stabilized by extensive cross-linking [149].

Tropoelastin gene structure

Elastin, unlike collagen, is a single gene-copy protein. The human tropoelastin gene was initially localized to chromosome 2 (2q31-qter)

[150]. More recent data, using *in situ* hybridization on metaphase chromosomes and PCR with tropoelastin-specific primers on a human–rodent hybrid cell line, located the gene on chromosome 7 (7q11.1–q21.1) [151]. It now seems likely that the segment of DNA on chromosome 2 represents a pseudo-gene [152].

The complete nucleotide sequence of the coding regions of human elastin and its genomic organization have been reported [153, 154]. The human tropoelastin gene consists of 34 exons in about 45 kb of DNA [155]. Full-length tropoelastin mRNA is approximately 3.5 kb, of which 2358 nucleotides are translated to 786 amino acids. The remaining 1.2 kb of mRNA constitutes the 3′ untranslated region. The specific function of this region is unknown, but it is highly conserved between species [153], and like in procollagens it may have a role in determining the coordinate regulation of gene expression and in the regulation of mRNA stability [22]. The number of nucleotides in each coding exon is a multiple of three, although unlike collagen, exon boundaries are often split codons [156]. This structure allows for alternative splicing of exons producing an in-frame mRNA transcript. The translated exons vary in size between 27 and 186 bp. The exon to intron size ratio is 1 : 19, which is low compared with collagen which has a ratio of 1 : 8. The majority of exons code for either a hydrophobic or an alanine-rich cross-link region within the protein, and these exons alternate throughout the gene [156]. There are five characterized polymorphisms in human tropoelastin, three are single base-pair changes [157, 158] and two are more complex polymorphic systems arising from recombinants associated with AluI repeat elements [159].

The promoter sequence of tropoelastin, 5′ to the translation start site has also been characterized [160]. There is no 'TATA' box, although there are consensus sequences for two 'CCAAT' boxes and for a number of regulatory *cis*-elements, including multiple binding sites for the transcription factors Sp1 and Ap-1 [155]. Additional delineation of the regulatory *cis*-elements in 2.2 kb of 5′ flanking sequence indicates the presence of three putative glucocorticoid-responsive elements, and sequence variants of cAMP-responsive regulatory elements and TPA-inducible elements (12-O-tetradecanoyl phorphol-13-acetate) [161]. Examination of tropoelastin promoter activity, using a chimeric tropoelastin chloramphenicol acetyltransferase construct, identified five major functional domains, two of which were down-regulatory elements (−2260 to −1553 and −986 to −476), two were up-regulatory (−1553 to −986 and −459 to −129) and the fifth was the basic promoter (−128 to −1). The first 128 nucleotides of the 5′ flanking sequence, which included three Sp1 sites, have been demonstrated to be necessary for tropoelastin gene expression [161]. Unlike the procollagens, no regulatory *cis*-elements have been identified within either the first intron or first exon of the tropoelastin gene.

The absence of a 'TATA' box and the fact that there are multiple initiation sites for tropoelastin transcription suggest that the promoter of the tropoelastin gene belongs to the class of promoters from the 'housekeeping' genes [155]. This is unusual since housekeeping genes are often considered to be constitutively expressed, e.g. enzymes of intermediary metabolism, whereas elastin is developmentally and tissue-specifically regulated, and has historically been considered to be a protein which is not normally synthesized in adults [162]. However, more recent evidence points to a basal level of elastin gene expression throughout life [163, 164].

Tropoelastin isoforms

Despite there being only a single gene for tropoelastin, multiple protein isoforms arise from alternative splicing of tropoelastin primary RNA. The isolation of bovine nuchal ligament elastin poly(A) + RNA and the synthesis of complementary DNA (cDNA) suggested that there were at least three differentially spliced tropoelastin mRNA species [165]. Similarly, three different tropoelastin cDNA species were isolated from a cDNA library derived from foetal human aorta [156] and five tropoelastin cDNA species were isolated from a human skin fibroblast cDNA library [166]. The exons which have been shown to be alternatively spliced in human tropoelastin are 22, 23, 24, 26A, 32 and 33 [154]. For exons 22, 23, 32 and 33 the whole exon is subject to alternative splicing; however, exons 24 and 26A are spliced alternatively within the exon. At present, no differential role for the alternatively spliced tropoelastins have been elucidated, either during development or in pathological conditions in humans. However, a developmental pattern of alternative spliced transcripts has been observed for bovine tropoelastin [167], and rat tropoelastin exhibits both developmental- and tissue-specific differences in alternative splicing [168].

Several different tropoelastin products have been isolated from organ culture and cell-free mRNA translation studies [169, 170], and these have subsequently been demonstrated to arise from different mRNA variants and not from differentially processed proteins [171]. At present, however, protein products for some of the mRNA variants have not been isolated. This may be because the tropoelastins have similar molecular weights, which are not resolved by electrophoresis. Alternatively certain mRNA products may not be translated, indicating post-transcriptional regulation of tropoelastin production.

Tropoelastin biosynthesis

Tropoelastin is synthesized in a similar manner to procollagens and other extracellular proteins. DNA is transcribed in the nucleus and the primary RNA transcript is spliced prior to localization in the cytoplasm where translation occurs. The nascent polypeptide is targeted to the endoplasmic reticulum by a signal peptide of 26 amino acids [172]. The signal peptide is proteolytically cleaved once tropoelastin is localized in the endoplasmic reticulum. Within the rough endoplasmic reticulum, some proline residues are hydroxylated by prolyl 4-hydroxylase, although unlike collagen this step does not affect the stability of the molecule [173] and it has been suggested that this occurs 'accidentally' in cells which are concomitantly synthesizing procollagen [174]. There are apparently no other post-translational modifications prior to secretion from the cell, which occurs approximately 20 min after the initiation of synthesis. Tropoelastins have a molecular weight of about 70 kD [170, 175, 176]. There is a direct correlation between the rate of tropoelastin biosynthesis and the tropoelastin mRNA levels in tissues [177, 178], indicating that the rate of transcription of tropoelastin mRNA and its stability are important determinants of the tropoelastin synthesis rate.

Non-polar amino acids, particularly glycine, valine, alanine and proline, comprise 75% of tropoelastin [147]. Many of these non-polar amino acids occur in hydrophobic domains of the protein, which have few intermolecular bonds. These hydrophobic regions alternate with hydrophilic regions, rich in alanine as well as lysine residues, which participate in cross-link formation [179, 180].

Once secreted from the cell, tropoelastins are thought to bind to a membrane glycoprotein (molecular weight 67 kD), which has been described as an elastin receptor [149]. It possesses a binding site for hydrophobic sequences in tropoelastin [181] and apparently 'chaperones' tropoelastin to the microfibrils where the molecules align and lysyl oxidase converts the majority of ε-amino groups of lysine residues to aldehydes [92]. These moieties then participate in Schiff base and aldol condensation reactions to generate cross-links. Over a few days these cross-links isomerize into stable quaternary pyridinium structures, namely desmosine and isodesmosine, to generate a stably cross-linked three-dimensional fibrous network which has a high degree of extensibility [179, 180].

It is unclear which cells are responsible for tropoelastin synthesis in the lung. Evidence points to the interstitial fibroblast as the major cell [176]; however, during alveoli formation pulmonary smooth muscle cells synthesize tropoelastin [182], as do pulmonary arterial endothelial cells [175]. Thus a number of cells are apparently responsible for synthesizing tropoelastin dependent upon the structural location of the matrix component for which the tropoelastin is destined.

Elastin degradation

Elastin may be susceptible to degradation at several sites in the biosynthetic pathway; intracellularly during synthesis, during tropoelastin secretion and matrix assembly, and as elastin in the insoluble cross-linked extracellular matrix. Approximately 1% of newly synthesized tropoelastin is degraded intracellularly during biosynthesis [183], although the exact site of this degradation is uncertain. Soluble tropoelastin is susceptible to degradation by a number of non-specific proteases, including: elastase, trypsin, chymotrypsin, thermolysin, cathepsin G and stromelysin [184]. The relevance of these enzymes *in vivo* is still uncertain, but the susceptibility of soluble tropoelastin to degradation raises the possibility that degradation may be a modulator of tropoelastin deposition.

Cross-linked insoluble elastin is highly resistant to degradation and, so far, only one class of enzymes, the elastases, causes demonstrable proteolysis. Elastases are serine proteinases contained in platelets and produced by a large number of cells including neutrophils, macrophages, monocytes, smooth muscle cells and fibroblasts. The production of elastases by fibroblasts and smooth muscle cells suggests that the same cells responsible for synthesizing elastin are also capable of degrading it, thereby indicating a role for degradation in normal remodelling associated with growth. However, very little is known about the source and role of elastases in maintaining normal pulmonary architecture and this is an important area meriting investigation. *In vivo* studies suggest that elastin turnover is extremely low in adult animals [162], and cross-linked elastin has a half-life in humans of 74 years [185].

Role of tropoelastin in lung development and during ageing

Elastin has been proposed to play a key role during lung development and alveolarization [94]. In rat lung the appearance of tropoelastin mRNA [186, 187] precedes tropoelastin synthesis [188] and deposition [189]. During alveolarization elastin is deposited to form a fish-net structure, where the apertures in the net represent the mouths of newly forming alveoli. A deficiency in elastin deposition during foetal development has been proposed to underlie pulmonary hypoplasia associated with oligohydramnios [190].

Tropoelastin mRNA levels decreased in rat by 75% between 1 and 9 months of age, and thereafter remained constant [164]. Similarly, in human skin fibroblasts from donors of different ages the tropoelastin mRNA levels remained constant for several decades of life prior to decreasing in subjects aged 60 years or greater [159]. Tropoelastin synthesis remained constant for 30 population doublings in skin fibroblasts aged *in vitro*, before decreasing twofold [183]. These data support the view that the tropoelastin gene is continually transcribed but that synthesis and deposition into the extracellular matrix may be regulated post-transcriptionally.

Regulation of tropoelastin gene expression

The main determinant of tropoelastin gene expression is probably transcriptional. A direct correlation has been demonstrated between the rate of tropoelastin biosynthesis and the tropoelastin mRNA levels in tissues [177, 178]. This indicates that the rate of transcription of tropoelastin mRNA and its stability are important determinants of the elastin synthesis rate [191, 192].

Tropoelastin synthesis may be subject to feedback control and currently two pieces of indirect evidence support this notion. The first comes from studies with monensin, a calcium ionophore, which blocked tropoelastin translocation from the proximal to the distal Golgi apparatus, causing a decrease in tropoelastin steady-state mRNA levels, probably via reducing transcription [193]. The second comes from experiments on pulmonary fibroblast cultures where fragments of elastin have been shown to exert feedback control to regulate tropoelastin synthesis [194].

Currently, most of the agents that affect elastin synthesis mediate their effect through alterations in the steady-state level of tropoelastin

Table 13.11 Some agents which may regulate tropoelastin production *in vitro*

Agent	Effect on synthesis	Mechanism	Cells	Reference
1,25-Dihydroxy-vitamin D$_3$	Decrease	Decrease steady-state mRNA levels	Bovine fibroblasts, smooth muscle cells	[278]
Ascorbate	Decrease	—	Rabbit aorta smooth muscle cells	[279]
Glucocorticoids	Decrease	Decrease steady-state mRNA levels	Isolated chick aortas	[177]
Heparin	Increase	Increase steady-state mRNA levels	Rat lung fibroblasts	[280]
Hypoxia	Decrease	Decrease steady-state mRNA levels	Bovine lung smooth muscle cells	[281]
IGF-I	Increase	Increase steady-state mRNA levels	Rat lung fibroblasts	[282]
IL-1β	Decrease	Decrease steady-state mRNA levels	Rat lung fibroblasts	[283]
SMEF*	Increase	—	Pulmonary artery smooth muscle cells	[143]
TGF-β	Increase	Increase steady-state mRNA levels	Rat lung fibroblasts	[284]
TNFα	Decrease	Decrease steady-state mRNA levels	Human skin fibroblasts	[285]

* SMEF, smooth muscle-derived elastogenic factor.

mRNA (Table 13.11); however, the precise mechanism is uncertain and some of these agents may also affect post-translational processes. The administration of IGF-I *in vivo* to aged rats has been shown to affect lungs and aorta differently, increasing mRNA levels in aorta but having no effect in the lungs [164]. This raises the important point that the effects of cytokines on young animals or cultured cells may not reflect their physiological action in diseased or aged individuals, and care must be exercised in interpreting these data.

Pathologies associated with elastin

At present, the only disorder associated with specific mutations in the tropoelastin gene is supravalvular aortic stenosis [194a]. However, there are a number of other disorders in which elastic fibres are affected. These include cutis laxa, pseudoxanthoma elasticum and the Buschke–Ollendorff syndrome [160, 195]. In individuals with cutis laxa there is a reduction in the number of elastic fibres in tissues, and cultured skin fibroblasts from these patients have decreased steady-state levels of tropoelastin mRNA. Emphysema is often apparent in individuals with cutis laxa, an observation consistent with the role of the elastic fibres in the pulmonary parenchyma.

Pseudoxanthoma elasticum is characterized by excess fragmentation and calcification of elastic fibres in the dermis. In the Buschke–Ollendorff syndrome there is an excessive accumulation of elastin in tissues, and increased steady-state levels of tropoelastin mRNA are observed in cultured fibroblasts from individuals with this condition. Deficient tropoelastin expression in foetal lung may give rise to pulmonary hypoplasia associated with oligohydramnios [190]. However, in these disorders no specific defect at the molecular level has been elucidated. None the less alterations in elastin synthesis and degradation are involved in at least three major pulmonary diseases which are briefly discussed below.

Emphysema

This disease is characterized by abnormal, permanent enlargement of the airspaces distal to the bronchioles, accompanied by destruction of their walls and with no obvious fibrosis [196]. Degradation of elastin and associated elastic fibres in the lung is considered to be the major event which gives rise to the end-stage condition [141]. Currently, the most widely accepted hypothesis to explain the pathogenesis of emphysema is the so-called 'protease/antiprotease imbalance' hypothesis. Briefly, this proposes that under normal circumstances pulmonary architecture is maintained due to a balance between the degradative enzymes (elastases, collagenases, etc.) and their many inhibitors; but under certain conditions this fine balance may be thrown into disequilibrium. If protease activity increases then lung tissue may be destroyed and emphysema develops; similarly if protease activity is diminished a fibrosis-like disorder may result. There are two major factors which may contribute to emphysema: first, deficiencies in the protease inhibitor α_1-antitrypsin [197]; and second, cigarette smoke [141]. An α_1-antitrypsin deficiency is present in a small subset of patients prone to emphysema. These individuals have a mutation in the gene for α_1-antitrypsin [198], which is the main tissue inhibitor of elastase [199]. Cigarette smoke may induce emphysema by several different pathways, including the direct oxidation of tissue components and by neutrophil recruitment and accumulation within lung tissue. Direct oxidation, generally mediated by free radical species within the cigarette smoke, may directly damage both elastin and collagen fibres [200, 201]. In addition, the insult of cigarette smoke recruits both neutrophils and macrophages into the lung. Neutrophils release oxidants and neutrophil elastase, a potent protease capable of degrading both elastin and collagen, into the interstitial space. Neutrophils are capable of inactivating directly α_1-antitrypsin. Similarly, macrophages release their own proteases and generate hydrogen peroxide. At present the relative roles of these processes in the pathogenesis of emphysema are unclear. However, considerable effort has been directed at using either elastase inhibitors [202] or replacement therapy for α_1-antitrypsin deficiency [203] as therapeutic rationales in emphysema.

As a consequence of the fragmentation and destruction of a functional elastic network in the lung there is some concomitant resynthesis of elastin; however, this newly synthesized elastin is deposited in a disorganized and non-functional manner [204, 205] and therefore normal pulmonary architecture is not maintained. This inappropriately directed synthesis may further contribute to the destructive nature of emphysema as the lung tries ineffectively to remodel this newly deposited elastin.

Pulmonary fibrosis

Elastin, in general, is not considered in the pathogenesis of pulmonary fibrosis, although evidence from experimental models of bleomycin-induced pulmonary fibrosis suggested that there were increases in steady-state levels of tropoelastin mRNA, tropoelastin synthesis and elastin content [206, 207]. The increased elastin production is likely to be deposited in a deranged manner in the alveolar wall, thus further disrupting pulmonary architecture. A number of the putative agents in the pathogenesis of pulmonary fibrosis (e.g. TGF-β, IGF-I) exert direct effects on tropoelastin gene expression *in vitro* (see Table 13.11). Therefore, it is conceivable that the pathways which may be responsible for elevating collagen production could also, through the same mediators, result in increased elastin deposition.

Pulmonary hypertension

During the induction of pulmonary hypertension both elastin and collagen are deposited in the pulmonary artery. The agents which induce tropo-elastin gene expression (see Table 13.11) have also been implicated as mediators in the pathogenesis of pulmonary hypertension, and therefore it is again likely that common pathways result in both collagen and elastin deposition in the vessel wall.

The way forward in lung research

It is evident that at present no genetic mutations have been established in the genes for collagens or elastin, which directly result in pulmonary disease. It is most likely that the involvement of both collagens and elastin in pulmonary diseases, such as fibrosis and emphysema, results from an imbalance in either their gene expression or metabolism. We have outlined in this chapter some of the major factors which may regulate both their gene expression and metabolism. Clearly these regulatory processes occur at many different levels. However, given current knowledge on the molecular biology of collagens and elastin there are some useful avenues which are worth pursuing experimentally to investigate these diseases.

A better understanding of the regulatory *cis*-elements and their *trans*-acting factors will enable researchers to clarify the pathways which are active in regulating gene expression of these molecules. This knowledge will also help to understand and elucidate the pathogenesis of pulmonary diseases associated with the extracellular matrix. Several approaches may be useful. First, 'footprinting' of the putative regulatory *cis*-elements will reveal if these sequences are binding *trans*-acting regulatory factors. Second, mutagenesis of the regulatory *cis*-elements and the expression of the mutated gene in either transfected cells or transgenic mice may give insight to the complex patterns of regulation. Third, the application of *in situ* hybridization techniques to reveal which genes are being actively transcribed in individuals with pulmonary disease may also lead to a better understanding of these disorders. Finally, linkage analysis of affected families should be carried out to exclude the role of the genes for the interstitial collagens, elastin and some of the putative *trans*-acting regulatory factors (e.g. TGF-β, PDGF, IGF-I) in pulmonary fibrosis and pulmonary hypertension and to map any disease-associated loci. The application of this strategy to emphysema is less promising especially given the role that cigarette smoking has in the pathogenesis of the disease. This last approach appears daunting especially if full analysis of the genome were to occur; however, using the polymerase chain reaction this task becomes both manageable and possibly fruitful. This approach has proven worthwhile in elucidating the gene responsible for Marfan's syndrome [208−211] and as long as good candidate families are identified there is no reason to suspect that this approach should not be profitable for other disorders.

It is evident that a considerable amount of information is still needed on the regulation of collagen and elastin gene expression in the normal lung, but given the current pace of research, there should be some progress towards understanding the diseases causing an alteration in the components of the pulmonary extracellular matrix.

Acknowledgements

We are indebted to our many colleagues for helpful comments and discussions. Work from the authors' laboratory was supported by grants from the Medical Research Council of Great Britain.

References

1 van der Rest M, Garrone R. Collagen family of proteins. *FASEB J* 1991; 5: 2814−23.

2 Miller EJ, Gay S. Collagen structure and function. In: Cohen IK, Diegelmann RF, Lindblad WJ, eds. *Wound Healing: Biochemical and Clinical Aspects*. Philadelphia: WB Saunders, 1992: 130−51.

3 Kielty CM, Hopkinson I, Grant ME. Collagen: The collagen family: Structure, assembly and organization in the extracellular matrix. In: Royce PM, Steinmann B, eds. *Connective Tissue and Its Heritable Disorders*. New York: Wiley-Liss, 1993: 103−47.

4 Miller EJ. The structure of fibril forming collagens. *Ann N Y Acad Sci* 1985; 460: 1−13.

5 Gay S, Miller EJ. What is collagen, what is not? *Ultrastruct Pathol* 1983; 4: 365−77.

6 Yoshioka H, Zhang H, Ramirez F *et al*. Synteny between the loci for a novel FACIT-like collagen locus (D6S228E) and α1 (IX) collagen (COL9A1) on 6q12−q14 in humans. *Genomics* 1992; 13: 884−86.

7 Marchant JK, Linsenmayer TF, Gordon MK. cDNA analysis of a cornea-specific collagen. *Proc Natl Acad Sci USA* 1991; 88: 1560−4.

8 Piez KA. Molecular and aggregate structures of the collagens. In: Piez KA, Reddi AH, eds. *Extracellular Matrix Biochemistry*. New York: Elsevier, 1984: 1−39.

9 Lapiere CM, Nusgens B, Pierard GE. Interaction between collagen type I and III in conditioning bundles organisation. *Connect Tissue Res* 1977; 5: 21−9.

10 Romanic AM, Adachi E, Kadler KE, Hojima Y, Prockop DJ. Copolymerization of pNcollagen III and collagen I. pNcollagen III decreases the rate of incorporation of collagen I into fibrils, the amount of collagen I incorporated, and the diameter of the fibrils formed. *J Biol Chem* 1991; 266: 12703−9.

11 Adachi E, Hayashi T. *In vitro* formation of hybrid fibrils of type V collagen and type I collagen. Limited growth of type I collagen into thick fibrils by type V collagen. *Connect Tissue Res* 1986; 14: 257−66.

12 Eyre DR, Wu JJ, Woods PE, Weis MA. The cartilage collagens and joint degeneration. *Br J Rheumatol* 1991; 30 (Suppl. 1): 10−15.

13 Paulsson M. Basement membrane proteins: structure, assembly, and cellular interactions. *Crit Rev Biochem Mol Biol* 1992; 27: 93−127.

14 Shaw LM, Olsen BR. FACIT collagens: diverse molecular bridges in extracellular matrices. *Trends Biochem Sci* 1991; 16: 191−4.

15 Kirk JME, Heard BE, Kerr I, Turner-Warwick M, Laurent GJ. Quantitation of types I and III collagen in biopsy lung samples from patients with cryptogenic fibrosing alveolitis. *Collagen Relat Res* 1984; 4: 169−82.

16 Mays PK, Bishop JE, Laurent GJ. Age-related changes in the proportion of types I and III collagen. *Mech Ageing Dev* 1988; 45: 203−12.

17 Burgeson RE. The collagens of skin. *Curr Probl Dermatol* 1987; 17: 61−75.

18 Ramirez F, Di Liberto M. Complex and diversified regulatory programs control the expression of vertebrate collagen genes. *FASEB J* 1990; 4: 1616−23.

19 Sandell LJ, Boyd CD. Conserved and divergent sequence and functional elements within collagen genes. In: Sandell LJ, Boyd CD, eds. *Extracellular Matrix Genes.* New York: Academic Press, 1990: 1−56.

20 Vuorio E, de Crombrugghe B. The family of collagen genes. *Annu Rev Biochem* 1990; 59: 837−72.

21 Chu M-L, Prockop DJ. Collagen: Gene structure. In: Royce PM, Steinmann B, eds. *Connective Tissue and Its Heritable Disorders.* New York: Wiley-Liss, 1993: 149−65.

22 Carter BZ, Malter JS. Regulation of mRNA stability and its relevance to disease. *Lab Invest* 1991; 65: 610−21.

23 Yamada Y, Avvedimento VE, Mudryj M *et al.* The collagen gene: evidence for its evolutionary assembly by amplification of a DNA segment containing an exon of 54 bp. *Cell* 1980; 22: 887−92.

24 Thomas JT, Cresswell CJ, Rash B *et al.* The human collagen X gene. *Biochem J* 1991; 280: 617−23.

25 Sandell LJ, Morris N, Robbins JR, Goldring MB. Alternatively spliced type II procollagen mRNAs define distinct populations of cells during vertebral development: differential expression of the amino-peptide. *J Cell Biol* 1991; 114: 1307−19.

26 Uitto J, Chu M-L. Regulation of collagen gene expression in human skin fibroblasts and its alterations in disease. In: Olsen BR, Nimni ME, eds. *Collagen,* Vol IV. Boca Raton, FL: CRC Press, 1989: 109−24.

27 Khillan JS, Schmidt A, Overbeek PA, de Crombrugghe B, Westphal H. Developmental and tissue-specific expression directed by the α2 type I collagen promoter in transgenic mice. *Proc Natl Acad Sci USA* 1986; 83: 725−9.

28 Sokolov BP, Mays PK, Khillan JS, Prockop DJ. Tissue- and development-specific expression in transgenic mice of a type I procollagen (COL1A1) minigene construct with 2.3 kb of the promoter region and 2 kb of the 3'-flanking region. Specificity is independent of the putative regulatory sequences in the first intron. *Biochemistry* 1993; 32: 9242−9.

29 Soininen R, Huotari M, Hostikka SL, Prockop DJ, Tryggvason K. The structural genes for α1 and α2 chains of human type IV collagen are divergently encoded on opposite DNA strands and have an overlapping promoter region. *J Biol Chem* 1988; 263: 17217−20.

30 Burbelo PD, Bruggeman LA, Gabriel GC, Klotman PE, Yamada Y. Characterization of a *cis*-acting element required for efficient transcriptional activation of the collagen IV enhancer. *J Biol Chem* 1991; 266: 22297−302.

31 Bornstein P, Sage H. Regulation of collagen gene expression. *Prog Nucleic Acids Res Mol Biol* 1989; 37: 67−106.

32 Liska DJ, Slack JL, Bornstein P. A highly conserved intronic sequence is involved in transcriptional regulation of the α1(I) collagen gene. *Cell Regul* 1990; 1: 487−98.

33 Baker R, Lynch J, Ferguson L, Priestley L, Sykes B. PCR detection of five

restriction site dimorphisms at the type I collagen loci COL1A1 and COL1A2. *Nucleic Acids Res* 1991; 19: 4315.

34 Strobel D, Tsuneyoshi T, Kuivaniemi H *et al*. Three new polymorphisms at the COL1A2 locus. *Matrix* 1992; 12: 87–91.

35 Lee B, D'Alessio M, Vissing H, Ramirez F, Steinmann B, Superti-Furga A. Characterization of a large deletion associated with a polymorphic block of repeated dinucleotides in the type III procollagen gene (COL3A1) of a patient with Ehlers–Danlos syndrome type IV. *Am J Hum Genet* 1991; 48: 511–7.

36 Mays PK, Tromp G, Kuivaniemi H, Ryynanen M, Prockop DJ. A 15 base-pair AT-rich variable number tandem repeat in the type III procollagen gene (COL3A1) as an informative marker for 2q31-2q32.3. *Matrix* 1992; 12: 44–9.

37 Nimni ME, Harkness RD. Molecular structure and functions of collagen. In: Nimni ME, ed. *Collagen. I. Biochemistry*. Boca Raton, FL: CRC Press, 1988: 1–77.

38 Kivirikko KI, Myllyla R. Biosynthesis of the collagens. In: Piez KA, Reddi AH, eds. *Extracellular Matrix Biochemistry*. New York: Elsevier, 1984: 83–118.

39 Gelman RA, Poppke DC, Piez KA. Collagen fibril formation *in vitro*. The role of the non-helical terminal regions. *J Biol Chem* 1979; 254: 11741–5.

40 Risteli L, Risteli J. Noninvasive methods for detection of organ fibrosis. In: Rojkind M, ed. *Connective Tissue in Health and Disease*. Boca Raton, FL: CRC Press, 1990: 61–98.

41 Bassuk JA, Berg RA. Protein disulphide isomerase, a multifunctional endoplasmic reticulum protein. *Matrix* 1989; 9: 244–58.

42 Kivirikko KI, Myllyla R, Pihlajaniemi T. Protein hydroxylation: prolyl 4-hydroxylase, an enzyme with four cosubstrates and a multi-functional subunit. *FASEB J* 1989; 3: 1609–16.

43 Bansal M, Ananthanarayanan VS. The role of hydroxyproline in collagen folding. *Biopolymers* 1988; 27: 299–312.

44 Steinmann B, Rao VH, Gitzelmann R. Intracellular degradation of newly synthesised collagen is conformation dependent. *FEBS Lett* 1981; 133: 142–4.

45 Berg RA, Prockop DJ. The thermal transition of a non-hydroxylated form of collagen. Evidence for a role for hydroxyproline in stabilizing the triple-helix of collagen. *Biochem Biophys Res Commun* 1973; 52: 115–20.

46 Kuhn K. The classical collagens: types I, II and III. In: Mayne R, Burgeson RE, eds. *Structure and Functions of Collagen Types*. New York: Academic Press; 1987: 1–42.

47 Gerard S, Puett D, Mitchell WM. Kinetics of collagen fold formation in human type I procollagen and the effects of disulfide bonds. *Biochemistry* 1981; 20: 1857–65.

48 Bienkowski RS. Intracellular degradation of newly synthesized collagen. In: Knecht E, Grisolia S, eds. *Current Trends in Intracellular Degradation*. New York: Springer International, 1989: 423–43.

49 Bienkowski RS. Degradation of newly synthesized collagen. *Collagen Relat Res* 1984; 4: 399–412.

50 Berg RA, Schwartz ML, Rome LH, Crystal RG. Lysosomal function in the degradation of defective collagen in cultured lung fibroblasts. *Biochemistry* 1984; 23: 2134–8.

51 Mays PK, McAnulty RJ, Laurent GJ. Age-related changes in lung collagen metabolism: a role for degradation in regulating lung collagen production. *Am Rev Respir Dis* 1989; 140: 410–6.

52 Berg RA. Intracellular turnover of collagen. In: Mecham RP, ed. *Regulation of Matrix Accumulation*. New York: Academic Press, 1986: 29–52.

53 Laurent GJ. Dynamic state of collagen: pathways of collagen degradation *in vivo*

and their possible role in the regulation of collagen mass. *Am J Physiol* 1987; 252: C1--9.

54 Hojima Y, McKenzie J, van der Rest M, Prockop DJ. Type I procollagen *N*-proteinase from chick embryo tendons. *J Biol Chem* 1989; 264: 11336−45.

55 Hojima Y, van der Rest M, Prockop DJ. Type I procollagen carboxy-terminal proteinase from chick embryo tendons. *J Biol Chem* 1985; 260: 15996−16003.

56 Aycock RS, Raghow R, Stricklin GP, Seyer JM, Kang AH. Post-transcriptional inhibition of collagen and fibronectin synthesis by a synthetic homolog of a portion of the carboxyl-terminal propeptide of human type I collagen. *J Biol Chem* 1986; 261: 14355−60.

57 Wu CH, Donovan CB, Wu GY. Evidence for pretranslational regulation of collagen synthesis by procollagen peptides. *J Biol Chem* 1986; 261: 10482−4.

58 Trelstad RL, Hayashi K. Tendon collagen fibrillogenesis. *Dev Biol* 1979; 71: 228−42.

59 Birk DE, Trelstad RL. Extracellular compartments in tendon morphogenesis: collagen fibril, bundle and macroaggregate formation. *J Cell Biol* 1986; 103: 231−40.

60 Kadler KE, Hojima Y, Prockop DJ. Collagen fibrils *in vitro* grow from pointed tips in the C- to N-terminal direction. *Biochem J* 1990; 268: 339−43.

61 Ricard-Blum S, Ville G. Collagen cross-linking. *Cell Mol Biol* 1988; 34: 581−90.

62 Yamauchi M, Mechanic GL. Cross-linking of collagen. In: Nimni ME, ed. *Collagen. Volume I. Biochemistry*. Boca Raton, FL: CRC Press, 1988: 157−72.

63 Matrisian LM. Metalloproteinases and their inhibitors in matrix remodelling. *Trends Genet* 1990; 6: 121−5.

64 Woessner JF. Matrix metalloproteinases and their inhibitors in connective tissue remodelling. *FASEB J* 1991; 5: 2145−54.

65 Stricklin GP, Hibbs MS. Biochemistry and physiology of mammalian collagenases. In: Nimni ME, ed. *Collagen. Volume I. Biochemistry*. Boca Raton, FL: CRC Press, 1988: 187−205.

66 Danielsen CC. Thermal stability of human-fibroblast-collagenase-cleavage products of type-I and type-III collagens. *Biochem J* 1987; 247: 725−9.

67 Ten Cate AR. Morphological studies of fibrocytes in connective tissue undergoing rapid remodelling. *J Anat* 1972; 112: 401−14.

68 Etherington DJ. Proteinases in connective tissue breakdown. In: *Protein Degradation in Health and Disease*. Ciba Foundation Symposium 1980: 75, 87−103.

69 Slack JL, Liska DJ, Bornstein P. An upstream regulatory region mediates high-level, tissue-specific expression of the human α1(I) collagen gene in transgenic mice. *Mol Cell Biol* 1991; 11: 2066−74.

70 Cedar H. DNA methylation and gene activity. *Cell* 1988; 53: 3−4.

71 Barsh GS, Rousch CL, Gelinas RE. DNA and chromatin structure of the human α1(I) collagen gene. *J Biol Chem* 1984; 259: 14906−13.

72 Breindl M, Harbers K, Janeisch R. Retrovirus-induced lethal mutation in collagen I gene of mice is associated with an altered chromatin structure. *Cell* 1984; 38: 9−16.

73 Adams RLP. DNA methylation: the effect of minor bases on DNA−protein interactions. *Biochem J* 1990; 265: 309−20.

74 Rhodes K, Breindl M. Developmental changes in the methylation status of regulatory elements in the murine α1(I) collagen gene. *Gene Express* 1992; 2: 59−69.

75 Chan H, Hartung S, Breindl M. Retrovirus-induced interference with collagen I gene expression in Mov13 fibroblasts is maintained in the absence of DNA methylation. *Mol Cell Biol* 1991; 11: 47−54.

76 Thompson JP, Simkevich CP, Holness MA, Kang AH, Raghow R. *In vitro*

methylation of the promoter and enhancer of proα1(I) collagen gene leads to its transcriptional inactivation. *J Biol Chem* 1991; 266: 2549−56.

77 Fouser L, Sage EH, Clark J, Bornstein P. Feedback regulation of collagen gene expression: a Trojan horse approach. *Proc Natl Acad Sci USA* 1991; 88: 10158−62.

78 Katayama K, Seyer JM, Raghow R, Kang AH. Regulation of extracellular matrix production by chemically synthesized subfragments of type I collagen carboxy peptide. *Biochemistry* 1991; 30: 7097−104.

79 Wu CH, Walton CM, Wu GY. Propeptide-mediated regulation of procollagen synthesis in IMR-90 human lung fibroblast cell cultures. *J Biol Chem* 1991; 266: 2983−7.

80 Goldstein RH, Fine A, Farnsworth LJ, Poliks C, Polgar P. Phorbol ester-induced inhibition of collagen accumulation by human lung fibroblasts. *J Biol Chem* 1990; 265: 13623−8.

81 Elias JA, Gustilo K, Baeder W, Freundlich B. Synergistic stimulation of fibroblast prostaglandin production by recombinant interleukin-1 and tumour necrosis factor. *J Immunol* 1987; 138: 3812−16.

82 Heino J, Heinonen T. Interleukin-1β prevents the stimulatory effect of transforming growth factor-β on collagen gene expression in human skin fibroblasts. *Biochem J* 1990; 271: 827−30.

83 Varga J, Olsen A, Herhal J, Constantine G, Rosenbloom J, Jimenez SA. Interferon-γ reverses the stimulation of collagen but not fibronectin gene expression by transforming growth factor-β in normal human fibroblasts. *Eur J Clin Invest* 1990; 20: 487−93.

84 Mauviel A, Heino J, Kahari V-M *et al.* Comparative effects of interleukin-1 and tumor necrosis factor-α on collagen production and corresponding procollagen mRNA levels in human dermal fibroblasts. *J Invest Dermatol* 1991; 96: 243−9.

85 Rossi P, Karsenty G, Roberts AB, Roche NS, Sporn MB, de Crombrugghe B. A nuclear factor 1 binding site mediates the transcriptional activation of a type I collagen promoter by transforming growth factor-β. *Cell* 1988; 52: 405−14.

86 Raghow R, Postlethwaite AE, Keski-Oja J, Moses HL, Kang AH. Transforming growth factor-β increases steady-state levels of type I procollagen and fibronectin messenger RNAs posttranscriptionally in cultured human dermal fibroblasts. *J Clin Invest* 1987; 79: 1285−8.

87 McAnulty RJ, Campa JS, Cambrey AD, Laurent GJ. The effect of transforming growth factor β on rates of procollagen synthesis and degradation *in vitro*. *Biochem Biophys Acta* 1991; 1091: 231−5.

88 Prockop DJ, Kivirikko KI, Tuderman L, Guzman NA. The biosynthesis of collagen and its disorders. *N Engl J Med* 1979; 301: 13−23, 77−85.

89 Bassuk JA, Berg RA. Correlation of the steady-state RNA levels among the α-subunit of prolyl 4-hydroxylase and the α1 and α2 chains of type I collagen during growth of chicken embryo tendon fibroblasts. *Biochem Biophys Res Commun* 1991; 174: 169−75.

90 Yeowell HN, Murad S, Pinnell SR. Hydralazine differentially increases mRNAs for the α and β subunits of prolyl 4-hydroxylase whereas it decreases proα1(I) collagen mRNAs in human skin fibroblasts. *Arch Biochem Biophys* 1991; 289: 399−404.

91 Bienkowski RS, Cowan MJ, McDonald JA, Crystal RG. Degradation of newly synthesized collagen. *J Biol Chem* 1978; 253: 4356−63.

92 Kagan HM, Trackman PC. Properties and function of lysyl oxidase. *Am J Respir Cell Mol Biol* 1991; 5: 206−10.

93 Mercer RR, Crapo JD. Spatial distribution of collagen and elastin fibers in the lungs. *J Appl Physiol* 1990; 69: 756−65.

94 Rucker RB, Dubick MA. Elastin metabolism and chemistry: potential roles in lung development and structure. *Environ Health Perspectives* 1984; 55: 179–91.

95 Knudson RJ. Physiology of the aging lung. In: Crystal RG, West JB, eds. *The Lung: Scientific Foundations*. New York: Raven Press, 1991: 1749–59.

96 Byers PH. Brittle bones-fragile molecules: disorders of collagen gene structure and expression. *Trends Genet* 1990; 6: 293–300.

97 Lee B, D'Alessio M, Ramirez F. Modifications in the organization and expression of collagen genes associated with skeletal disorders. *Crit Rev Eukr Gene Exp* 1991; 1: 173–87.

98 Prockop DJ. Mutations in collagen genes as a cause of connective-tissue diseases. *N Engl J Med* 1992; 326: 540–6.

99 Prockop DJ. Mutations that alter the primary structure of type I collagen: the perils of a system for generating large structures by the principle of nucleated growth. *J Biol Chem* 1990; 265: 15349–52.

100 Barsh GS, Byers PH. Reduced secretion of structurally abnormal type I procollagen in a form of osteogenesis imperfecta. *Proc Natl Acad Sci USA* 1981; 78: 5142–6.

101 Williams CJ, Prockop DJ. Synthesis and processing of a type I procollagen containing shortened pro-α1(I) chains by fibroblasts from a patient with osteogenesis imperfecta. *J Biol Chem* 1983; 258: 5915–21.

102 Prockop DJ, Kivirikko KI. Heritable diseases of collagen. *N Engl J Med* 1984; 311: 376–86.

103 Kuivaniemi H, Tromp G, Prockop DJ. Mutations in collagen genes: causes of rare and some common diseases in humans. *FASEB J* 1991; 5: 2052–60.

104 Vogel BE, Doelz R, Kadler KE, Hojima Y, Engel J, Prockop DJ. A substitution of cysteine for glycine 748 of the α1 chain produces a kink at this site in the procollagen I molecule and an altered *N*-proteinase cleavage site over 225 nm away. *J Biol Chem* 1988; 263: 19249–55.

105 Clark JG, Kuhn III C, Uitto J. Lung collagen in type IV Ehlers–Danlos syndrome: ultrastructural and biochemical studies. *Am Rev Respir Dis* 1980; 122: 971–8.

106 Snider GL. Interstitial lung disease: pathogenesis, pathophysiology, and clinical presentation. In: Schwarz MI, King TE, eds. *Interstitial Lung Disease*. Philadelphia: BC Decker Inc., 1988: 1–13.

107 Harrison NK, Laurent GJ. Lung collagen metabolism: the link between inflammation and pulmonary fibrosis. In: Selman Lama M, Barrios R, eds. *Interstitial Pulmonary Diseases: Selected Topics*. Boca Raton, FL: CRC Press, 1990: 47–74.

108 Crystal RG. Ferrans VJ, Basset F. Biologic basis of pulmonary fibrosis. In: Crystal RG, West JB, eds. *The Lung: Scientific Foundations*. New York: Raven Press, 1991: 2031–46.

109 Fine A, Goldstein RH, Snider GL. Animal models of pulmonary fibrosis. In: Crystal RG, West JB, eds. *The Lung: Scientific Foundations*. New York: Raven Press, 1991: 2047–57.

110 Thrall RS, Barton RW, D'Amanto DA, Sulavik SB. Differential cellular analysis of bronchoalveolar lavage fluid obtained at various stages during the development of bleomycin-induced pulmonary fibrosis in the rat. *Am Rev Respir Dis* 1982; 126: 488–92.

111 Thet LA, Parra SC, Shelbourne JD. Sequential changes in lung morphology during the repair of acute oxygen-induced lung injury in adult rats. *Exp Lung Res* 1986; 11: 209–28.

112 Phan SH, Thrall RS, Ward PA. Bleomycin-induced pulmonary fibrosis in rats: biochemical demonstration of increased rate of collagen synthesis. *Am Rev Respir Dis* 1980; 121: 501–6.

113 Kelley J. Cytokines of the lung. *Am Rev Respir Dis* 1990; 141: 765–88.

114 Kovacs EJ. Fibrogenic cytokines: the role of immune mediators in the develop-

ment of scar tissue. *Immunol Today* 1991; 12: 17–23.

115 Elias JA, Kotloff R, Ray P. Cytokines in pulmonary inflammation. In: Fishman AP, ed. *Update: Pulmonary Diseases and Disorders*. New York: McGraw-Hill Inc., 1992: 93–114.

116 Broekelmann TJ, Limper AH, Colby TV, McDonald JA. Transforming growth factor β1 is present at sites of extracellular matrix gene expression in human pulmonary fibrosis. *Proc Natl Acad Sci USA* 1991; 88: 6642–6.

117 Khalil N, O'Connor RN, Unruh HW *et al*. Increased production and immuno-histochemical localization of transforming growth factor β in idiopathic pulmonary fibrosis. *Am J Respir Cell Mol Biol* 1991; 5: 155–62.

118 Hoyt DG, Lazo JS. Alterations in pulmonary mRNA encoding procollagens, fibronectin and transforming growth factor β precede bleomycin-induced pulmonary fibrosis in mice. *J Pharmacol Exp Ther* 1988; 246: 765–71.

119 Raghow R, Irish P, Kang AH. Coordinate regulation of transforming growth factor β gene expression and cell proliferation in hamster lungs undergoing bleomycin-induced pulmonary fibrosis. *J Clin Invest* 1989; 84: 1836–42.

120 Snyder LS, Hertz MI, Peterson MS *et al*. Acute lung injury: pathogenesis of intraalveolar fibrosis. *J Clin Invest* 1991; 88: 663–73.

121 Shaw RJ, Benedict SH, Clark RAF, King TE. Pathogenesis of pulmonary fibrosis in interstitial lung disease: Alveolar macrophage PDGF(B) gene activation and up-regulation by interferon gamma. *Am Rev Respir Dis* 1991; 143: 167–73.

122 Fabisiak JP, Evans JN, Kelley J. Increased expression of PDGF-B (*c-sis*) mRNA in rat lung precedes DNA synthesis and tissue repair during chronic hypoxia. *Am J Respir Cell Mol Biol* 1989; 1: 181–9.

123 Bitterman PB, Rennard SI, Hunninghake GW, Crystal RG. Human alveolar macrophage growth factor for fibroblasts: regulation and partial characterization. *J Clin Invest* 1982; 70: 806–22.

124 Bitterman PB, Adelberg S, Crystal RG. Mechanisms of pulmonary fibrosis: spontaneous release of the alveolar-macrophage-derived growth factor in the interstitial lung disorders. *J Clin Invest* 1983; 72: 1801–13.

125 Rom WN, Basset P, Fells GA, Nukiwa T, Trapnell BC, Crystal RG. Alveolar macrophages release an insulin-like growth factor 1-type molecule. *J Clin Invest* 1988; 82: 1685–93.

126 Raghu G, Striker LJ, Hudson LD, Striker GE. Extracellular matrix in normal and fibrotic human lungs. *Am Rev Respir Dis* 1985; 131: 281–9.

127 Laurent GJ, McAnulty RJ. Protein metabolism during bleomycin-induced pulmonary fibrosis in rabbits. *In vivo* evidence for collagen accumulation because of increased synthesis and decreased degradation of newly synthesized collagen. *Am Rev Respir Dis* 1983; 128: 82–8.

128 Kirk JME, Bateman ED, Haslam PL, Laurent GJ, Turner-Warwick M. Serum type III procollagen peptide concentration in cryptogenic fibrosing alveolitis and its clinical relevance. *Thorax* 1984; 39: 726–32.

129 Low RB, Cutroneo KR, Davis GS, Giancola BS. Lavage type III procollagen N-terminal peptides in human pulmonary fibrosis and sarcoidosis. *Lab Invest* 1983; 48: 755–63.

130 Raghu G, Masta S, Meyers D, Narayanan AS. Collagen synthesis by normal and fibrotic human lung fibroblasts and the effect of transforming growth factor-β. *Am Rev Respir Dis* 1989; 140: 95–100.

131 Harrison NK, Argent AC, McAnulty RJ, Black C, Corrin B, Laurent GJ. Collagen synthesis and degradation by systemic sclerosis lung fibroblasts. *Chest* 1991; 99 (Suppl.): 71–2S.

132 MacMillan JM. Familial pulmonary fibrosis. *Dis Chest* 1951; 20: 426–36.

133 Rubin EH, Lubliner R. Hamman–Rich syndrome. Review of the literature and

analysis of 15 cases. *Medicine* 1957; 36: 397–463.

134 Bitterman PB, Rennard SI, Keogh BA, Wewers MD, Adelberg S, Crystal RG. Familial idiopathic pulmonary fibrosis. Evidence of lung inflammation in unaffected family members. *N Engl J Med* 1986; 314: 1343–7.

135 Musk AW, Zilko PJ, Manners P, Kay AH, Kamboh MI. Genetic studies in familial fibrosing alveolitis. Possible linkage with immunoglobin allotypes (Gm). *Chest* 1986; 89: 206–10.

136 King TE. Idiopathic pulmonary fibrosis. In: Schwarz MI, King TE, eds. *Interstitial Lung Disease*. Philadelphia: BC Decker Inc., 1988: 139–69.

137 Geddes DM, Brewerton DA, Webley M *et al*. Alpha-1-antitrypsin phenotypes in fibrosing alveolitis and rheumatoid arthritis. *Lancet* 1977; ii: 1049–50.

138 Turton CWG, Morris LM, Lawler SD, Turner-Warwick M. HLA in cryptogenic fibrosing alveolitis. *Lancet* 1978; i: 507–8.

139 Laurent GJ. Lung collagen: more than scaffolding. *Thorax* 1986; 41: 418–28.

140 Davidson JM. Biochemistry and turnover of lung interstitium. *Eur Respir J* 1990; 3: 1048–68.

141 Shock A, Laurent GJ. Leucocytes and pulmonary disorders: mobilization, activation and role in pathology. *Mol Aspects Med* 1990; 11: 425–526.

142 Keeley FW. Dynamic responses of collagen and elastin to vessel wall perturbation. In: Gotlieb AI, Langille BL, Federoff S, eds. *Atherosclerosis*. New York: Plenum Press, 1991: 101–14.

143 Mecham RP, Whitehouse LA, Wrenn DS *et al*. Smooth muscle-mediated connective tissue remodeling in pulmonary hypertension. *Science* 1987; 237: 423–6.

144 Crouch EC. Molecular diversity of basement membrane collagen: elucidation of the Goodpasture's epitope. *Am J Respir Cell Mol Biol* 1991; 5: 99–100.

145 Gunwar S, Ballester F, Kalluri R *et al*. Glomerular basement membrane. Identification of dimeric subunits of the noncollagenous domain (hexamer) of collagen IV and the Goodpasture antigen. *J Biol Chem* 1991; 266: 15318–24.

146 Gunwar S, Bejarano PA, Kalluri R *et al*. Alveolar basement membrane: molecular properties of the noncollagenous domain (hexamer) of collagen IV and its reactivity with Goodpasture autoantibodies. *Am J Respir Cell Mol Biol* 1991; 5: 107–12.

147 Sage H, Gray WR. Studies on the evolution of elastin-I. Phylogenetic distribution. *Comp Biochem Physiol* 1979; 64B: 313–27.

148 Cleary EG, Gibson MA. Elastin-associated microfibrils and microfibrillar proteins. *Int Rev Connect Tissue Res* 1983; 10: 97–209.

149 Mecham RP. Elastin synthesis and fiber assembly. *Ann N Y Acad Sci* 1991; 624: 137–46.

150 Emmanuel BS, Cannizzaro L, Ornstein-Goldstein N *et al*. Chromosomal localization of the human elastin gene. *Am J Hum Genet* 1985; 37: 873–82.

151 Fazio MJ, Mattei M-G, Passage E *et al*. Human elastin gene: new evidence for localization to the long arm of chromosome 7. *Am J Hum Genet* 1991; 48: 696–703.

152 Levi-Minzi SA, Wynder KL, Christiano AM *et al*. The chromosomal localization of the human tropoelastin gene: a revisit. *Biophys J* 1992; 61: A77 [Abstract].

153 Indik Z, Yeh H, Ornstein-Goldstein N, Rosenbloom J. Structure of the elastin gene and alternative splicing of elastin mRNA. In: Sandell L, Boyd C, eds. *Extracellular Matrix Genes*. San Diego, CA: Academic Press, 1990: 221–50.

154 Rosenbloom J, Bashir M, Yeh H *et al*. Regulation of elastin gene expression. *Ann N Y Acad Sci* 1991; 624: 116–36.

155 Bashir MM, Indik Z, Yeh H *et al*. Characterization of the complete human elastin gene: delineation of unusual features in the 5'-flanking region. *J Biol Chem* 1989; 264: 8887–91.

156 Indik Z, Yeh H, Ornstein-Goldstein N *et al*. Alternative splicing of human elastin mRNA indicated by sequence analysis of cloned genomic and complementary DNA. *Proc Natl Acad Sci USA* 1987; 84: 5680−4.

157 Kainulainen K, Rosenbloom J, Peltonen L. Two polymorphisms for the human elastin gene. *Nucleic Acids Res* 1990; 18: 3114.

158 Tromp G, Christiano A, Goldstein N *et al*. A to G polymorphism in ELN gene. *Nucleic Acids Res* 1991; 19: 4314.

159 Christiano AM, Boyd CD. Two complex polymorphic systems in the human tropoelastin gene. *Clin Res* 1992; 39: 511A [Abstract].

160 Rosenbloom J, Bashir MM, Kahari V-M, Uitto J. Elastin genes and regulation of their expression. *Crit Rev Eukr Gene Exp* 1991; 1: 145−56.

161 Kahari V-M, Fazio MJ, Chen YQ, Bashir MM, Rosenbloom J, Uitto J. Deletion analyses of 5′-flanking region of the human elastin gene. Delineation of functional promoter and regulatory *cis*-elements. *J Biol Chem* 1990; 265: 9485−90.

162 Slack HGB. Metabolism of elastin in the adult rat. *Nature* 1954; 174: 512−3.

163 Fazio MJ, Olsen DR, Kuivaniemi H *et al*. Isolation and characterization of human elastin cDNAs, and age-associated variation in elastin gene expression in cultured skin fibroblasts. *Lab Invest* 1988; 58: 270−7.

164 Foster JA, Rich CB, Miller M, Benedict MR, Richman RA, Florini JR. Effect of age and IGF-1 administration on elastin gene expression in rat aorta. *J Gerontol* 1991; 45: B113−8.

165 Yeh H, Ornstein-Goldstein N, Indik Z *et al*. Sequence variation of bovine elastin mRNA due to alternative splicing. *Collagen Relat Res* 1987; 7: 235−47.

166 Fazio MJ, Olsen DR, Kauh EA *et al*. Cloning of full-length elastin cDNAs from a human skin fibroblast recombinant cDNA library: further elucidation of alternative splicing utilizing exon-specific oligonucleotides. *J Invest Dermatol* 1988; 91: 458−64.

167 Yeh H, Anderson N, Ornstein-Goldstein N *et al*. Structure of the bovine elastin gene and S1 nuclease analysis of alternative splicing of elastin mRNA in the bovine nuchal ligament. *Biochemistry* 1989; 28: 2365−70.

168 Heim RA, Pierce RA, Deak SB, Riley DJ, Boyd CD, Stolle CA. Alternative splicing of rat tropoelastin mRNA is tissue-specific and developmentally regulated. *Matrix* 1991; 11: 359−66.

169 Foster JA, Rich CB, Fletcher S, Karr SR, Przybyla A. Translation of chick aorta elastin messenger ribonucleic acid. Comparison to elastin synthesis in chick aorta organ culture. *Biochemistry* 1980; 19: 857−64.

170 Burnett W, Eichner R, Rosenbloom J. Correlation of functional elastin messenger ribonucleic acid levels and rate of elastin synthesis in the developing chick aorta. *Biochemistry* 1980; 19: 1106−11.

171 Wrenn DS, Parks WC, Whitehouse LA *et al*. Identification of multiple tropoelastins secreted by bovine cells. *J Biol Chem* 1987; 262: 2244−9.

172 Davidson JM, Giro MG. Control of elastin synthesis: molecular and cellular aspects. In: Mecham RP, ed. *Regulation of Matrix Accumulation*. New York: Academic Press, 1986: 177−216.

173 Uitto J, Hoffmann H-P, Prockop DJ. Synthesis of elastin and procollagen by cells from embryonic aorta: differences in the role of hydroxyproline and effects of proline analogs on the secretion of the two proteins. *Arch Biochem Biophys* 1976; 173: 187−200.

174 Rosenbloom J. Elastin: biosynthesis, structure, degradation and role in disease processes. *Connect Tissue Res* 1982; 10: 73−91.

175 Mecham RP, Madaras J, McDonald JA, Ryan U. Elastin production by cultured calf pulmonary artery endothelial cells. *J Cell Physiol* 1983; 116: 282−8.

176 Campagnone R, Regan J, Rich CB *et al*. Pulmonary fibroblasts: a model system

for studying elastin synthesis. *Lab Invest* 1987; 56: 224−30.

177 Burnett W, Finnigan-Bunick A, Yoon K, Rosenbloom J. Analysis of elastin gene expression in the developing chick aorta using cloned elastin cDNA. *J Biol Chem* 1982; 257: 1569−72.

178 Davidson JM, Shibahara S, Boyd C, Mason ML, Tolstoshev P, Crystal RG. Elastin mRNA levels during foetal development of sheep nuchal ligament and lung: hybridization to complementary and cloned DNA. *Biochem J* 1984; 220: 653−63.

179 Sandberg LB, Soskel NT, Leslie JG. Elastin structure, biosynthesis, and relation to disease states. *N Engl J Med* 1981; 304: 566−79.

180 Eyre DR, Paz MA, Gallop PM. Cross-linking in elastin and collagen. *Annu Rev Biochem* 1984; 53: 717−48.

181 Wrenn DS, Griffin GL, Senior RM, Mecham RP. Characterization of biologically active domains on elastin: identification of a monoclonal antibody to a cell recognition site. *Biochemistry* 1986; 25: 5172−6.

182 Noguchi A, Reddy R, Kursar JD, Parks WC, Mecham RP. Smooth muscle isoactin and elastin in fetal bovine lung. *Exp Lung Res* 1989; 15: 537−52.

183 Sephel GC, Davidson JM. Elastin production in human skin fibroblast cultures and its decline with age. *J Invest Dermatol* 1986; 86: 279−85.

184 Starcher BC. Elastin and the lung. *Thorax* 1986; 41: 577−85.

185 Campbell E, Pierce J, Endicott S, Shapiro S. Evaluation of extracellular matrix turnover: methods and results for normal lung parenchymal elastin. *Chest* 1991; 99 (Suppl.): 49S.

186 Bruce MC. Developmental changes in tropoelastin mRNA levels in rat lung: evaluation by *in situ* hybridization. *Am J Respir Cell Mol Biol* 1991; 5: 344−50.

187 Foster JA, Curtiss SW. The regulation of lung elastin synthesis. *Am J Physiol* 1990; 259: L13−23.

188 Dubick MA, Rucker RB, Cross CE, Last JA. Elastin metabolism in rodent lung. *Biochim Biophys Acta* 1981; 672: 303−6.

189 Powell JT, Whitney PL. Postnatal development of rat lung: changes in lung lectin, elastin, acetylcholinesterase and other enzymes. *Biochem J* 1980; 188: 1−8.

190 Haidar A, Ryder TA, Wigglesworth JS. Failure of elastin development in hypoplastic lungs associated with oligohydramnios: an electron microscopic study. *Histopathology* 1991; 18: 471−3.

191 Parks WC, Secrist H, Wu LJ, Mecham RP. Developmental regulation of tropoelastin isoforms. *J Biol Chem* 1988; 263: 4416−23.

192 Pollock J, Baule VJ, Rich CB, Ginsburg CD, Curtiss SW, Foster JA. Chick tropoelastin isoforms: from the gene to the extracellular matrix. *J Biol Chem* 1990; 265: 3697−702.

193 Frisch SM, Davidson JM, Werb Z. Blockage of tropoelastin secretion by monensin represses tropoelastin synthesis at a pretranslational level in rat smooth muscle cells. *Mol Cell Biol* 1985; 5: 253−8.

194 Foster JA, Rich CB, Miller MF. Pulmonary fibroblasts: an *in vitro* model of emphysema: regulation of elastin gene expression. *J Biol Chem* 1990; 265: 15544−9.

194a Curran ME, Atkinson DL, Ewart AK *et al*. The elastin gene is disrupted by a translocation associated with supravalvular aortic stenosis. *Cell* 1993; 73: 159−68.

195 Uitto J, Christiano AM, Kahari V-M, Bashir MM, Rosenbloom J. Molecular biology and pathology of human elastin. *Biochem Soc Trans* 1991; 19: 824−9.

196 Snider GL, Kleinerman J, Thurlbeck WM, Bengali ZH. The definition of emphysema. Report of a National Heart, Lung, and Blood Institute, Division of

Lung Diseases Workshop. *Am Rev Respir Dis* 1985; 132: 182−5.

197 Hutchison DCS. Natural history of alpha-1-protease inhibitor deficiency. *Am J Med* 1988; 84 (Suppl. 6A): 3−12.

198 Brantly M, Nukiwa T, Crystal RG. Molecular basis of alpha-1-antitrypsin deficiency. *Am J Med* 1988; 84 (Suppl. 6A): 13−31.

199 Bieth JG. Elastases: catalytic and biological properties. In: Mecham RP, ed. *Regulation of Matrix Accumulation*. New York: Academic Press, 1986: 217−320.

200 Rao NV, Hoidal JR, Gray BH. Oxidised halogens degrade elastin: a potential mechanism for smoking-induced emphysema. In: Mittman C, ed. *Pulmonary Emphysema and Proteolysis*. New York: Academic Press, 1987: 407−12.

201 Riley DJ, Kerr JS. Oxidant injury of the extracellular matrix: potential role in the pathogenesis of pulmonary emphysema. *Lung* 1985; 163: 1−13.

202 Eriksson S. The potential role of elastase inhibitors in emphysema treatment. *Eur Respir J* 1991; 4: 1041−3.

203 Gadek JE, Klein HG, Holland PV, Crystal RG. Replacement therapy of α1-antitrypsin deficiency: reversal of protease−antiprotease imbalance within the alveolar structures of P_iZ subjects. *J Clin Invest* 1981; 68: 1158−65.

204 Kuhn C, Yu S-Y, Chraplyvy M, Linder HE, Senior RM. The induction of emphysema with elastase. II. Changes in connective tissue. *Lab Invest* 1976; 34: 372−80.

205 Fukuda Y, Masuda Y, Ishizaki M, Masugi Y, Ferrans VJ. Morphogenesis of abnormal elastic fibers in lungs of patients with panacinar and centriacinar emphysema. *Hum Pathol* 1989; 20: 652−9.

206 Starcher BC, Kuhn C, Overton JE. Increased elastin and collagen content in the lungs of hamsters receiving an intratracheal injection of bleomycin. *Am Rev Respir Dis* 1978; 117: 299−305.

207 Raghow R, Lurie S, Seyer JM, Kang AH. Profiles of steady-state levels of messenger RNAs coding for type I procollagen, elastin, and fibronectin in hamster lungs undergoing bleomycin-induced interstitial pulmonary fibrosis. *J Clin Invest* 1985; 76: 1733−9.

208 Kainulainen K, Pulkkinen L, Savolainen A, Katila I, Peltonen L. Location on chromosome 15 of the gene defect causing Marfan syndrome. *N Engl J Med* 1990; 323: 935−9.

209 McKusick VA. The defect in Marfan syndrome. *Nature* 1991; 352: 279−81.

210 Tsipouras P. Marfan syndrome: a mystery solved. *J Med Genet* 1992; 29: 73−4.

211 Sarfarazi M, Tsipouras P, Del Mastro R *et al.* A linkage map of 10 loci flanking the Marfan syndrome locus on 15q: results of an International Consortium Study. *J Med Genet* 1992; 29: 75−80.

212 Roman J, McDonald JA. Fibronectins. In: Crystal RG, West JB, eds. *The Lung: Scientific Foundations*. New York: Raven Press, 1991: 399−411.

213 Juul SE, Wight TN, Hascall VC. Proteoglycans. In: Crystal RG, West JB, eds. *The Lung: Scientific Foundations*. New York: Raven Press, 1991: 413−20.

214 Roberts CR. Lung proteoglycans in health and disease. In: Selman Lama M, Barrios R, eds. *Interstitial Pulmonary Diseases: Selected Topics*. Boca Raton, FL: CRC Press, 1990: 99−135.

215 Beck K, Hunter I, Engel J. Structure and function of laminin: anatomy of a multidomain glycoprotein. *FASEB J* 1990; 4: 148−60.

216 Sage EH, Bornstein P. Extracellular proteins that modulate cell−matrix interactions. SPARC, Tenascin, and Thrombospondin. *J Biol Chem* 1991; 266: 14831−4.

217 Timpl R, Aumailley M, Gerl M *et al.* Function and structure of the laminin−nidogen complex. *Ann N Y Acad Sci* 1990; 580: 311−23.

218 Ruoslahti E. Integrins. *J Clin Invest* 1991; 87: 1−5.

219 Erle DJ, Pytela R. How do integrins integrate? The role of cell adhesion receptors in differentiation and development. *Am J Respir Cell Mol Biol* 1992; 6: 459−60.

220 Sakai LY, Keene DR, Engvall E. Fibrillin, a new 350 kD glycoprotein, is a component of extracellular microfibrils. *J Cell Biol* 1986; 103: 2499−509.

221 Mays C, Rosenberry TL. Characterisation of pepsin-resistant collagen-like tail subunit fragments of 18S and 14S acetylcholinesterase from *Electrophorus electricus*. *Biochemistry* 1981; 20: 1810−17.

222 Strang CJ, Slayter HS, Lachmann PJ, Davis AE. Ultrastructure and composition of bovine conglutinin. *Biochem J* 1986; 234: 381−9.

223 Reid KBM. Complete amino acid sequences of the three collagen-like regions present in subcomponent C1q of the first component of human complement. *Biochem J* 1979; 179: 367−71.

224 Drickamer K, Dordal MS, Reynolds L. Mannose-binding proteins isolated from rat liver contain carbohydrate-recognition domains linked to collagenous tails. *J Biol Chem* 1986; 261: 6878−87.

225 Hawgood S. Pulmonary surfactant apoproteins: a review of protein and genomic structure. *Am J Physiol* 1989; 257: L13−22.

226 Rust K, Grosso L, Zhang V *et al*. Human surfactant protein D: SP-D contains a C-type lectin carbohydrate recognition domain. *Arch Biochem Biophys* 1991; 290: 116−26.

227 Gotte L. Molecular morphology of elastin. *Front Matrix Biol* 1980; 8: 33−53.

228 Adams SL. Collagen gene expression. *Am J Respir Mol Cell Biol* 1989; 1: 161−8.

229 Bennett VD, Weiss IM, Adams SL. Cartilage-specific 5′-end of chick α2(I) collagen mRNAs. *J Biol Chem* 1989; 264: 8402−9.

230 Ryan MC, Sandell LJ. Differential expression of a cysteine-rich domain in the amino-terminal propeptide of type II (cartilage) procollagen by alternative splicing of mRNA. *J Biol Chem* 1990; 265: 10334−9.

231 Nah H-D, Upholt WB. Type II collagen mRNA containing an alternatively spliced exon predominates in the chick limb prior to chondrogenesis. *J Biol Chem* 1991; 266: 23446−52.

232 Saitta B, Stokes DG, Vissing H, Timpl R, Chu M-L. Alternative splicing of the human α2(VI) collagen gene generates multiple mRNA transcripts which predict three protein variants with distinct carboxyl termini. *J Biol Chem* 1990; 265: 6473−80.

233 Saitta B, Timpl R, Chu M-L. Human α2(VI) collagen gene. Heterogeneity at the 5′-untranslated region generated by an alternate exon. *J Biol Chem* 1992; 257: 6188−96.

234 Svoboda KK, Nishimura I, Sugrue SP, Ninomiya Y, Olsen BR. Embryonic chicken cornea and cartilage synthesize type IX collagen molecules with different amino-terminal domains. *Proc Natl Acad Sci USA* 1988; 85: 7496−500.

235 Trueb J, Trueb B. Two splice variants of collagen XII share a common 5′-end. *Biochim Biphys Acta* 1992; 1171: 97−8.

236 Tikka L, Pihlajaniemi T, Henttu P, Prockop DJ, Tryggvason K. Gene structure for the α1 chain of a human short-chain collagen (type XIII) with alternatively spliced transcripts and translation termination codon at the 5′ end of the last exon. *Proc Natl Acad Sci USA* 1988; 85: 7491−5.

237 Bernard MP, Myers JC, Chu M-L, Ramirez F, Eikenberry EF, Prockop DJ. Structure of a cDNA for the proα2 chain of human type I procollagen. Comparison with chick cDNA for proα2(I) identifies structurally conserved features of the protein and the gene. *Biochemistry* 1983; 22: 1139−45.

238 Bernard MP, Chu M-L, Myers JC, Ramirez F, Eikenberry EF, Prockop DJ. Nucleotide sequences of complementary deoxyribonucleic acids for the proα1(I) chain of human type I procollagen. Statistical evaluation of structures that are

conserved during evolution. *Biochemistry* 1983; 22: 5213–23.

239 Kuivaniemi H, Tromp G, Chu M-L, Prockop DJ. Structure of a full-length cDNA clone for preproα2(I) chain of human type I procollagen. *Biochem J* 1988; 252: 633–40.

240 Tromp G, Kuivaniemi H, Stacey A *et al*. Structure of a full-length cDNA clone for the preproα1(I) chain of human type I procollagen. *Biochem J* 1988; 253: 919–22.

241 Ala-Kokko L, Kontusaari S, Baldwin CT, Kuivaniemi H, Prockop DJ. Structure of cDNA clones coding for the entire preproα1(III) chain of human type III procollagen. *Biochem J* 1989; 260: 509–16.

242 Geesin JC, Darr D, Kaufman R, Murad S, Pinnell SR. Ascorbic acid specifically increases type I and type III procollagen messenger RNA levels in human skin fibroblasts. *J Invest Dermatol* 1988; 90: 420–4.

243 Tan EML, Dodge GR, Sorger T *et al*. Modulation of extracellular matrix gene expression by heparin and endothelial cell growth factor in human smooth muscle cells. *Lab Invest* 1991; 64: 474–82.

244 Kurata S-I, Hata R-I. Epidermal growth factor inhibits transcription of type I collagen genes and production of type I collagen in cultured human skin fibroblasts in the presence or absence of L-ascorbic acid 2-phosphate, a long-acting vitamin C derivative. *J Biol Chem* 1991; 266: 9997–10003.

245 Federspiel SJ, DiMari SJ, Howe AM, Guerry-Force ML, Haralson MA. Extracellular matrix biosynthesis by cultured fetal rat lung epithelial cells. III. Effects of chronic exposure to epidermal growth factor on growth, differentiation, and collagen biosynthesis. *Lab Invest* 1991; 64: 463–73.

246 Tseng SCG, Savion N, Stern R, Gospodarowicz D. Fibroblast growth factor modulates synthesis of collagen in cultured vascular endothelial cells. *Eur J Biochem* 1982; 122: 355–60.

247 Pardes JB, Martin TA, Helfman T, Ochoa S, Takagi H, Falanga V. Transcription of alpha1(I) procollagen by human dermal fibroblasts is directly downregulated by fibrinogen fragments and fibrin substrates. *J Invest Dermatol* 1993; 100: 549 [Abstract].

248 Cockayne D, Sterling KM, Shull S, Mintz KP, Illeyne S, Cutroneo KR. Glucocorticoids decrease the synthesis of type I procollagen mRNAs. *Biochemistry* 1986; 25: 3202–9.

249 Goldstein RH, Poliks CF, Pilch PF, Smith BD, Fine A. Stimulation of collagen formation by insulin and insulin-growth factor I in cultures of human lung fibroblasts. *Endocrinology* 1989; 124: 964–70.

250 Jimenez SA, Freundlich B, Rosenbloom J. Selective inhibition of human diploid fibroblast collagen synthesis by interferons. *J Clin Invest* 1984; 74: 1112–6.

251 Rosenbloom J, Feldman G, Freundlich B, Jimenez SA. Transcriptional control of human diploid fibroblast collagen synthesis by γ-interferon. *Biochem Biophys Res Commun* 1984; 123: 365–72.

252 Clark JG, Dedon TF, Wayner EA, Carter WG. Effects of interferon-γ on expression of cell surface receptors for collagen and deposition of newly synthesized collagen by cultured human lung fibroblasts. *J Clin Invest* 1989; 83: 1505–11.

253 Mauviel A, Evans CH, Uitto J. Leukoregulin down-regulates type I collagen mRNA levels and promoter activity in human dermal fibroblasts and counteracts the up-regulation elicited by transforming growth factor β. *Biochem J* 1992; 284: 629–32.

254 Hildebran JN, Chrin L, Kelley J. Effect of macrophage-derived competence factor on lung fibroblast protein and collagen synthesis. *Am Rev Respir Dis* 1986; 133: A257 (Abstr).

255 Ernst M, Schmid C, Froesch ER. Enhanced osteoblast proliferation and collagen

gene expression by estradiol. *Proc Natl Acad Sci USA* 1988; 85: 2307—10.

256 Kream BE, Rowe DW, Gworek SC, Raisz LG. Parathyroid hormone alters collagen synthesis and procollagen mRNA levels in fetal rat calvaria. *Proc Natl Acad Sci USA* 1980; 77: 5654—8.

257 Kelley J. Collagen. In: Massaro D, ed. *Lung Cell Biology*. New York: Marcel Dekker Inc., 1989: 821—66.

258 Barile FA, Ripley-Rouzier C, Siddiqi Z-E-A, Bienkowski RS. Effects of prostaglandin E_1 on collagen production and degradation in human fetal lung fibroblasts. *Arch Biochem Biophys* 1988; 265: 441—6.

259 Baum BJ, Moss J, Breul SD, Berg RA, Crystal RG. Effect of cyclic AMP on the intracellular degradation of newly synthesized collagen. *J Biol Chem* 1980; 255: 2843—7.

260 Goldstein RH, Polgar P. The effect and interaction of bradykinin and prostaglandins on protein and collagen production by lung fibroblasts. *J Biol Chem* 1982; 257: 8630—3.

261 Varga J, Diaz-Perez A, Rosenbloom J, Jimenez SA. PGE_2 causes a coordinate decrease in the steady-state levels of fibronectin and types I and III procollagen mRNAs in normal human dermal fibroblasts. *Biochem Biophys Res Commun* 1987; 147: 1282—8.

262 Oikarinen H, Oikarinen AI, Tan EML *et al.* Modulation of procollagen gene expression by retinoids. Inhibition of collagen production by retinoic acid accompanied by reduced type I procollagen messenger ribonucleic acid levels in human skin fibroblast cultures. *J Clin Invest* 1985; 75: 1545—53.

263 Solis-Herruzo JA, Brenner DA, Chojkier M. Tumor necrosis factor α inhibits collagen gene transcription and collagen synthesis in cultured human fibroblasts. *J Biol Chem* 1988; 263: 5841—5.

264 Lichtler A, Stover ML, Angilly J, Kream B, Rowe DW. Isolation and characterization of rat α1(I) collagen promoter. Regulation by 1,25-dihydroxyvitamin D. *J Biol Chem* 1989; 264: 3072—7.

265 Barker DF, Hostikka SL, Zhou J *et al.* Identification of mutations in the COL4A5 collagen gene in Alport syndrome. *Science* 1990; 248: 1224—7.

266 Christiano AM, Greenspan DS, Hoffman GG, *et al.* A missense mutation in type VII collagen in two affected siblings with recessive dystrophic epidermolysis bullosa. *Nat Genet* 1993; 4: 62—6.

267 Superti-Furga A, Gugler E, Gitzelmann R, Steinmann B. Ehlers—Danlos syndrome type IV: a multi-exon deletion in one of the two COL3A1 alleles affecting structure, stability, and processing of type III procollagen. *J Biol Chem* 1988; 263: 6226—32.

268 Weil D, Bernard M, Combates N *et al.* Identification of a mutation that causes exon skipping during collagen pre-mRNA splicing in an Ehlers—Danlos syndrome variant. *J Biol Chem* 1988; 263: 8561—4.

269 Kontusaari S, Tromp G, Kuivaniemi H, Romanic AM, Prockop DJ. A mutation in the gene for type III procollagen (COL3A1) in a family with aortic aneurysms. *J Clin Invest* 1990; 86: 1465—73.

270 Ala-Kokko L, Baldwin CT, Moskowitz RW, Prockop DJ. Single base mutation in the type II procollagen gene (COL2A1) as a cause of primary osteoarthritis associated with a mild chondrodysplasia. *Proc Natl Acad Sci USA* 1990; 87: 6565—8.

271 Chu M-L, Williams CJ, Pepe G, Hirsch JL, Prockop DJ, Ramirez F. Internal deletion in a collagen gene in a perinatal lethal form of osteogenesis imperfecta. *Nature* 1983; 304: 78—80.

272 Spotila LD, Constantinou CD, Sereda L, Ganguly A, Riggs LB, Prockop DJ. Mutation in a gene for type I procollagen (COL1A2) in a woman with post-menopausal osteoporosis: evidence for phenotypic and genotypic overlap with

mild osteogenesis imperfecta. *Proc Natl Acad Sci USA* 1991; 88: 5423−7.

273 Lee B, Vissing H, Ramirez F, Rogers D, Rimoin D. Identification of the molecular defect in a family with spondyloepiphyseal dysplasia. *Science* 1989; 244: 978−80.

274 Zhou J, Mochizuki T, Smeets H, Antignac C, Laurila P, de Paepe A, Tryggvason K, Reeders ST. Deletion of the paired a5(IV) and a6(IV) collagen genes in inherited smooth muscle tumors. *Science* 1993; 261: 1167−9.

275 Ahmad NN, Ala-Kokko L, Knowlton RG *et al.* Stop codon in the procollagen II gene (COL2A1) in a family with the Stickler syndrome (arthroophthalmopathy). *Proc Natl Acad Sci USA* 1991; 88: 6624−7.

276 Beighton P, De Paepe A, Hall JG *et al.* Molecular nosology of heritable disorders of connective tissue. *Am J Med Genet* 1992; 42: 431−48.

277 Kivirikko KI. Collagens and their abnormalities in a wide spectrum of diseases. *Annals of Medicine* 1993; 25: 113−26.

278 Hinek A, Botney MD, Mecham RP, Parks WC. Inhibition of tropoelastin expression by 1,25-dihydroxyvitamin D_3. *Connect Tissue Res* 1991; 26: 155−66.

279 Faris B, Ferrera R, Toselli P, Nambu J, Gonnerman WA, Franzblau C. Effect of varying amounts of ascorbate on collagen, elastin and lysyl oxidase synthesis in aortic smooth muscle cells. *Biochim Biophys Acta* 1984; 797: 71−5.

280 McGowan SE, Liu R, Harvey CS. Effects of heparin and other glycosaminoglycans on elastin production by cultured neonatal rat lung fibroblasts. *Arch Biochem Biophys* 1993; 302: 322−31.

281 Durmowicz AG, Badesch DB, Parks WC, Mecham RP, Stenmark KR. Hypoxia-induced inhibition of tropoelastin synthesis by neonatal calf pulmonary artery smooth muscle cells. *Am J Respir Cell Mol Biol* 1991; 5: 464−9.

282 Noguchi A, Nelson T. IGF-1 stimulates tropoelastin synthesis in neonatal rat pulmonary fibroblasts. *Pediatr Res* 1991; 30: 248−51.

283 Berk JL, Franzblau C, Goldstein RH. Recombinant interleukin-1β inhibits elastin formation by a neonatal rat lung fibroblast subtype. *J Biol Chem* 1991; 266: 3192−7.

284 McGowan SE, McNamer R. Transforming growth factor-β increases elastin production by neonatal rat lung fibroblasts. *Am J Respir Cell Mol Biol* 1990; 3: 369−76.

285 Kahari VM, Chen YQ, Bashir MM, Rosenbloom J, Uitto J. Tumor necrosis factor-alpha down-regulates human elastin gene expression: Evidence for the role of AP-1 in the suppression of promoter activity. *J Biol Chem* 1992; 267: 26134−141.

14 Transepithelial transport of secretory immunoglobulins

ELIZABETH SZTUL

Introduction

The mucosal surfaces are constantly exposed to external antigens including bacteria and viruses. In order to assist clearance of such agents, a complex system of lung defences has evolved to retain sterility of the bronchial tree. One of the major components of this defence system is the secretory immunoglobulins. It is well recognized that systemic deficiency of immunoglobulin is associated with recurrent and persistent respiratory infections. Nevertheless, in many patients with such problems, circulating immunoglobulins appear essentially normal. However, a specialized transport system has evolved at mucosal surfaces to facilitate immunoglobulin secretion, although our knowledge of this process has (to date) been relatively scant. Understanding the process of antibody secretion and transport may be critical for determining why some subjects retain healthy lungs, while others develop recurrent or persistent diseases related to inhaled antigens and infectious agents.

Mucosal immunity

Secretory antibodies provide a major defence, which protects the mucosal surfaces of the body against infectious microorganisms and environmental antigens present in ingested food and inhaled air. Polymeric immunoglobulin A (pIgA) is the predominant immunoglobulin isotype mediating this secretory immunity. The primary function of pIgA is believed to be to bind and induce aggregation and subsequent clearance of microorganisms from the mucosal surface thereby preventing their invasion. The polymeric nature of pIgA is essential to its function, as it results in an increased avidity for antigens and enhances its crosslinking properties. pIgA binds directly to foreign antigens, thereby neutralizing them and preventing their adhesion to mucosal surfaces, rather than binding complement effectively and promoting phagocytosis like some other immunoglobulins. Thus, pIgA plays a fundamental role in the primary immune response by facilitating the non-inflammatory clearance of foreign antigens from mucosal surfaces.

Dimeric IgA (dIgA) is synthesized by immunoglobulin-secreting

261

plasma cells which differentiate from potential pIgA-producing cells found at the mucosa-associated lymphoid tissues (for reviews see refs. 1 and 2). These cells are located predominantly in the submucosal lamina propria, where they secrete dIgA into the interstitial fluid adjacent to the basolateral surface of the mucosal epithelium (Fig. 14.1). dIgA consists of two individual IgA monomers joined by a small protein (J chain) resulting in a linked dimeric molecule. This assembly takes place within the plasma cell and the dimer is released preformed. For the dIgA to exert its role in the primary immune response, it must then be released into the antigen-containing milieu and thus must be trans-

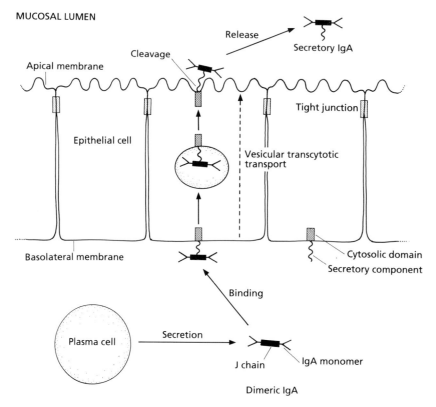

Fig. 14.1 Transfer of dIgA from submucosal lamina propria into epithelial lumen. dIgA is secreted by plasma cells and binds to pIgA-receptor (pIgA-R, a molecule composed of an extracellular portion, called the secretory component, and a transmembrane-cytoplasmic domain) on the basolateral membrane of epithelial cells. This ligand–receptor complex is internalized and transported across the cell via vesicular transport. After the dIgA–pIgA-R complex reaches the apical membrane, the pIgA-R is cleaved forming a secretory IgA molecule composed of the entire dIgA and the secretory component fragment of the pIgA-R.

ported from the site of synthesis within the lamina propria, through the layer of epithelial cells and into the mucosal lumen.

Direct measurements have indicated that pIgA is the major immunoglobulin isotype secreted into the mucosal lumen, even though IgG is the major immunoglobulin present on the basolateral surface of the epithelium [3], suggesting that a selective pathway exists which transports pIgA exclusively into the external secretions. (Direct transfer of molecules from the submucosa to the lumen is prevented by the presence of epithelial tight junctions which form a seal between the 'inside' and 'outside' of epithelia.) All epithelial cells lining mucosal surfaces throughout the body (e.g. the gastrointestinal and respiratory tracts, the ocular tissue, the salivary glands, the urinary tract, the uterus and the skin) exhibit a similar pathway of selective transport of pIgA into external secretions. In all these tissues, the majority of transported pIgA appears to be synthesized by local submucosal IgA-secreting plasma cells. However, a proportion of IgA produced at these sites is also released into blood and these molecules seem to be cleared from the systemic circulation by another epithelial organ, the liver.*

Comparison of pIgA found in external secretions with that produced by plasma cells revealed that the secretory IgA was associated with an additional polypeptide chain, termed the secretory component (SC), which seemed to be acquired during transport across the mucosal epithelium [7]. Subsequent work has conclusively shown that the specific transport of pIgA from the basolateral side of mucosal epithelium to its apical surface is mediated by a specific Fc-α receptor, the pIgA-receptor (pIgA-R) [8] and occurs via vesicular transcytotic transport. Part of this receptor is the SC polypeptide which remains with the dIgA after secretion into the epithelial fluid.

Polymeric IgA receptor

pIgA receptors from rat liver [9], rabbit liver and rabbit mammary gland [10] have been cloned and sequenced. The basic structure of the rabbit liver pIgA-R is shown in Fig. 14.2. The protein consists of 773 amino acids which can be divided into an 18 amino acid N-terminal signal peptide (which is removed shortly after translation giving a mature protein with 755 amino acids), a 629 amino acid extracellular domain (which is later cleaved to form the SC), a 23 amino acid transmembrane segment and a 103 amino acid cytoplasmic tail. The extracellular dIgA-binding domain consists of five (100−115 amino acids long) domains,

---

* The level of hepatic pIgA clearance is related to the level of expression of pIgA-R in hepatocytes and varies with species [4, 5]. Rats, rabbits and chickens synthesize high quantities of hepatic pIgA-R and transport substantial amounts of pIgA into bile. Humans synthesize very little hepatic pIgA-R and show limited biliary excretion of pIgA [6].

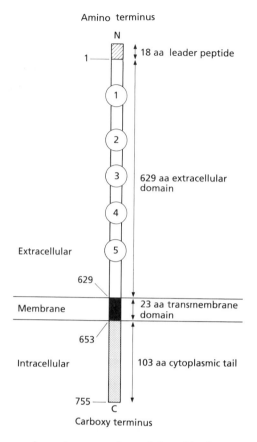

Fig. 14.2 Structure and membrane topology of the rabbit liver pIgA-R. The hatched region represents the leader peptide, the solid segment is the transmembrane domain and the shaded fragment is the cytoplasmic tail. Amino acid (aa) 629 is the last residue within the extracellular domain, while amino acid 653 is the first residue of the cytoplasmic tail. The circles denote the five immunoglobulin-like domains.

which are homologous with each other and with immunoglobulin variable regions [11]. The pIgA-R is clearly a member of the immunoglobulin gene family which includes, in addition to the immunoglobulins, other immunoglobulin-binding proteins such as the major histocompatibility antigens [12] and the T-cell receptor [13].

The rat and rabbit pIgA-R protein sequences show a low level of homology (36% identity) within the extracellular domains, but a significantly higher level (60% identity) in their cytoplasmic domain [9]. The higher level of homology in the cytoplasmic domain may be related to the conservation of specific signals required for correct delivery of the receptor to distinct cellular membranes. Although the extracellular domains are, on the whole, poorly conserved, the longest stretch of conserved amino acids (SVSITCYYP) is found within that domain, close to the N-terminus. It has been postulated that this region of the receptor might be involved in the non-covalent binding of IgA dimers. It has been shown previously by biochemical analyses that the first N-terminal immunoglobulin-like domain of the pIgA-R (see Fig. 14.2, loop 1) is crucial for the binding of dIgA [14, 15], while domains two and three may stabilize the interaction [16] but are not required for dIgA binding [17]. In addition, domain one can be disulphide bonded to the α-chain in one of the monomer subunits of the dIgA molecule [18]. The affinity binding constant of $\sim 5 \times 10^{10}$ M^{-1} for pIgA-R and dIgA indicates that binding is practically irreversible (at pH 5−8) and comparable in magnitude with that observed for antigen−antibody interactions.

Biosynthesis of the pIgA-R has been examined in a variety of epithelial or epithelial origin cells: e.g. a cell line derived from a human colon adenocarcinoma [19], rabbit mammary cells [20, 21], a cell line derived from the rabbit mammary gland [22] and rabbit and rat liver [23−25]; the entire pathway is shown diagrammatically in Fig. 14.3.

pIgA-R is synthesized on ribosomes bound to the endoplasmic reticulum (ER) membrane as a single-span, type 1 (i.e. amino terminus is extracellular while carboxy terminus is cytoplasmic) transmembrane protein. It is glycosylated at the time of translation by the addition of at least five oligosaccharide chains to its asparagine residues.* The receptor is transported from the ER to the Golgi complex (step 1, Fig. 14.3) presumably via small vesicles [27]. In the liver, the ER to Golgi transport occurs within approximately 15 min after synthesis; however, depending on the cell type, this interval can extend as long as 1−2 h [28]. During transit through the Golgi, the oligosaccharide chains are processed by trimming of mannose residues and then terminally glycosylated [29].

The terminally glycosylated protein is then transported to a specialized portion of the Golgi complex, the trans-Golgi network (TGN) [30] and sorted into basolateral membrane delivery vesicles (BMDV, step 2, Fig. 14.3). The vesicles then move from the Golgi region of the cell to the basolateral membrane (step 3, Fig. 14.3). The vesicles fuse with the basolateral membrane and the receptor is inserted into and rapidly distributes uniformly over the basolateral surface of the cell [31]. The receptor is now in contact with blood plasma and may bind circulating dIgA (step 4, Fig. 14.3), although even receptor which does not bind ligand is efficiently endocytosed and subsequently transcytosed. At this point, and also irrespective of ligand binding [23, 32], the pIgA-R undergoes phosphorylation, predominantly on serine and to a lesser extent on threonine residues [33]. Phosphorylation probably occurs at the basolateral membrane, in a similar way to other membrane receptors which autophosphorylate following ligand binding [34]. Nevertheless, the possi-

---

* Human receptor has five to seven N-linked chains [26] while rabbit pIgA-R contains two N-linked oligosaccharide chains [14].

† Clathrin-coated vesicles contain regular lattices made of the protein clathrin on their cytoplasmic surfaces.

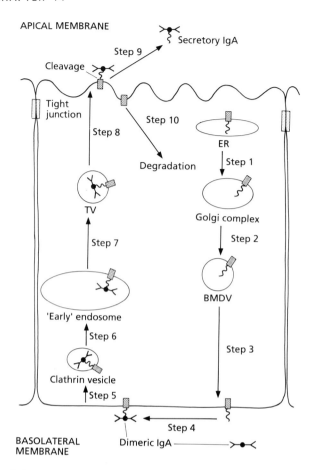

APICAL MEMBRANE

Secretory IgA

Step 9

Cleavage

Tight junction

Step 10

Step 8

ER

Step 1

Degradation

TV

Golgi complex

Step 7

Step 2

'Early' endosome

BMDV

Step 6

Clathrin vesicle

Step 3

Step 5

Step 4

BASOLATERAL
MEMBRANE

Dimeric IgA

Fig. 14.3 Cellular compartments traversed by pIgA-R. pIgA-R is synthesized as a transmembrane core glycosylated protein in the endoplasmic reticulum (ER) and transported (step 1) to the Golgi complex where it is terminally glycosylated. It is then sorted into specific transport vesicles (step 2) and transported (step 3) to the basolateral membrane where it is phosphorylated. The receptor can bind dIgA (step 4) and is endocytosed via clathrin-coated vesicles (step 5) and delivered to 'early' endosomes (step 6) where it is sorted into TVs (step 7). The vesicles translocate the receptor to the apical membrane (step 8). Following insertion into the apical membrane, the ectodomain of the pIgA-R is cleaved and secretory IgA is released (step 9) into lumenal secretion. The transmembrane–cytosolic tail fragment of the receptor enters a degradative pathway (step 10). The figure is not to scale.

bility exists that pIgA-R phosphorylation is a later, perhaps endosomal event, related to sorting into the transcytotic pathway. This latter view is consistent with the finding that a non-phosphorylated mutant of the pIgA-R (see below) is correctly endocytosed but not targeted into the transcytotic pathway.

The phosphorylated (and a small proportion of non-phosphorylated) receptor as well as the dIgA bound to the receptor are then internalized into clathrin-coated vesicles† and delivered to 'early' endosomes (step 6,

Fig. 14.3). After sorting within the 'early' endosome the receptor is incorporated into transcytotic vesicles (TVs; step 7, Fig. 14.3), which are translocated from the basolateral to the apical membrane where they fuse (step 8, Fig. 14.3) with the apical membrane, resulting in the insertion of the receptor (±dIgA) into the apical membrane. The inserted receptor is then cleaved within its exoplasmic domain by an apical membrane protease [35] to give an N-terminal soluble portion and a C-terminal transmembrane segment. The cleaved fragment without IgA (the SC) or the fragment with bound IgA (called secretory IgA molecule) is then released (step 9, Fig. 14.3) as a soluble protein into various secretions (e.g. bile, saliva, milk) while the fragment containing the trans-membrane segment and the cytosolic tail appears to be endocytosed and transported (step 10, Fig. 14.3) to lysosomes for degradation [36]. Based on the heterogeneity of amino acids found on the C-terminus of secreted pIgA-R fragments [37], it has been proposed that multiple proteases might be involved either in the original cleavage or in subsequent C-terminal processing, although their nature remains unknown.

Transcytotic pathway

Although IgA transport across the respiratory epithelium has not been studied directly, it is believed that the transcytotic pathway in the cells lining the respiratory tree is analogous to that seen in other epithelial cells, most notably, the hepatocyte in which the transepithelial transport of pIgA has been extensively analysed. In the rat liver, which transfers pIgA from blood to bile [8], the cellular pathway traversed by dIgA during transcytosis and the characterization of the compartment in which sorting of various internalized molecules occurs were studied morpho-logically [38−42]. As shown in Fig. 14.4, different circulating ligands, including dIgA, bind to their respective receptors exposed on the hepatic basolateral cell membrane and enter hepatocytes via clathrin-coated vesicles that form from the basolateral membrane. The endocytosed vesicles contain pIgA-R as well as other receptors such as the asialo-glycoprotein receptor (ASGP-R), the transferrin receptor (T-R) and the epidermal growth factor receptor (EGF-R). All proteins are delivered together to a shared 'early endosome' [43], a membrane-bound compart-ment consisting of vesicles and tubules, adjacent to the basolateral cell surface.* This compartment, also called CURL (Compartment of Uncoup-ling of Receptors and Ligands) is responsible for sorting the various endo-cytosed receptors into distinct pathways.

Three well-defined pathways originate from the 'early' endosome

---

* It must be mentioned that in polarized epithelial cells endocytosis occurs from both the basolateral and apical membrane and, therefore, two endosomal systems are present, one near each of the membrane domains [44]. In liver, pIgA is endocytosed exclusively from the basolateral surface.

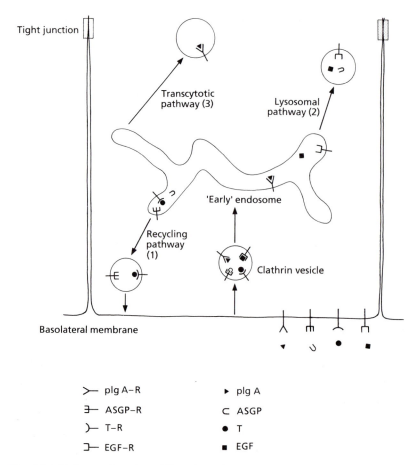

Tight junction

Transcytotic
pathway (3)

Lysosomal
pathway (2)

'Early' endosome

Recycling
pathway
(1)

Clathrin vesicle

Basolateral membrane

$\succ\!\!-$ plg A–R   ▶ plg A

$\exists\!-$ ASGP–R   C ASGP

$\succ\!\!-$ T–R   ● T

$\exists\!-$ EGF–R   ■ EGF

Fig. 14.4 Endosomal sorting of ligands and receptors. Ligands and receptors enter the cell by clathrin-coated vesicles and are delivered to an endosomal sorting compartment, the 'early' endosome. The acidic interior of this compartment may cause the dissociation of ligands from their cognate receptors. From this compartment some receptors (pathway 1) are recycled back to the same membrane (e.g. ASGP-R, T-R); some are delivered to lysosomes (pathway 2; e.g. EGF-R) and some are packaged into TVs (pathway 3; e.g. pIgA-R). The majority of dissociated ligands are transported to lysosomes (e.g. ASGP, EGF) while bound ligands can either recycle (e.g. transferrin) or transcytose (e.g. dIgA).

(Fig. 14.4). First, a recycling pathway which returns some proteins (e.g. T-R) to the basolateral membrane; second, a lysosomal pathway which transports some proteins (e.g. EGF-R) to late endosomes and eventually to lysosomes for degradation; and third, a transcytotic pathway which transports some proteins (e.g. pIgA-R) to the opposite cell membrane domain. Sorting of the pIgA-R from other proteins destined to be either recycled or degraded is thought to occur in tubular projections of the CURL, from which TVs seem to form [31]. Although the low pH of endosomes can cause the dissociation of ligands such as ASGP or EGF from their receptors and their consequent delivery to lysosomes, it does not induce the dissociation of pIgA from the pIgA-R and, consequently, both the receptor and the bound ligand are sorted into TVs.*

TVs are small (approximately 100 nm) and do not appear to be coated by either clathrin or other electron-dense material. Transcytosis of vesicles from the basolateral to the apical membrane occurs via a microtubule-dependent mechanism [32] since addition of microtubule disrupting agents (such as colchicine or nocadazole) to cells blocks vesicular movement towards the apical membrane and results in the accumulation of TVs near the basolateral membrane [45].

Sorting signals

Considering the complicated cellular pathway traversed by pIgA-R, it remains of great interest and importance to elucidate the molecular machinery responsible for this correct multistep targeting. Specifically, it is necessary to define the molecular interactions that take place during the transport of pIgA-R from the site of biosynthesis in the ER to the basolateral membrane and then, from the basolateral to the apical membrane. Two levels of sorting complexity need to be implicated in the overall transcytotic targeting process: sorting of the receptor into a correct vesicle (i.e. the packaging of pIgA-R into BMDVs or into TVs) and sorting of the vesicles leading to specific fusion with an appropriate target membrane (e.g. the fusion of TVs with the apical membrane).

It is believed currently that sorting of a specific protein into a particular cellular pathway is mediated by structural features (sorting signals) contained within the protein, which are recognized and acted upon by a complementary cellular sorting 'machinery' [46]. Sorting signals can be composed of relatively short, contiguous amino acid sequences such as leader peptides [47] or the endoplasmic reticulum retention signal [48], non-contiguous sequences which interact to form a specific three-dimensional structure, or specific post-translational modifications such as addition of mannose-6-phosphate residue to lysosomal enzymes targeted from TGN to lysosomes [49].

Sorting of vesicles is much less well understood but is generally believed to utilize a similar molecular mechanism based on the interaction between specific components present on the vesicular surface and their cognate 'receptors' present on the target membrane. The identity of such molecules is currently unknown.

The new techniques of molecular biology provide tools whereby the

---

* pIgA can also be transcytosed in liver by a 'receptor-switching' mechanism: when human pIgA, which contains exposed galactose residues, is injected intravenously into rats, it is removed from circulation by binding to the ASGP-R. Following endocytosis, pIgA dissociates from ASGP-R in the acidic environment of the endosome and binds to the pIgA-R, which transcytoses it across the hepatocyte [50].

identity of the sorting signals and the mechanisms of sorting processes can be elucidated.

Sorting of polymeric IgA receptor

To define sorting signals present within the pIgA-R and responsible for the correct targeting of the protein between distinct cellular compartments, a transfected cell culture system has been utilized in which molecular manipulations of the pIgA-R can be correlated with either normal or altered receptor sorting. Madin−Darby canine kidney (MDCK) cells can be cultured on permeable filter supports and form polarized monolayers that mimic the *in vivo* epithelial architecture (see Fig. 14.1) [51, 52]. The cellular membrane of cells growing on such filters is divided into two distinct domains: the basolateral, which rests on the support filter, and the apical domain. The monolayer forms tight junctions between polarized cells and is impermeable to macromolecules.

When the complementary DNA encoding rabbit liver pIgA-R is expressed in these cells, the synthesized receptor follows the same processing pathway as shown in Fig. 14.3. The exogenous receptor is synthesized in the ER as a core glycosylated precursor, transported through the Golgi complex (where it undergoes terminal glycosylation) and the TGN to the basolateral membrane, where it is phosphorylated, then endocytosed, specifically sorted into the transcytotic pathway and routed to the apical membrane where it is cleaved and released as a soluble fragment into the apical medium [53]. The receptor functions normally in MDCK cells, since when its ligand (dIgA) is added to the basolateral domain of transfected cells (the surface containing the pIgA-R), the ligand is endocytosed and the majority (60%) is subsequently transcytosed to the apical membrane while some (30%) recycles to the basolateral membrane and can be re-endocytosed and transcytosed. In contrast, ligand added to the apical surface of cells, while endocytosed, cannot be transcytosed [28, 54]. This cell system can therefore be used to define distinct sorting regions contained within the pIgA-R by manipulating the pIgA-R sequence expressed by the cells. In this chapter we will consider the sorting of pIgA-R during exit from the TGN, during formation of clathrin-coated vesicles and during formation of TVs (steps 2, 5 and 7 in Fig. 14.3).

It should be mentioned that prior to these sorting events, targeting of pIgA-R to the ER membrane occurs. This event is mediated by the association of the nascent pIgA-R leader peptide (18 amino acids long, see Fig. 14.2) with the signal recognition particle (SRP), which specifically targets the nascent chain for insertion into the ER membrane. During subsequent translation, the newly synthesized polypeptide is translocated through the ER membrane. Although leader peptides do not show extensive sequence homology [47], they all contain certain 'typical' structures such as one or more positively charged amino acids at the N-terminus followed by a continuous stretch of six to 12 uncharged, hydrophobic amino acids. The 18 amino acid leader peptide of rat pIgA-R shows the expected amino acid arrangement with a positively charged arginine at position −17 and an eight amino acid hydrophobic segment from −16 to −8 [9].

pIgA-R and other proteins destined for distinct (apical or basolateral) membrane domains are all inserted into the ER membrane and are not sorted during transport from the ER to the TGN [55], although some proteins are retained by specific sequences in the ER [48, 56] and in the Golgi complex [57].

Basolateral sorting

All newly synthesized proteins are delivered to the TGN and therein are sorted and packaged into distinct vesicular carriers, which deliver them to the appropriate (apical or basolateral) cell membrane domain. To define regions of the pIgA-R required for basolateral sorting, various mutants were constructed, expressed in MDCK cells and their sorting analysed. The nature of these mutants and their phenotypes are shown diagrammatically in Fig. 14.5.

The importance of the cytoplasmic tail in correct basolateral sorting is easily apparent; a mutant pIgA-R (654t pIgA-R; mutant A) lacking almost the entire 103 amino acid cytoplasmic tail, except for two membrane proximal amino acids (residues 653 and 654), was delivered from the TGN to the apical membrane [58]. Similarly, a mutant (anchor minus pIgA-R; mutant B) lacking both the cytoplasmic tail and the transmembrane anchor segment was secreted apically, indicating that the cytosolic domain of the receptor (residues 653−755) contains sorting signal(s) for basolateral targeting [59].

More recent work [60] has localized the basolateral sorting signal of the pIgA-R to a 14 amino acid (residues 654−669) region of the cytoplasmic tail proximal to the membrane-spanning segment. This region of the tail is sufficient for correct targeting since a mutant (669t pIgA-R; mutant C) containing residues 654−669 of the tail and lacking all other tail residues was still correctly sorted to the basolateral surface. Furthermore, removal of this region (Δ655−668 pIgA-R; mutant D) resulted in missorting of the pIgA-R from the TGN to the apical membrane.

The importance of this 14 amino acid region in targeting proteins to the basolateral membrane has been demonstrated further with the protein placental alkaline phosphatase. This protein normally sorts to the apical membrane of the cell [61]. However, when the protein was linked to the 14 amino acid sequence of pIgA-R, the alkaline phosphatase was sorted in the opposite direction to the basolateral membrane [60]. These data also suggest that basal sorting signals are dominant and can override signals for apical membrane targeting.

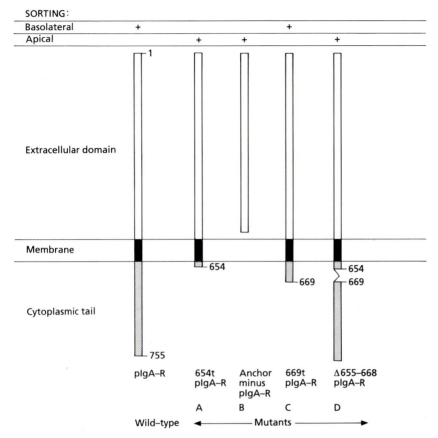

SORTING:

	Basolateral	Apical
	+	
		+ +
	+	+

Fig. 14.5 Basolateral sorting signals in the pIgA-R. The wild-type pIgA-R is shown on the left; the solid rectangle represents the transmembrane pIgA-R domain, with the extracellular sequences on top and the cytoplasmic tail on the bottom (not to scale). The wild-type pIgA-R is sorted from the TGN to the basolateral membrane. Various mutants of pIgA-R (A through D) were constructed and tested for sorting from the TGN to either the basolateral or the apical membrane.

The 14 amino acid segment shows no sequence homology to any protein sequence reported previously, suggesting that the cellular sorting machinery functions not by recognizing a particular primary amino acid sequence, but rather by acting upon a folded structure containing a specific motif. Although the exact structure recognized during sorting has not yet been defined, it should be noted that the 14 amino acid segment is highly conserved (11 of 14 residues are identical) between the rat, rabbit and human pIgA-R and that it contains a highly charged segment (residues 655−662) and a hydrophobic segment (residues 663−668). Whether this charge−hydrophobicity separation is required for correct sorting remains to be elucidated. Nevertheless, it is believed that the 14 amino acid segment either directly or indirectly prevents pIgA-R sorting into the apical membrane pathway, thus resulting in the entry of the receptor into a 'default' basolateral membrane pathway.

This 'basal membrane' sorting signal is not related to the signal required for correct endocytosis since 669t pIgA-R (mutant C), which is sorted basolaterally (correctly) from the TGN is not endocytosed, while Δ 655−668 pIgA-R (mutant D) which is sorted apically (incorrectly) is endocytosed normally.

The molecular and biochemical mechanism of TGN sorting and the molecules mediating recognition and selection are currently unknown.

Transcytotic sorting

pIgA-R has to be sorted from other proteins at two distinct stages of transcytosis: during the formation of the clathrin-coated vesicle prior to endocytosis and during the formation of TVs prior to transcytosis (see Fig. 14.3, steps 5 and 7).

Mutagenesis studies have shown that distinct portions of the cytosolic tail of pIgA-R are required for endocytosis and transcytosis [62, 63]. As shown in Fig. 14.6, deleting the C-terminal 30 amino acids of the pIgA-R tail (residues 726−755) generated a receptor (725t pIgA-R; mutant A) which was poorly endocytosed, presumably due to an impaired ability to be clustered into clathrin-coated vesicles. However, once endocytosed, the mutant was sorted into TVs correctly and transcytosed. A similar phenotype was exhibited by a mutant pIgA-R construct (ser 734 pIgA-R; mutant B) in which the highly conserved tyrosine 734 residue (positioned 21 amino acids from the C-terminus) was replaced by serine. Presumably this tyrosine forms part of the structural motif in which a β-turn is formed around correctly placed aromatic residues [64, 65] and which is required for endocytosis.

While the C-terminal 30 amino acids of the tail are involved in controlling endocytosis, the middle of the cytoplasmic tail appears to be required for correct sorting into the transcytotic pathway. Deletion of 38 amino acid residues (residues 670−707) within the middle of the tail (Δ 670−707 pIgA-R; mutant C) causes the receptor to be endocytosed correctly but targeted from the 'early' endosome to lysosomes (for degradation) instead of into the transcytotic pathway. The deleted region, therefore, either contains targeting sequences recognized actively by the sorting machinery, or alternatively, the deletion disrupts a sequence preventing sorting to lysosomes.

In addition to the 670−707 segment, distinct targeting information is provided by a serine residue at position 664 of the tail. As mentioned previously, the pIgA-R is phosphorylated predominantly on serine residues. Mutagenesis of serine 664 to alanine (an amino acid which is not a substrate for phosphorylation) produces a receptor (ala 664 pIgA-R; mutant D) which is endocytosed correctly but whose post-endocytotic sorting is affected. Instead of being transcytosed, the receptor continu-

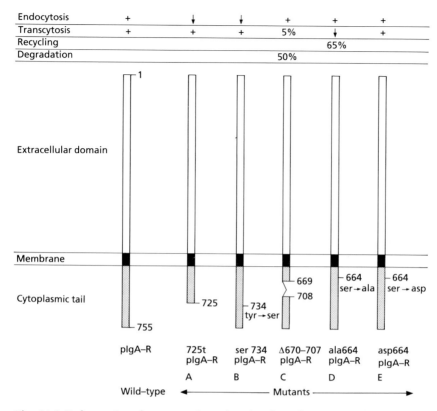

Fig. 14.6 Endocytosis and transcytosis sorting signals in the pIgA-R. The wild-type
pIgA-R is shown on the left; the solid rectangle represents the transmembrane
pIgA-R domain, with the extracellular sequences on top and the cytoplasmic tail on
the bottom (not to scale). The wild-type pIgA-R is endocytosed via clathrin-coated
vesicles and correctly sorted into transcytotic vesicles. Various mutants of pIgA-R (A
through E) were constructed and tested for correct endocytosis and transcytosis.
Mutants C and D showed a high level of missorting into the lysosomal or the
recycling pathway, respectively. Arrows indicate reduced level of endocytosis or
transcytosis as compared to wild-type pIgA-R.

ously recycles back to the basolateral membrane. It has been shown that
a negatively charged residue (not necessarily a serine) at position 664 is
required for correct transcytotic sorting by constructing a pIgA-R (asp
664 pIgA-R; mutant E) in which serine 664 was replaced by aspartic
acid, a residue which mimics the negative charge of a phosphorylated
serine. This results in a receptor that is efficiently endocytosed and
transcytosed. The negatively charged phosphorylated serine residue (or
its functional analogue, aspartic acid) is therefore required for correct
transcytotic sorting.

It should be pointed out that serine 664 is one of the 14 amino acid
residues required for basolateral sorting (residues 655−668; mutant D,
Fig. 14.5). However, the negative charge of phosphorylated serine 664 is
not used during basolateral sorting because ala 664 pIgA-R (mutant D in

Fig. 14.6) is sorted correctly to the basolateral membrane (i.e. presence of phosphorylated serine is not required), but is sorted incorrectly from the transcytotic pathway to the recycling pathway (i.e. presence of phosphorylated serine or an analogue is required).

These data suggest that distinct structural domains of pIgA-R cytoplasmic tail are recognized during sorting from the TGN or during sorting from the early endosome and, by inference, that different cellular sorting machinery is required at each stage.

Conclusions

pIgA-R functions to transport pIgA from the site of its synthesis within the submucosal layer underlying the epithelial tissue, across the epithelial cellular layer, to the epithelial lumen. The receptor is synthesized as a transmembrane protein and initially delivered from an internal Golgi compartment to the basolateral membrane. There it binds pIgA (Fc portion) and the complex is internalized and translocated across the cell in specialized vesicular carriers, the TVs. The structural features which control the passage of pIgA-R through the biosynthetic and transcytotic pathways have been defined (at least at the amino acid level), while the cellular machinery which acts upon these signals remains unknown. A study of this process will significantly add to our knowledge of general protein traffic phenomena and to our understanding of secretory immunity in particular.

References

1 Underdown BJ, Schiff JM. Immunoglobulin A: strategic defense initiative at the mucosal surface. *Annu Rev Immunol* 1986; 4: 389–417.

2 Mestecky J, McGhee JR. Immunoglobulin A (IgA): molecular and cellular interactions involved in IgA biosynthesis and immune response. *Adv Immunol* 1987; 40: 153–245.

3 Tomasi TB, Bienenstock J. Secretory immunoglobulins. *Adv Immunol* 1968; 9: 1–96.

4 Delacroix DL, Furtado-Barreira G, de Hemptinne B, Goodswaard J, Dive C, Vaerman JP. The liver in the IgA secretory immune system. Dogs, but not rats and rabbits, are suitable models for human studies. *Hepatology* 1983; 3: 980–8.

5 Delacroix DL, Furtado-Barreira G, Rahier J, Vaerman JP. Immunohistochemical localization of secretory component in the liver of guinea pigs, dogs versus rats, rabbits and mice. *Scand J Immunol* 1984; 19: 425–34.

6 Jonard PP, Rambaud JC, Dive C, Vaerman JP, Galian A, Delacroix DL. Secretion of immunoglobulins and plasma proteins from the jejunal mucosa. Transport rate and origin of polymeric IgA. *J Clin Invest* 1984; 74: 525–35.

7 Tomasi TB, Tan EM, Solomon A, Prendergast RA. Characteristics of an immune system common to certain external secretions. *J Exp Med* 1985; 121: 101–24.

8 Underdown BJ. In: Metzger H, ed. Transcytosis by the Receptor for Polymeric Immunoglobulin. *Fc Receptors and the Action of Antibodies*. American Society for Microbiology, Washington, D.C. 1990: 74–93.

9 Banting G, Brake B, Braghetta P, Luzio JP, Stanley KK. Intracellular targeting signals of polymeric immunoglobulin receptors are highly conserved between species. *FEBS Lett* 1989; 254: 177–83.

10 Mostov KE, Friedlander M, Blobel G. The receptor for transepithelial transport of IgA and IgM contains multiple immunoglobulin-like domains. *Nature* 1984; 308: 37–43.

11 Hunkapiller T, Hood L. Diversity of the immunoglobulin gene superfamily. *Adv Immunol* 1989; 44: 1–63.

12 Moller G. Molecular genetics of class I and II MHC antigens. *Immunol Rev* 1985; 84: 125–36.

13 Hedrick SM, Cohen D, Nielsen EA, Davis MM. Isolation of cDNA clones encoding T cell-specific membrane-associated proteins. *Nature* 1984; 308: 149–53.

14 Frutiger S, Hughes GJ, Hanley WC, Jaton JC. Rabbit secretory components of different allotypes vary in their carbohydrate content and their sites of N-linked glycosylation. *J Biol Chem* 1988; 263: 8120–5.

15 Beale D. Tryptic digestion of bovine secretory IgA at elevated temperature and in urea. Isolation of SC domain which is covalently bound to IgA dimer and binds non-covalently to IgM. *Int J Biochem* 1989; 21: 549–54.

16 Beale D. Cyanogen bromide cleavage of bovine secretory component and its tryptic fragments. *Int J Biochem* 1988; 20: 873–9.

17 Deitcher DL, Mostov KE. Alternate splicing of rabbit polymeric immunoglobulin receptor. *Mol Cell Biol* 1986; 6: 2712–15.

18 Underdown BJ, DeRose J, Plaut A. Disulfide bonding of secretory component to a single monomer subunit in human secretory IgA. *J Immunol* 1977; 118: 1816–21.

19 Mostov KE, Blobel G. A transmembrane precursor of secretory component. *J Biol Chem* 1982; 257: 11816–21.

20 Kuhn LC, Kraehenbuhl JP. The membrane receptor for polymeric immuno-globulins is structurally related to secretory component. Isolation and characteriz-ation of membrane secretory component from rabbit liver and mammary gland. *J Biol Chem* 1981; 256: 12490–5.

21 Solari R, Kraehenbuhl JP. Biosynthesis of the IgA antibody receptor: A model for the transepithelial sorting of a membrane glycoprotein. *Cell* 1984; 36: 61–71.

22 Schaerer E, Verrey F, Racine L, Tallichet C, Reinhardt M, Kraehenbuhl J-P. Polarized transport of the polymeric immunoglobulin receptor in transfected rabbit mammary epithelial cells. *J Cell Biol* 1990; 110: 987–98.

23 Musil LS, Baenziger JR. Intracellular transport and processing of secretory com-ponent in cultured rat hepatocytes. *Gastroenterology* 1987; 93: 1194–204.

24 Sztul ES, Howell KE, Palade GE. Biogenesis of the polymeric IgA receptor in rat hepatocytes. 1. Kinetic studies of its intracellular forms. *J Cell Biol* 1985; 100: 1248–54.

25 Sztul ES, Howell KE, Palade GE. Biogenesis of the polymeric IgA receptor in rat hepatocytes. II. Localization of its intracellular forms by cell fractionation studies. *J Cell Biol* 1985; 100: 1255–61.

26 Mizoguchi A, Mizoguchi T, Kobata A. Structure of the carbohydrate moieties of secretory component purified from human milk. *J Biol Chem* 1982; 257: 9612–21.

27 Wieland FT, Gleason ML, Serafini TA, Rothman FE. The rate of bulk flow from the endoplasmic reticulum to the cell surface. *Cell* 1987; 50: 289–300.

28 Mostov KE, Deitcher DL. Polymeric immunoglobulin receptor expressed in MDCK cells transcytoses IgA. *Cell* 1986; 46: 613–21.

29 Kornfeld R, Kornfeld S. Assembly of asparagine-linked oligosaccharides. *Annu Rev Biochem* 1985; 54: 631–64.

30 Griffiths G, Simons K. The trans Golgi network: sorting at the exit site of the Golgi complex. *Science* 1986; 234: 438−43.

31 Geuze HJ, Slot JW, Strous GJ *et al*. Intracellular receptor sorting during endocytosis: comparative immunoelectron microscopy of multiple receptors in rat liver. *Cell* 1984; 37: 195−204.

32 Mullock BM, Jones RS, Peppard J, Hinton RH. Effect of colchicine on the transfer of IgA across hepatocytes into bile in isolated perfused liver. *FEBS Lett* 1980; 120: 278−82.

33 Larkin JM, Sztul ES, Palade GE. Phosphorylation of the rat hepatic polymeric IgA receptor. *Proc Natl Acad Sci USA* 1986; 83: 4759−63.

34 Yarden Y, Ullrich A. Growth factor receptor tyrosine kinases. *Annu Rev Biochem* 1988; 57: 443−78.

35 Musil LS, Baenziger JR. Proteolytic processing of rat liver membrane secretory component cleavage activity is localized to bile canalicular membranes. *J Biol Chem* 1988; 263: 15799−808.

36 Solari RE, Schaerer E, Tallichet C, Braiterman LT, Hubbard AL, Kraehenbuhl JP. Cellular location of the cleavage event of the polymeric immunoglobulin receptor and fate of its anchoring domain in the rat hepatocyte. *Biochem J* 1989; 257: 759−68.

37 Eiffert H, Quentin E, Decker J *et al*. Die primarstruktur der menschlichen frien sekretkomponente und die anordnung der disulfidbrücken. *Physiol Chem* 1984; 364: 1489−95.

38 Orlans E, Peppard J, Fry JF, Hinton RH, Mullock BM. Secretory component as the receptor for polymeric IgA on hepatocytes. *J Exp Med* 1979; 50: 1557−81.

39 Schiff JM, Fisher MM, Underdown BJ. Receptor-mediated biliary transport of immunoglobulin A and asialoglycoprotein: sorting and missorting of ligands revealed by two radiolabeling methods. *J Cell Biol* 1984; 98: 79−89.

40 Jackson GDF, Lemaitre-Coelho I, Vaerman JP, Bazin H, Beckers A. Rapid disappearance from serum of intravenously injected rat myeloma IgA and its secretion into bile. *Eur J Immunol* 1978; 8: 123−6.

41 Hoppe CA, Connolly TP, Hubbard AL. Transcellular transport of polymeric IgA in the rat hepatocyte: biochemical and morphological characterization of the transport pathway. *J Cell Biol* 1985; 101: 2113−23.

42 Limet JN, Quinart J, Schneider Y, Courtoy PIJ. Receptor-mediated endocytosis of polymeric IgA and galactosylated serum albumin in rat liver. *Eur J Biochem* 1985; 146: 539−48.

43 Goldstein JL, Brown MSS, Anderson RW, Russell DW, Schneider WJ. Receptor-mediated endocytosis. *Annu Rev Cell Biol* 1985; 1: 1−40.

44 Parton RG, Prydz K, Bomsel M, Simons K, Griffiths G. Meeting of the apical and basolateral endocytic pathways of the Madin−Darby canine kidney cell in late endosomes. *J Cell Biol* 1989; 109: 3259−72.

45 Hunziker W, Male P, Mellman I. Differential microtubule requirements for transcytosis in MDCK cells. *EMBO J* 1990; 9: 3515−25.

46 Breitfeld P, Casanova JE, Harris JM, Simister NE, Mostov KE. Expression and analysis of the polymeric immunoglobulin receptor. *Methods Cell Biol* 1989; 32: 329−37.

47 Kaiser CA, Preuss D, Grisafi P, Botstein D. Many random sequences functionally replace the secretion signal sequence of yeast invertase. *Science* 1987; 235: 312−17.

48 Munro S, Pelham HRB. A C-terminal signal prevents secretion of luminal ER proteins. *Cell* 1987; 48: 899−907.

49 Kornfeld S, Mellman I. The biogenesis of lysosomes. *Annu Rev Cell Biol* 1989; 5: 483−526.

50 Schiff JM, Fisher M, Jones AL, Underdown BJ. Human IgA as a heterovalent ligand: switching from the asialoglycoprotein receptor to secretory component during transport across the rat hepatocyte. *J Cell Biol* 1986; 102: 920−31.

51 Simons K, Fuller SD. Cell surface polarity in epithelia. *Annu Rev Cell Biol* 1985; 1: 243−88.

52 Simons K, Wandinger-Ness A. Polarized sorting in epithelia. *Cell* 1990; 62: 207−10.

53 Casanova JE, Breitfeld PP, Ross SA, Mostov KE. Phosphorylation of the polymeric immunoglobulin receptor is required for its efficient transcytosis. *Science* 1990; 248: 742−5.

54 Breitfeld PP, Harris JM, Mostov KE. Post-endocytotic sorting of the ligand for the polymeric immunoglobulin receptor in Madin−Darby canine kidney cell. *J Cell Biol* 1989; 109: 475−86.

55 Rindler MJ, Ivanov IE, Plesken H, Rodriguez-Boulan E, Sabatini DD. Viral glyco-proteins destined for apical or basolateral plasma membrane domains traverse the same Golgi apparatus during their intracellular transport in Madin−Darby canine kidney cells. *J Cell Biol* 1984; 98: 1304−19.

56 Pelham HRB. Evidence that luminal ER proteins are sorted from secreted proteins in a post-ER compartment. *EMBO J* 1988; 7: 913−18.

57 Machamer CE, Rose J. A specific transmembrane domain of a coronavirus E1 glycoprotein is required for its retention in the Golgi region. *J Cell Biol* 1987; 105: 1205−14.

58 Mostov KE, De Bruyn Kops A, Deitcher DL. Deletion of the cytoplasmic domain of the polymeric immunoglobulin receptor prevents basolateral localization and endocytosis. *Cell* 1986; 47: 359−64.

59 Mostov KE, Breitfeld P, Harris JM. An anchor-minus form of the polymeric immunoglobulin receptor is secreted predominantly apically in Madin−Darby canine kidney cells. *J Cell Biol* 1987; 105: 2031−6.

60 Casanova JE, Apodaca G, Mostov KE. An autonomous signal for basolateral sorting in the cytoplasmic domain of the polymeric immunoglobulin receptor. *Cell* 1991; 66: 65−75.

61 Lisanti MP, Sargiacomo M, Graeve I, Saltiel AR, Rodriguez-Boulan ER. Polarized apical distribution of glycosyl-phosphatidylinositol-anchored proteins in a renal epithelial cell line. *Proc Natl Acad Sci USA* 1988; 85: 9557−61.

62 Breitfeld PP, Casanova JE, McKinnon WC, Mostov KE. Deletions in the cyto-plasmic domain of the polymeric immunoglobulin receptor differentially affect endocytic rate and postendocytic traffic. *J Biol Chem* 1990; 265: 13750−7.

63 Hunziker W, Mellman I. Expression of macrophage-lymphocyte Fc receptors in MDCK cells: polarity and transcytosis differ for isoforms with or without coated pit localization domains. *J Cell Biol* 1989; 109: 3291−302.

64 Lazarovitz J, Roth M. A single amino acid change in the cytoplasmic domain allows the influenza virus hemagglutinin to be endocytosed through coated pits. *Cell* 1988; 53: 743−52.

65 Collawn JF, Stangel M, Kuhn LA *et al.* Transferrin receptor internalization sequence YXRF implicates a tight turn as the structural recognition motif for endocytosis. *Cell* 1990; 63: 1061−72.

15 Heat shock proteins

LAN JORNOT AND ALAIN F. JUNOD

Introduction

The heat shock proteins (HSPs), more appropriately called stress proteins (SPs), are a very highly conserved group of proteins found in every organism in response to heat as well as to many other forms of stress: viral infection, irradiation, heavy metal ions, ethanol, oxidants, etc. [1−4].

This phenomenon was discovered in 1962 by Ritossa [5] who observed chromosomal puffing in *Drosophila* exposed to heat. Subsequently, molecular biologists were able to clone the gene for SPs and to isolate and purify the proteins synthesized following heat shock. For a long time, however, these proteins remained without a well-defined biological function. The only unquestionable fact was the association between the production of these proteins and the phenomenon of thermotolerance, with the following sequence: heat shock, inhibition of overall protein synthesis at the translational level (less marked in mammalian cells than in prokaryotes), activation of transcription of SP genes and selective translation of the related proteins, development of thermotolerance (resistance to a second thermal stress) and progressive return to basal conditions. In the past 10 years, however, there has been a rapid expansion of knowledge related to the roles of these various proteins under physiological as well as under experimental conditions.

The stress proteins

Because these proteins are generally recognized by autoradiography of a sodium dodecylsulphate (SDS)−polyacrylamide gel following incubation in the presence of a labelled amino acid (generally [^{35}S]methionine), the different SPs are labelled as a function of their molecular mass, hence the 28, 32, 47, 58, 70 (or 72 and 73), 90 and 110 kD SP or families of SP (Fig. 15.1). Isoforms of SPs of similar molecular mass can also be separated as a function of their isoelectric point by the use of two-dimensional gel electrophoresis (Fig. 15.2). There is also a group of so-called glucose-regulated proteins (GRPs), sensitive to glucose deprivation, with a wide range of molecular weights: 75, 80 and 100 kD.

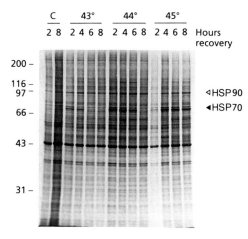

Fig. 15.1 One-dimensional gel analysis of the proteins synthesized in normal (C) and heat-shocked endothelial cells. Human umbilical vein endothelial cells on 60-mm plastic dishes were grown in RPMI 1640 containing 10% foetal calf serum, $30 \mu g \, ml^{-1}$ endothelial cell growth supplement and $10 \mu g \, ml^{-1}$ heparin. At confluence, the cells were incubated at either 43, 44 or 45°C for 30 min, and then returned to 37°C for 2, 4, 6 and 8 h. The cells were labelled with $[^{35}S]$methionine $(20 \mu Ci \, ml^{-1})$ for the last hour of recovery in methionine-free RPMI supplemented with 10% fetal calf serum. Fifty micrograms of radiolabelled proteins were analysed per lane on 10% SDS—polyacrylamide gel, and the proteins were visualized by autoradiography. Major SP at 90 (SP 90) and 70 (SP 70) kD are designated. SP 90 is only weakly induced; in contrast, a major induction of SP is seen at 70 kD. The positions of the molecular mass markers are indicated at the left of the figure (from top to bottom): myosin (200 kD), β-galactosidase (116 kD), phosphorylase B (97 kD), bovine serum albumin (66 kD), ovalbumin (42 kD), bovine carbonic anhydrase (31 kD). From Jornot L, Mirault ME, Junod AF, *Am J Respir Cell Mol Biol* 1991; 5: 265–75.

Finally, it is important to mention that bacteria, mycobacteria and parasites contain antigens structurally related to SPs, among which the 65 kD SP or GroEL and the 70 kD SP DnaK-related proteins are especially important in view of their relationship with the immune response in mammalians and humans in particular.

We shall examine only and succinctly the SPs found in mammalians. There are many reviews devoted to this topic [1–4, 6], and the reader can refer especially to the last review by Welch [6] for detailed references.

'Usual' stress proteins

Ubiquitins

Seventy-six amino acid proteins, first synthesized in response to heat as well as to the administration of amino acid analogues as a polymer called polyubiquitin and consisting of tandem repeats of the protein coding sequences. They can attach in an adenosine triphosphate (ATP)-

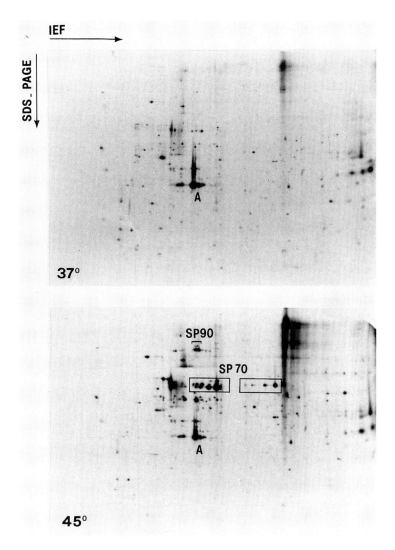

Fig. 15.2 Two-dimensional gel analysis of the proteins synthesized in normal (37°C) and heat-shocked (45°C) endothelial cells. Porcine aortic endothelial cells on 60-mm plastic dishes were grown in RPMI 1640 containing 10% foetal calf serum. At confluence, the cells were exposed to a 45°C heat shock for 30 min and allowed to recover at 37°C for 6 h. The cells were labelled with 50 μCi ml^{-1} of [^{35}S]methionine in methionine-free RPMI for the last hour of recovery. Following the labelling period, the cells were solubilized in two-dimensional gel electrophoresis sample buffer and the labelled proteins were analysed on pH 3–10 isoelectric focusing gels (IEF) followed by electrophoresis on 10% SDS–polyacrylamide gel. Autoradiographs of the gels are presented with the acidic end to the left. The different isoforms of the major SPs at 90 and 70 kD are shown. For reference, actin is indicated by 'A' (41 kD; pI 5.3). Cell lysates containing equal amounts of radioactivity were loaded.

dependent process to cytosolic proteins and mark them for further degradation. Their role in the transcription of the 72–73 kD SP has not yet been characterized with certainty.

The 28 kD SP

These low molecular weight phosphoproteins are made up of at least four major isoforms. They are found around the Golgi cisternae, but are relocalized within the nucleus upon heat exposure. They seem to be somewhat related to steroids since their amount increases in the presence of oestrogen or progesterone receptors.

The 32 kD SP

This SP is identical to haem oxygenase, an enzyme involved in the degradation of the haem moiety of haemoglobin. Its production is not heat-inducible, but related to the presence of heavy metals, iodoacetamide, ultraviolet light and H_2O_2 [7]. Glutathione depletion appears to be linked to its expression.

The 47 kD SP

This is a recently discovered basic SP, found so far in chicken fibroblasts. It appears to be a membrane glycoprotein that binds to collagen.

The 58 kD SP

This is present in mitochondria and may be important in the assembly of proteins produced in the cytoplasm and subsequently translocated into mitochondria. There is a strong homology between this SP and the GroEL protein of *Escherichia coli*.

The 72 and 73 kD SP (or HSP 70 and HSP 72 or HSP 70 family)

This is a heterogeneous group of both constitutively expressed (73 kD) and induced (72 kD) SPs; the 72 kD SP is made up of several isoforms, separated as a function of their charge by their isoelectric point. These two groups of proteins, although highly related, correspond to different genes. They appear, however, to serve similar functions, and it is customary therefore to refer to them as the 72–73 kD SPs or HSP 70 family.

Primate cells appear to differ from other mammalian cells in the sense that they synthesize both the 72 and 73 kD SPs under normal conditions. This constitutive expression of the 72 kD SP synthesis is related to the cell cycle (synthesis of 72 kD SP at the G_1/S level of the cell cycle); it is also increased following cell transformation, transfection with either of the two oncogenes, E1A or *myc*, or infection by viruses (adenovirus, polyomavirus, simian virus 40, etc.). In unstressed cells, the 72−73 kD SPs are capable, in the presence of ATP, of binding to the clathrin coat and removing the clathrin triskelions, thus facilitating the fusion of endocytotic vesicles with other cytoplasmic organelles.

They also play a role in the ATP-dependent protein translocation across intracellular membranes and in the protection of nascent incompletely folded proteins. In stressed cells, these SPs, once synthesized, localize in the nucleus, especially in the nucleolus; this coincides with the shutdown of the nucleolar function, i.e. RNA synthesis and ribosomal assembly. During recovery from stress, the SPs leave the nucleus and accumulate within the cytoplasm in association with the ribosomes. They are thought to bind to denatured or unfolded proteins in an ATP-dependent process and to facilitate the removal of these proteins.

The 90 kD SP

This is a constitutively expressed protein which, under stress, is massively synthesized and phosphorylated. It can be associated with the viral oncogene protein pp60^{src} and other oncogene proteins, with, as a consequence, loss of the tyrosine kinase function of this protein. This function is restored when the complex reaches the plasma membrane and is dissociated. It is also associated with the steroid receptor and can bind to the 8S/9S form of this receptor [8, 9]. Under these conditions, the 90 kD SP prevents the binding of the receptor to DNA and gene activation. In the presence of a steroid, however, the 90 kD SP dissociates from the complex and the steroid receptor can then exhibit its activity. The 90 kD SP also plays a role in the activation of the factor eIF-2-α for the initiation of protein synthesis in ribosomes.

The 110 kD SP

This constitutively expressed protein increases its synthesis fivefold following stress. It could play a role in messenger RNA (mRNA) formation and processing.

Glucose-regulated proteins

The GRP 75

Located in the mitochondria, it has a high affinity for ATP and exhibits an immunological cross-reactivity with antibodies raised against the 72−73 kD SPs. It serves a role in the assembly of proteins within the mitochondria.

The GRP 80 (or GRP 78 or BiP)

This is a constitutively expressed protein, present in the endoplasmic reticulum (ER). It has 50% homology with the 70 kD SP. In fact, it is identical to immunoglobulin (Ig) heavy chain-binding protein (BiP), a protein present in the lumen of ER and capable of binding with the heavy (H) and light (L) chains of maturing IgG. This function of mediation for the proper assembly of the H and L chains into their dimeric form has also been reported to occur for other proteins. They are considered therefore to function in an ATP-dependent fashion to stabilize and promote the correct oligomeric assembly of proteins migrating through the ER. They may also play a role in the recognition and removal of proteins secreted into the ER, but unable to move further [10, 11].

The GRP 100

This protein is homologous with the 90 kD SP and is localized in the ER and Golgi. It is thought to exert a regulatory action with other macromolecules in these sites.

Transcriptional and post-transcriptional regulation of SP synthesis

Transcriptional control

Heat shock element and its interaction with heat shock factor

The molecular signal(s) responsible for the pleiotropic triggering of heat shock response under diverse stress situations is presently unknown, but its main target seems to reside at the transcriptional level. In all the organisms examined, the induction of heat shock genes in response to a temperature upshift is mediated by the binding of a transcriptional activator, the heat shock factor (HSF), to a highly conserved short DNA sequence located within the promoter region and referred to as the heat shock element (HSE). The HSE was originally defined by the 14 base pairs (bp) inverted repeat consensus sequence, 5'-CnnGAAnnTTCnnG-3', where n denotes less strongly conserved nucleotides that nevertheless may be involved in important DNA−protein interactions [12, 13]. Subsequent analyses of numerous HSEs have more precisely defined the HSE as contiguous arrays of variable numbers of the 5 bp sequence nGAAn arranged in alternating orientations [14]. The presence of this element located about 80−150 bp upstream of the start site of RNA transcription is the most definitive evidence that the gene encodes an SP.

At least two nGAAn units are needed for high affinity binding of the HSF, and these may be arranged either head-to-head (nGAAnnTTCn) or tail-to-tail (nTTCnnGAAn) [15]. The fact that HSEs with different arrays of 5 bp units may be equally bound by an HSF is suggestive of an oligomeric nature of the HSF protein. It is currently believed that each subunit of an HSF multimer binds to a single nGAAn unit, and the binding to successive units is highly cooperative [16, 17]. It is not clear, however, whether HSF exists *in vivo* primarily as a trimeric, hexameric, or even larger complex.

Biochemical features of HSF

Different groups have reported the isolation, to apparent homogeneity, of different putative HSFs. Wiederrecht *et al.* [18] purified a 70 kD polypeptide from *Drosophila* and *Saccharomyces cerevisiae* which, after electrophoresis and renaturation, bound specifically to the HSE region in a pattern indistinguishable from that of the native protein. Also in yeast, Sorger and Pelham [19] have identified a 150 kD protein that gives rise upon mild digestion with papain to a 70 kD fragment, which retains DNA-binding activity. In humans, HSF has been isolated from HeLa cells and characterized as an 83 kD molecule [20]. More recently, Gallo *et al.* [21] have purified to near homogeneity by affinity chromatography the *Schizosaccharomyces pombe* HSF and have shown that this protein has an apparent molecular size of approximately 108 kD.

The gene encoding HSF was first isolated from *S. cerevisiae* (S-HSF) [22, 23]. It exists as a single-copy gene with no close homologue and is essential for viability of this organism at all temperatures. HSF genes have also been isolated from *Drosophila* (D-HSF) [24], the yeast *Kluyveromyces lactis* (K-HSF) [25] and recently from human cells (H-HSF) [26, 27]. Despite the strong phylogenetic conservation of the HSE sequence, HSF proteins from different species have only limited sequence similarity. For example, S-HSF and K-HSF share only 18 amino acid identity. The similarity is confined to the DNA-binding domain and to the region involved in trimerization.

Activation of HSF by heat shock and other stresses

Upon heat shock, a pre-existing pool of unactivated HSF is converted into an active form capable of efficiently stimulating transcription. In *Drosophila*, *S. pombe* and human cells, HSF binds to DNA only after heat shock [21]. Both H-HSF and S-HSF become highly phosphorylated following heat shock. In all organisms, a correlation between transcriptional activation and heat shock-dependent phosphorylation of HSF has been observed. Thus, it appears that activation of mammalian HSF by heat requires at least two distinct steps: first, the induction of DNA binding to create an HSF bound to heat shock promoters; second, the phosphorylation of HSF to create a complex with high transcriptional activity [28]. It is noteworthy that HSF prepared from unshocked HeLa cells can be induced to bind DNA *in vitro* by exposing cell extracts at elevated temperatures [28].

Besides heat treatment, other stresses including exposure of cells to heavy metal ions such as cadmium, amino acid analogues such as azetidine, oxidants such as H_2O_2 [29], a hypoxic atmosphere [30] or nitroso-urea antitumour drugs [31] have been shown to cause activation of HSF. Although the HSE-binding activity induced by these agents appears to be identical to HSF induced by heat shock, as determined by comparison of mobility in gel retention assays and sequence specificity of DNA binding, there is evidence suggesting multiple pathways for stress-induced activation of HSF. The most notable evidence follows from the time course of activation of HSF binding and SP 70 gene transcription after the onset of the stress conditions. The response is rapid during heat stress (<20 min) but occurs only after considerable delay following azetidine treatment (30−60 min) or during hypoxia (120 min). Additionally, while *de novo* synthesis of HSF is not required for transcriptional activation by heat and heavy metals, the activation of HSF by antitumoral agents is dependent upon *de novo* protein synthesis [32].

Unresolved issues

Two most important unresolved problems are: 1, the identification of the intracellular signals that activate HSF, leading to the pleiotropic transcriptional activation of SP genes; and 2, the determination of the mechanism by which HSF activates transcription. How does such a factor sense all these stress agents? Perturbations in protein conformation [33] or changes in the translational capacity of the cell [34] have been proposed as the triggering mechanism by which the response is activated. Evidence to support the first model has been provided from experiments using agents known to affect protein conformation, such as hydrogen ions, urea or non-ionic detergents [35]. On the other hand, activation of HSF *in vitro* was inhibited in a concentration-dependent manner by glycerol and ^2H_2O, two reagents widely used to stabilize protein structure.

The mechanism by which HSF activates transcription also remains obscure. Any of several steps required for RNA synthesis could potentially be a rate-limiting step, and, presumably, the active HSF−HSE complex acts catalytically to accelerate the rate of that step. In uninduced *Drosophila* cells, a molecule of RNA polymerase II is already present near the transcription start of the SP 70 promoter [36]. Moreover, this promoter-associated RNA polymerase II molecule is transcriptionally engaged with the formation of a nascent RNA chain of approximately 25 nucleotides, but is apparently arrested at that point and unable to penetrate further into the SP 70 gene without heat induction [37, 38]. This suggests that

HSF may act by accelerating the rate of RNA polymerase release from this arrested configuration. HSF may also have a catalytic role in the recruitment and initiation of additional RNA polymerase molecules.

Post-transcriptional regulation of SP synthesis

Along with the transcriptional regulation discussed above, several different mechanisms have evolved to ensure that the SPs will be produced as rapidly as possible after a shift to high temperature, and quickly become the major products of protein synthesis in the cell. Regulatory mechanisms acting at the levels of RNA processing, mRNA translation and degradation have been shown to exert a profound effect on SP gene expression during heat shock.

Effects of heat on RNA processing reactions

High temperatures have been shown to disrupt the splicing of intervening sequences from mRNA precursors in chickens [39] and mammals [40]. Although the precise nature of the heat-induced block in processing is unknown, it must occur early in the processing pathway since full-length intron-containing precursor RNAs accumulate with heat shock in *Drosophila* cells [41, 42], and in cell-free extracts of mammalian cells [43]. In *Xenopus* and human cells heat shock also results in the appearance of improperly terminated recombinant RNAs (rRNAs), because of either improper transcriptional termination or improper 3′ end processing [44, 45]. Finally, Bond [43], using extracts prepared from mammalian cells, showed that certain small ribonucleoprotein particles are altered at high temperatures and form aberrant splicing complexes. In this context, it is noteworthy that the human and mouse heat-inducible SP 70 genes do not contain intervening sequences, whereas closely related but constitutively expressed members of the SP 70 gene family in these organisms do [46].

Selective translation of heat shock messages

The preferential translation of SP mRNAs, concomitant with the repression of normal protein synthesis, during heat shock apparently results from: (1) specific recognition of SP mRNAs; and (2) inactivation or modification of a factor required for the translation of pre-existing mRNAs. From mutational analysis of heat shock genes and gene fusion experiments, it appears that a conserved sequence confined to the 5′ untranslated leader sequences of the SP mRNAs is required for heat shock translation [47, 48]. Although this conserved sequence is not yet precisely known, it is clear that messages will be translated during heat shock if, and only if, they possess this sequence. On the other hand,

Maroto and Sierra [49] have shown that, in lysates prepared from heat-shocked *Drosophila* embryos, translation of SP mRNAs is virtually unaffected by addition of cap analogues, as well as by addition of anti-bodies against cap-binding protein [50]. Taken together, these results permit a tentative model for regulation to be drawn: pre-existing mRNAs require cap-binding factor for efficient translation, possibly to unwind secondary structure in the message leader. Heat shock inactivates this factor. Since the 5' untranslated leader sequences of SP mRNAs are very rich in adenine (of the order of 45–49%), the message leader probably contains very little secondary structure. As a consequence, SP mRNAs are able to escape the requirement for cap-binding factor and are therefore translated.

Regulation of SP message degradation

Under normal temperatures, SP messages are extremely short-lived, and are much more stable after heat shock [51, 52]. Interestingly, the 3' untranslated region of the SP 70 message is AU-rich and contains sequence elements that resemble those implicated in the turnover of unstable messages in mammalian cells, such as c-*myc*, c-*fos* and various lymphokine mRNAs. Although the nucleotides responsible for destabilizing the SP 70 message have not been identified, it seems more than a coincidence that both the c-*myc* and c-*fos* messages are stabilized by heat shock in mammalian cells [53]. It appears that a highly conserved mechanism for the degradation of unstable messages is employed by SP mRNAs to reduce their constitutive levels of expression at normal temperatures, and that heat shock inactivates this mechanism, resulting in the remark-ably rapid and intense induction of SPs at high temperatures. The inacti-vation of this mechanism by heat shock, together with the transcriptional activation of the heat shock genes and the selective translation of SP mRNAs, allows the remarkably rapid and intense induction of SPs at high temperature.

SPs in respiratory medicine

Besides the well-established effects of SPs on thermotolerance (namely, resistance to a second heat exposure, a number of hours following an initial thermic stimulus) and the related properties of thermotolerant cells towards drugs, especially cytotoxic agents [54], there are a number of conditions where SPs can play a role in various ways, either as witness of an aggression or abnormal state or as potential causative agent.

SPs and the immune response [55−58]

Various relationships

A number of other different elements link the SPs to the immune response, in various ways. The main ones will be briefly summarized.

The role of SPs in the handling of proteins is somewhat similar to the processing of antigens. The observation that a binding protein to a peptide fragment containing the major epitope of pigeon cytochrome C reacted to a monoclonal antibody against 72−73 kD SPs, suggests a role of SPs in antigen processing [59, 60]. Peptide transport to the cell surface could also be one of the functions of some of the members of the SP 70 family (73 kD SP and GRP 78) and thereby they may participate in antigen presentation.

Together with the observation that increased SP levels have been found in certain tumour cells, there are reports that SPs, especially of the 90−100 kD family, could act as tumour antigens [61]. They may also be involved in the processing of other tumour antigens.

There are interesting relationships between cytokines and SPs. Thus, pretreatment with heat and the subsequent production of SPs offer some protection against the lytic effect of tumour necrosis factor (TNF)-α [62]. On the other hand, pretreatment with heat in combination with lipo-polysaccharides reduces the synthesis of the interleukin-1 (IL-1) β pre-cursor at the same time as the production of the 72−73 kD SPs is increased [63]. TNF-α administration is associated with an increased rate of phos-phorylation of SP 28 [64]. IL-2, when administered to T cells, causes an increase in 72−73 kD SPs, an effect shared by phytohaemagglutinin and the phorbol ester phorbol myristate acetate [65].

SPs as antigens of pathogens

SPs are major antigens of a large number of pathogens. It follows that these proteins become antigens that can participate in the immune response to these infectious agents [66−68]. Thus, antibodies against 72−73 kD SPs have been detected in patients infected by parasites (*Plasmodium, Leishmania, Schistosoma, Onchocerca treponema*, etc.) and by mycobacteria (*Mycobacterium leprae* and *M. tuberculosis*). Sixty-five kilodalton antigens, belonging to the 60 kD SP family and homologue of the GroEL proteins of *E. coli*, are found in *M. tuberculosis* and *M. leprae*, *Coxiella burnetii, Legionella pneumophila, Borrelia burgdorferi*, to quote only the main infectious agents. Interestingly enough, a member of the 60 kD SP family or GroEL, namely the 58 kD mitochondrial SP, which shows a strong amino acid homology with the mycobacterial 65 kD antigen, is also found in humans. *M. leprae* and *M. tuberculosis* also contain a 70 kD antigen, which was subsequently shown to belong to the SP 70 gene family.

T cells can be activated against the mycobacterial 65 kD antigen. In mice infected with *M. tuberculosis*, up to 20% of the T cells which respond to *M. tuberculosis* are specific for 65 kD SP. In fact, even in normal healthy subjects, T cells reactive to 65 kD SP have also been found, which suggests that the response to 65 kD SP can be directed against an epitope common to different infectious agents. It has even been considered that, in view of the wide occurrence of these antigens, the response to these SPs could be part of the general response or non-specific resistance against infection.

Because of the strong similarity between the 65 kD SP of *M. tuberculosis* and the human 60 kD SP, the experimental confirmation that T cells responded to epitopes shared by both human and mycobacterial 60−65 kD SPs was somewhat expected. Thus T cells of normal individuals can respond to self-epitopes of 65 kD SP. On the other hand, it appears that, in normals, self-epitopes of 65 kD SP are not present in a density high enough to activate T cells through the class II processing pathway, which can explain the tolerance to these self-antigens. The question as to whether these T cells could nevertheless become activated following infection remains open.

In another experiment, Koga *et al.* [69] demonstrated that murine T cells activated against mycobacterial 65 kD SP could lyse not only macrophages primed with this peptide, but also macrophages stressed by heat, viral infection or interferon-γ stimulation. It is therefore possible that T cells recognize epitopes shared by both mycobacteria and murine 65 kD SP. Furthermore, this result would also imply that the 65 kD SP synthesized under stress is processed and presented as antigens in the context of major histocompatibility complex (MHC) class I molecules.

It is obvious that all these experiments provide some substrate for the involvement of SPs in the development of autoimmune reactions, a topic which will be developed in the next section.

Sixty to sixty-five kilodalton SPs and autoimmune diseases

Sixty-five kilodalton mycobacterial antigen and rheumatoid arthritis [70, 71]. Monoclonal antibodies raised against mycobacterial 65 kD SP react with cellular elements of rheumatoid arthritis joints, especially synovial cells. Patients with rheumatoid arthritis also show high antibody titres to 65 kD SP. Finally, T cells obtained from synovial fluid have been shown to respond to mycobacterial 65 kD SP.

From an experimental point of view, rats having received Freund's adjuvant and a suspension of killed *M. tuberculosis* subsequently develop arthritis. T cells capable of recognizing the mycobacterial 65 kD SP antigen have also been shown to be arthritogenic under certain conditions.

Other autoimmune diseases. In other so-called autoimmune diseases, SPs have also been incriminated. Thus, peripheral blood monocytes in patients with systemic lupus erythematosus contain the 70 and 90 kD SPs, whereas antibodies against 70 and 90 kD SPs and ubiquitin are also detected in patients suffering from the same disease [72, 73]. Increased levels of mRNA encoding 70 kD SP are found in fibroblasts obtained from patients with scleroderma, whereas fibroblasts from controls show the same phenomenon only when serum activated [74]. A large fraction of patients with ankylosing spondylitis have antibodies against a 63 kD SP.

SPs and γ/δ T lymphocytes [75−78]

Gamma/delta T cells, a particular T-cell population characterized by the presence of a T-cell antigen receptor (TCR) made of γ- and δ-subunits (instead of the usual α/β-heterodimer receptor), have been recently shown to recognize mycobacterial antigens, whether under the form of purified protein derivatives (PPD) or purified recombinant *M. bovis* 65 kD SP. This observation is of interest because these T cells were not previously known to recognize well-defined ligands. Other authors have found that this T-cell population responds to *M. tuberculosis*, but not to its 65 kD antigen. Gamma/delta T cells usually comprise 1−5% of peripheral T cells, but appear to be concentrated in skin- and gut-associated lymphoid tissue. This property to recognize 65 kD SP as antigen is not restricted to γ/δ T cells, but is also shared by the α/β MHC class I-restricted T cells.

Recent experiments also reveal that γ/δ cells recognize autologous SPs, bringing one more line of evidence in favour of the role of SPs in the development of autoimmunity. In one patient out of 28 with polymyositis, inflammation appeared to be mediated by γ/δ T lymphocytes, whereas muscle fibres were highly reactive to 65 kD SP [79]. Finally, a subset of patients with sarcoidosis characterized by an expansion of the γ/δ T-cell population has been described [80]. Whether this finding is related to mycobacterial SP is not yet clear.

SPs and oxidant injury

The relationship between heat shock and oxidant injury or tolerance to oxidative stress has in general been of rather indirect nature. There are, however, several recent reports indicating that SPs can be synthesized as a consequence of exposure to oxidants.

Thus, Spitz *et al.* [81] have reported that a 70 kD SP was synthesized in Chinese hamster ovary cells following treatment with $0.1 \, \mathrm{mmol \, l^{-1}}$ H_2O_2. Pretreatment with H_2O_2 offered some protection against a new challenge with H_2O_2, but not against heat, whereas heat pretreatment, also associated with the production of SPs, was accompanied by tolerance to both heat and H_2O_2. Polla *et al.* [82] reported that H_2O_2 also induces SP production in human peripheral monocytes, but not in the U937 monocytoid cell line. We have found evidence of production of 70 kD SP in human umbilical vein endothelial cells (Fig. 15.3), together with the measurement of increased levels of mRNA for the 72 kD SP (Fig. 15.4) [83]. However, in comparison with the effect of heat, the action of H_2O_2 in the induction of SPs was much less intense, probably because of a much lower level of transcriptional activity (Fig. 15.5).

Interestingly, erythrophagocytosis by the U937 cells in the presence of vitamin D is also accompanied by the production of 32, 70 and 83–90 kD SPs, an effect prevented by a radioprotector capable of substituting for reduced glutathione [84]. It is noteworthy that the 32 kD SP or haem oxygenase is induced under the effect of H_2O_2 or, more generally, whenever cellular reduced glutathione levels are decreased.

Finally, expression of genes coding for SPs has been obtained from the liver of swine exposed to an ischaemia-reperfusion experimental model as well as from rat livers [85, 86].

Not all the stress conditions are associated with the expression of SPs. Neither hyperoxia [83] nor lipopolysaccharide administration [87] is followed by evidence of activation of genes coding for the 70 kD SP. On the other hand, bleomycin, a cytotoxic agent whose mode of action is also thought to be mediated by reactive oxygen intermediates, induces the 70 kD SP promoter in fibroblasts [88].

Miscellaneous conditions

SPs have been recognized in other conditions that can be encountered in respiratory medicine or physiology. Thus, rat cardiac myocytes, whenever exposed to an increased load, respond by the production of various SPs [89]. Aortic smooth muscle cells of hypertensive rats also induced the 70, 90 and 110 kD SPs at the transcriptional level [90]. Cells from various organs of exercising rats demonstrate enhanced synthesis of 65, 72 and 100 kD SPs [91]. Increased temperature as well as relative glucose deprivation or changes in intracellular Ca^{2+} could account for this phenomenon.

Finally, in some patients with the homozygous forms of α_1-antitrypsin deficiency and liver disease [92], evidence has been obtained for an increased production of the 70 and 90 kD SPs as well as of ubiquitin. Whether this response is causally related to the presence of abnormal α_1-antitrypsin is not yet known.

Conclusions

From the accidental discovery of chromosomal puffing of *Drosophila* to the most recent studies on SPs in autoimmune diseases, much progress

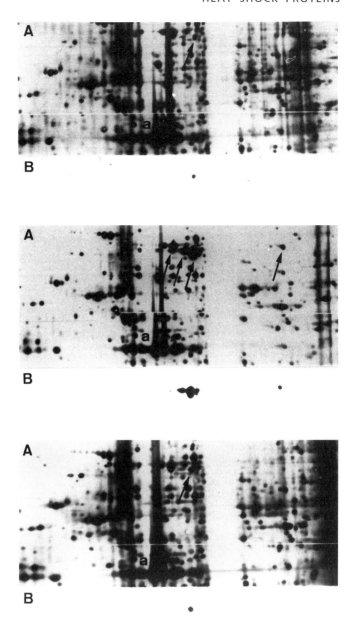

Fig. 15.3 Two-dimensional gel comparison of 70 kD SP (HSP 70) isoforms synthesized in heat-shocked and H_2O_2-treated cells and immunoblot analysis. Human umbilical vein endothelial cells were exposed to a 45°C heat shock for 30 min or $5 \, \text{mmol} \, l^{-1}$ for 20 min, and allowed to recover at 37°C for 8 h. The cells were labelled with $50 \, \mu\text{Ci} \, \text{ml}^{-1}$ of $[^{35}S]$methionine in methionine-free RPMI for the last hour of recovery. Cell lysates containing equal amounts of radioactivity were subjected to two-dimensional gel electrophoresis and immunoblot analysis. Shown are the autoradiographs of the regions of interest with the acidic end to the left (A panels) and the corresponding immunoblots (B panels) of control cells, heat-shocked and H_2O_2-treated cells. The arrows indicate the different isoforms of the 70 kD SP. For reference, actin is indicated by the letter 'a' (41 kD; pI 5.3).

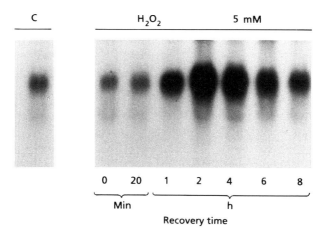

Fig. 15.4 Seventy kilodaltons SP (HSP 70) mRNA levels in normal (C) and H_2O_2-treated human endothelial cells. Human umbilical vein endothelial cells were treated with $5\,\mathrm{mmol\,l^{-1}}$ H_2O_2 for 20 min then allowed to recover at 37°C for 20 min, 1, 2, 4, 6 and 8 h. For each time point, 5 µg of total RNA was analysed by Northern hybridization. Shown is an autoradiograph of a typical RNA blot.

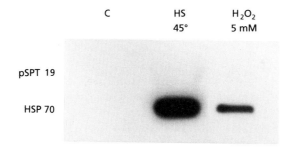

Fig. 15.5 Nuclear run-off transcription of the 70 kD SP (HSP 70) gene in human endothelial cells. Human umbilical vein endothelial cells were heated at 45°C for 30 min or exposed to $5\,\mathrm{mmol\,l^{-1}}$ H_2O_2 for 20 min, and allowed to recover for 1 h at 37°C. Nuclei were isolated from control (C) and treated cells by Triton-X100 lysis and nuclear transcripts were labelled with [α ^{32}P]uridine triphosphate and extracted. Aliquots of the RNA samples containing an identical amount of radioactivity were used for hybridization to an excess of 70 kD SP (HSP 70) DNA and, as control, plasmid pSPT 19 bound to Biodyne membrane. The relative abundance of the newly transcribed RNA of 70 kD SP (HSP 70) was about five times lower in H_2O_2-treated cells compared with heat-shocked cells.

has been accomplished. From a physiological point of view, SPs appear to play an important role in the recognition, assembly and transport of proteins and in the chaperoning of incompletely folded proteins. From a pathological viewpoint, the elicitation of increased productive SPs can be taken as the expression of exposure to stress, whatever its nature. Whether the production of SPs has a protective role in all the conditions studied is not yet determined. Finally, this chapter on the complex relationship between microbial and parasitic SPs or antigens, autologous

SPs and the immune response opens new ways of thinking on the pathogenesis of autoimmune disease.

References

1 Burdon RH. Heat shock and the heat shock proteins. *Biochem J* 1986; 240: 313−24.
2 Subjeck JR, Shyy TT. Stress protein systems of mammalian cells. *Am J Physiol* 1986; 250: C1−17.
3 Lindquist S, Craig EA. The heat-shock proteins. *Annu Rev Genet* 1988; 22: 631−77.
4 Morimoto RI, Tissières A, Georgopoulos C. The stress response, function of the proteins, and perspectives. In: Morimoto RI, Tissières A, Georgopoulos C, eds. *Stress Proteins in Biology and Medicine*. New York: Cold Spring Harbor Laboratory Press, 1990: 1−36.
5 Ritossa FM. A new puffing pattern induced by a temperature shock and DNP in *Drosophila*. *Experientia* 1962; 18: 571−3.
6 Welch WJ. The mammalian stress response: cell physiology and biochemistry of stress proteins. In: Morimoto RI, Tissières A, Georgopoulos C, eds. *Stress Proteins in Biology and Medicine*. New York: Cold Spring Harbor Laboratory Press, 1990: 223−78.
7 Keyse SM, Tyrrell RM. Heme oxygenase is the major 32-kDa stress protein induced in human skin fibroblasts by UVA radiation, hydrogen peroxide, and sodium arsenite. *Proc Natl Acad Sci USA* 1989; 86: 99−103.
8 Howard KJ, Holley SJ, Yamamoto KR, Distelhorst CW. Mapping the HSP90 binding region of the glucocorticoid receptor. *J Biol Chem* 1990; 265: 11928−35.
9 Picard D, Khursheed B, Garabedian MJ, Fortin MG, Lindquist S, Yamamoto KR. Reduced levels of hsp90 compromise steroid receptor action *in vivo*. *Nature* 1990; 348: 166−8.
10 Munro S, Pelham HR. An hsp70-like protein in the ER: identity with the 78 kd glucose-regulated protein and immunoglobulin heavy chain binding protein. *Cell* 1986; 46: 291−300.
11 Pelham HRB. Functions of the hsp70 protein family: an overview. In: Morimoto RI, Tissières A, Georgopoulos C, eds. *Stress Proteins in Biology and Medicine*. New York: Cold Spring Harbor Laboratory Press, 1990: 287−99.
12 Pelham HRB. A regulatory upstream promoter element in the *Drosophila* hsp70 heat-shock gene. *Cell* 1982; 30: 517−28.
13 Pelham HRB. Activation of heat shock genes in eukaryotes. *Trends Genet* 1985; 1: 31−5.
14 Amin J, Ananthan J, Voellmy R. Key features of heat shock regulatory elements. *Mol Cell Biol* 1988; 8: 3761−9.
15 Perisic O. Stable binding of *Drosophila* heat shock factor to head-to-head and tail-to-tail repeats of a conserved 5 bp recognition unit. *Cell* 1989; 59: 797−806.
16 Topol J, Ruden DM, Parker CS. Sequences required for *in vitro* transcriptional activation of a *Drosophila* hsp 70 gene. *Cell* 1985; 42: 527−37.
17 Xiao H, Perisic O, Lis JTT. Cooperative binding of *Drosophila* heat shock factor to arrays of a conserved 5 bp unit. *Cell* 1991; 64: 585−93.
18 Wiederrecht G, Shuey DJ, Kibbe WA, Parker CS. The *Saccharomyces* and *Drosophila* heat shock transcription factors are identical in size and DNA binding properties. *Cell* 1987; 48: 507−15.
19 Sorger PK, Pelham HRB. Purification and characterization of a heat-shock element binding protein from yeast. *EMBO J* 1987; 6: 3035−41.

20 Goldenberg CJ, Luo Y, Fenna M, Baler R, Weinmann R, Voellmy R. Purified human factor activates heat shock promoter in a HeLa cell-free transcription system. *J Biol Chem* 1988; 263: 19734−9.

21 Gallo GJ, Schuetz TJ, Kingston RE. Regulation of heat shock factor in *Schizosaccharomyces pombe* more closely resembles regulation in mammals than in *Saccharomyces cerevisiae*. *Mol Cell Biol* 1991; 11: 281−8.

22 Sorger PK, Pelham HRB. Yeast heat shock factor is an essential DNA-binding protein that exhibits temperature-dependent phosphorylation. *Cell* 1988; 54: 855−64.

23 Wiederrecht G, Seto D, Parker CS. Isolation of the gene encoding the *S. cerevisiae* heat shock transcription factor. *Cell* 1988; 54: 841−53.

24 Clos J, Westwood JT, Becker PB, Wilson S, Lambert K, Wu C. Molecular cloning and expression of a hexameric *Drosophila* heat shock factor subject to negative regulation. *Cell* 1990; 63: 1085−97.

25 Jakobsen BK, Pelham HRB. A conserved heptapeptide restrains the activity of the yeast heat shock transcription factor. *EMBO J* 1991; 10: 369−75.

26 Rabindran SK, Giorgi G, Clos J, Wu C. Molecular cloning and expression of a human heat shock factor, HSF 1. *Proc Natl Acad Sci USA* 1991; 88: 6906−10.

27 Schuetz TJ, Gallo GJ, Sheldon L, Tempst P, Kingston RE. Isolation of a cDNA for HSF2: evidence for two heat shock factor genes in humans. *Proc Natl Acad Sci USA* 1991; 88: 6911−15.

28 Larson JS, Schuetz TJ, Kingston RE. Activation *in vitro* of sequence-specific DNA binding by a human regulatory factor. *Nature* 1988; 335: 372−5.

29 Becker J, Mezger V, Courgeon AM, Best-Belpomme M. Hydrogen peroxide activates immediate binding of a *Drosophila* factor to DNA heat-shock regulatory element *in vivo* and *in vitro*. *Eur J Biochem* 1990; 189: 553−8.

30 Benjamin IJ, Kröger B, Williams RS. Activation of the heat shock transcription factor by hypoxia in mammalian cells. *Proc Natl Acad Sci USA* 1990; 87: 6263−7.

31 Kroes RA, Abravaya K, Seidenfeld J, Morimoto RI. Selective activation of human heat shock gene transcription by nitrosourea antitumor drugs mediated by isocyanate-induced damage and activation of heat shock transcription factor. *Proc Natl Acad Sci USA* 1991; 88: 4825−9.

32 Mosser DD, Theodorakis NG, Morimoto RI. Coordinate changes in heat shock element-binding activity and HSP70 gene transcription rates in human cells. *Mol Cell Biol* 1988; 8: 4736−44.

33 Ananthan J, Goldberg AL, Voellmy R. Abnormal proteins serve as eukaryotic stress signals and trigger the activation of heat shock genes. *Science* 1986; 232: 522−4.

34 VanBogelen RA, Neidhardt FC. Ribosomes as sensors of heat and cold shock in *Escherichia coli*. *Proc Natl Acad Sci USA* 1990; 87: 5589−93.

35 Mosser DD, Kotzbauer PT, Sarge KD, Morimoto RI. *In vitro* activation of heat shock transcription factor DNA-binding by calcium and biochemical conditions that affect protein conformation. *Proc Natl Acad Sci USA* 1990; 87: 3748−52.

36 Gilmour DS, Lis JT. RNA polymerase II interacts with the promoter region of the noninduced HSP 70 gene in *Drosophila melanogaster* cells. *Mol Cell Biol* 1986; 6: 3984−9.

37 Rougvie AE, Lis JT. The RNA polymerase II molecule at the 5′ end of the uninduced hsp70 gene of *D. melanogaster* is transcriptionally engaged. *Cell* 1988; 54: 795−804.

38 Rougvie AE, Lis JT. Postinitiation transcriptional control in *Drosophila melanogaster*. *Mol Cell Biol* 1990; 10: 6041−5.

39 Bond U, Schlesinger MJ. The chicken ubiquitin gene contains a heat shock promoter and expresses an unstable mRNA in heat shocked cells. *Mol Cell Biol*

1986; 12: 4602−10.

40 Kay RJ, Russnak RH, Jones D, Mathias C, Candido EPM. Expression of intron-containing *C. elegans* heat shock genes in mouse cells demonstrates divergence of 3′ splice site recognition sequences between nematodes and vertebrates, and an inhibitory effect of heat shock on the mammalian splicing apparatus. *Nucleic Acids Res* 1987; 15: 3723−41.

41 Yost HJ, Lindquist S. RNA splicing is interrupted by heat shock and is rescued by heat shock protein synthesis. *Cell* 1986; 45: 185−93.

42 Yost HJ, Lindquist S. Translation of unspliced transcripts after heat shock. *Science* 1988; 242: 1544−8.

43 Bond U. Heat shock but not other stress inducers leads to the disruption of a subset of snRNPs and inhibition of *in vitro* splicing in HeLa cells. *EMBO J* 1988; 7: 3509−18.

44 Labhart P, Reeder RH. Heat shock stabilizes highly unstable transcripts of the *Xenopus* ribosomal gene spacer. *Proc Natl Acad Sci USA* 1987; 84: 56−60.

45 Parker KA, Bond U. Analysis of pre-rRNAs in heat-shocked HeLa cells allows identification of the upstream termination site of human polymerase I transcription. *Mol Cell Biol* 1989; 9: 2500−12.

46 Dworniczak B, Mirault ME. Structure and expression of a human gene coding for a 71 kd heat shock 'cognate' protein. *Nucleic Acids Res* 1987; 15: 5181−97.

47 McGarry TJ, Lindquist S. The preferential translation of *Drosophila* hsp70 mRNA requires sequences in the untranslated leader. *Cell* 1985; 42: 903−11.

48 Klemenz R, Hultmark D, Gehring WJ. Selective translation of heat shock mRNA in *Drosophila melanogaster* depends on sequence information in the leader. *EMBO J* 1985; 4: 2053−60.

49 Maroto FG, Sierra JM. Translational control in heat-shocked *Drosophila* embryos. *J Biol Chem* 1988; 263: 15720−5.

50 Zapata JM, Maroto FG, Sierra JM. Inactivation of mRNA cap-binding protein complex in *Drosophila melanogaster* embryos under heat shock. *J Biol Chem* 1991; 266: 16007−14.

51 Theodorakis NG, Morimoto RI. Posttranscriptional regulation of HSP70 expression in human cells: effects of heat shock, inhibition of protein synthesis, and adenovirus infection on translation and mRNA stability. *Mol Cell Biol* 1987; 7: 4357−68.

52 Petersen RB, Lindquist S. Regulation of HSP70 synthesis by messenger RNA degradation. *Cell Regul* 1989; 1: 135−49.

53 Sadis S, Hickey E, Weber LA. Effect of heat shock on RNA metabolism in HeLa cells. *J Cell Physiol* 1988; 135: 377−86.

54 Hahn GM, Li GC. Thermotolerance, thermoresistance, and thermosensitization. In: Morimoto RI, Tissières A, Georgopoulos C, eds. *Stress Proteins in Biology and Medicine*. New York: Cold Spring Harbor Laboratory Press, 1990: 79−100.

55 Young RA, Elliott TJ. Stress proteins, infection, and immune surveillance. *Cell* 1989; 59: 5−8.

56 Kaufmann SHE. Heat shock proteins and the immune response. *Immunol Today* 1990; 11: 129−36.

57 Young RA. Stress proteins and immunology. *Annu Rev Immunol* 1990; 8: 401−20.

58 Young DB, Mehlert A, Smith DF. Stress proteins and infectious diseases. In: Morimoto RI, Tissières A, Georgopoulos C, eds. *Stress Proteins in Biology and Medicine*. New York: Cold Spring Harbor Laboratory Press, 1990: 131−65.

59 Lakey EK, Margoliash E, Pierce SK. Identification of a peptide binding protein that plays a role in antigen presentation. *Proc Natl Acad Sci USA* 1987; 84: 1659−63.

60 VanBuskirk A, Crump BL, Margoliash E, Pierce SK. A peptide binding protein having a role in antigen presentation is a member of the hsp70 heat shock family.

J Exp Med 1989; 170: 1799—809.

61 Ullrich SJ, Robinson EA, Law LW, Willingham M, Appella E. A mouse tumor-specific transplantation antigen is a heat shock related protein. *Proc Natl Acad Sci USA* 1986; 83: 3121—5.

62 Jäättalä M, Saksela K, Saksela E. Heat shock protects WEH1-164 target cells from the cytolysis by tumor necrosis factor alpha and beta. *Eur J Immunol* 1989; 19: 1413—17.

63 Schmidt JA, Abdulla E. Down-regulation of IL-1beta biosynthesis by inducers of the heat-shock response. *J Immunol* 1988; 141: 2027—34.

64 Arrigo APT. Tumor necrosis factor induces the rapid phosphorylation of the mammalian heat shock protein hsp28. *Mol Cell Biol* 1990; 10: 1276—80.

65 Ferris DK, Harel-Bellan A, Morimoto RI, Welch WJ, Farrar WL. Mitogen and lymphokine stimulation of heat shock proteins in T-lymphocytes. *Proc Natl Acad Sci USA* 1988; 85: 3850—4.

66 Kaufmann SHE, Schoel B, Wand-Württenberger A, Steinhoff U, Munk ME, Koga T. T-cells, stress proteins, and pathogenesis of mycobacterial infections. *Curr Top Microbiol Immunol* 1990; 155: 125—41.

67 Ottenhoff THM, Kaleab B, VanEmbden JAD, Thole JER, Kiessling R. The recombinant 65-kd heat shock protein of *Mycobacterium bovis* bacillus Calmette-Guerin/M. tuberculosis is a target molecule for CD4+ cytotoxic T lymphocytes that lyse human monocytes. *J Exp Med* 1988; 168: 1947—52.

68 Munk ME, Shinnick TM, Kaufmann SHE. Epitopes of the mycobacterial heat shock protein 65 for human T cells comprise different structures. *Immunobiology* 1990; 180: 272—7.

69 Koga T, Wand-Württenberger A, DeBruyn J, Munk ME, Schoel B, Kaufmann SHE. T cells against a bacterial heat shock protein recognize stressed macrophages. *Science* 1989; 245: 1112—15.

70 Winrow VR, McLean L, Morris CJ, Blake DR. The heat shock protein response and its role in inflammatory disease. *Ann Rheum Dis* 1990; 49: 128—32.

71 Gaston JSH, Life PF, Jenner PJ, Colston MJ, Bacon PA. Recognition of a mycobacteria-specific epitope in the 65-kD heat-shock protein by synovial fluid-derived T cell clones. *J Exp Med* 1990; 171: 831—41.

72 Deguchi Y, Negoro S, Kishimoto S. Heat-shock protein synthesis by human peripheral mononuclear cells from SLE patients. *Biochem Biophys Res Commun* 1987; 148: 1063—8.

73 Minota S, Cameron B, Welch WJ, Winfield JB. Autoantibodies to the constitutive 73-kD member of the hsp70 family of heat shock proteins in systemic lupus erythematosus. *J Exp Med* 1988; 168: 1475—80.

74 Deguchi Y, Shibata N, Kishimoto S. Elevated transcription of heat shock protein gene in scleroderma fibroblasts. *Clin Exp Immunol* 1990; 81: 97—100.

75 Born W, Happ MP, Dallas A *et al.* Recognition of heat shock proteins and gamma delta cell function. *Immunol Today* 1990; 11: 40—3.

76 O'Brien R, Happ MP, Dallas A, Palmer E, Kubo R, Born WK. Stimulation of a major subset of lymphocytes expressing T cell receptor gamma delta by an antigen derived from *Mycobacterium tuberculosis*. *Cell* 1975; 667: 674.

77 Haregewoin A, Soman G, Hom RC, Finberg RW. Human gamma delta+ T cells respond to mycobacterial heat-shock protein. *Nature* 1989; 340: 309—12.

78 Kabelitz D, Bender A, Schondelmaier S, Schoel B, Kaufmann SHE. A large fraction of human peripheral blood gamma/delta+ T cells is activated by *Mycobacterium tuberculosis* but not by its 65-kD heat shock protein. *J Exp Med* 1990; 171: 667—79.

79 Hohlfeld R, Engel A, Ii K, Harper MC. Polymyositis mediated by T lymphocytes that express the gamma/delta receptor. *N Engl J Med* 1991; 324: 877—81.

80 Balbi B, Moller DR, Kirby M, Holroyd KJ, Crystal RG. Increased numbers of T

lymphocytes with gammadelta-positive antigen receptors in a subgroup of individuals with pulmonary sarcoidosis. *J Clin Invest* 1990; 85: 1353−61.

81 Spitz DR, Dewey WC, Li GC. Hydrogen peroxide or heat shock induces resistance to hydrogen peroxide in Chinese hamster fibroblasts. *J Cell Physiol* 1987; 131: 364−73.

82 Polla BS, Healy AM, Wojno WC, Krane SM. Hormone 1alpha, 25-dihydroxyvitamin D₃ modulates heat shock response in monocytes. *Am J Physiol* 1987; 252: C640−9.

83 Jornot L, Mirault ME, Junod AF. Differential expression of HSP70 stress proteins in human endothelial cells exposed to heat shock and hydrogen peroxide. *Am J Respir Cell Mol Biol* 1991; 5: 265−75.

84 Clerget M, Polla BS. Erythrophagocytosis induces heat shock protein synthesis by human monocytes-macrophages. *Proc Natl Acad Sci USA* 1990; 87: 1081−5.

85 Schiaffonati L, Rappocchiolo E, Tacchini L, Cairo G, Bernelli-Zazzera A. Reprogramming of gene expression in postischemic rat liver: induction of proto-oncogenes and hsp 70 gene family. *J Cell Physiol* 1990; 143: 79−87.

86 Buchman TG, Cabin DE, Vickers S *et al.* Molecular biology of circulatory shock. Part II. Expression of four groups of hepatic genes is enhanced after resuscitation from cardiogenic shock. *Surgery* 1990; 108: 559−66.

87 Rinaldo JE, Gorry M, Strieter R, Cowan H, Abdolrasulnia R, Shepherd V. Effect of endotoxin-induced cell injury on 70-kD heat shock proteins in bovine lung endothelial cells. *Am J Respir Cell Mol Biol* 1990; 3: 207−16.

88 Moseley PL, York SJ, York J. Bleomycin induces the hsp 70 heat shock promoter in cultured cells. *Am J Respir Cell Mol Biol* 1989; 1: 89−93.

89 Delcayre C, Samuel JL, Marotte F, Best-Belpomme M, Mercadier JJ, Rappaport L. Synthesis of stress proteins in rat cardiac myocytes 2−4 days after imposition of hemodynamic overload. *J Clin Invest* 1988; 82: 460−8.

90 Kohane DS, Sarzani R, Schwartz JH, Chobanian AV, Brecher P. Stress-induced proteins in aortic smooth muscle cells and aorta of hypertensive rats. *Am J Physiol* 1990; 258: H1699−705.

91 Locke M, Noble EG, Atkinson BG. Exercising mammals synthesize stress proteins. *Am J Physiol* 1990; 258: C723−9.

92 Perlmutter DH, Schlesinger MJ, Pierce JA, Punsal PI, Schwartz AL. Synthesis of stress proteins is increased in individuals with homozygous PiZZ alpha1-antitrypsin deficiency and liver disease. *J Clin Invest* 1989; 84: 1555−61.

16 Molecular, cellular and genetic studies of atopic disease

BALARAM GHOSH AND DAVID G. MARSH

Introduction

Atopic allergy is a complex, immunological disease that is dependent on the ability of the individual to produce specific immunoglobulin E (IgE) antibody to environmental allergens [1]. Cross-linking of IgE on the surface of mast cells or basophils by allergens leads to degranulation and release of pharmacological mediators, such as histamine, leukotrienes, etc. The release of such mediators leads to inflammation which, in turn, leads to clinical symptoms of allergy, such as allergic rhinitis, asthma, atopic dermatitis, etc. A number of factors, both genetic and environmental, contribute towards the development of atopy. To understand the immunological basis of atopy, most of the recent studies focus on the molecular level, employing modern technologies of molecular biology and cell biology. These studies are also aimed at answering fundamental questions of immunology, such as the role of human leucocyte antigen (HLA)-D genes and T cells in human immune response.

The hallmark of the immune system is its ability to mount highly specific responses against virtually any foreign antigen, via its humoral and cellular arms. The antigen is taken up by antigen-presenting cells (APCs — dendritic cells, macrophages, B cells, etc.) and processed within endosomes into smaller fragments through proteolytic digestion and, in certain cases, through the breakage of disulphide bonds [2, 3]. A majority of $CD4^+$ helper T cells recognize and respond only to those fragments that appear on the surface of the APCs in association with class II major histocompatibility (Ia) molecules, encoded by major histocompatibility complex (MHC) genes (HLA-DR, DQ, DP in humans and I-A, I-E in mice). The initiation of an immune response involves the formation of a ternary complex comprised of an Ia molecule, an antigen fragment and a T-cell receptor (TCR; Fig. 16.1). During the past few years, a great deal of effort has been expended in understanding the molecular basis of this complex interaction, particularly the association of an Ia molecule with a peptide fragment. Bjorkman et al. [4, 5] have determined the three-dimensional structure of a human class I MHC molecule and, based on this structure, the homologous class II molecules have been modelled [6]. The salient feature of the structure is a 'cleft' formed by two

300

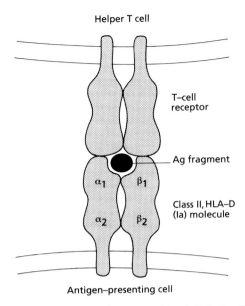

Fig. 16.1 The Ia−allergen−TCR complex. From Marsh DG, Zwollo P, Huang SK, Ghosh B, Ansari AA. *Cold Spring Harbor Symp Quant Biol* 1990; 54: 459−70.

antiparallel α-helices lying on a β-sheet (Fig. 16.2), which constitutes the binding site for an antigen peptide fragment of about 14 amino acids. It has also been shown that the peptide fragments can directly interact with the MHC molecules prior to presentation to TCRs [7−11]. The binding of a peptide fragment to an Ia molecule is a prerequisite·for an immune response to occur. Uncovering the basic principle underlying these complex interactions is very important in understanding human susceptibility to immunological diseases, including atopic allergy. Since

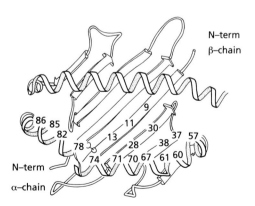

Fig. 16.2 The allergen-binding groove of a modelled HLA-DR molecule as viewed from the TCR. Numbered residues of DRβ chain are predicted to point into the groove. N-term is the amino terminus of the β-chain of HLA-DR. From Bjorkman PJ, Saper MA, Samraoui B, Bennett WS, Strominger JL, Wiley DC. *Nature* 1987; 329: 506−512, 512−18.

much of the earlier research has been extensively reviewed elsewhere [12–16], we will focus on recent findings concerning: 1, studies of allergens; 2, the roles of HLA-D genes, T cells and lymphokines in the human immune response; and 3, the genetics of atopy.

Studies of allergens

To understand the complex pathophysiological mechanisms of allergy, studies involving the structure and function of allergens are important. Allergens are usually proteins or glycoproteins of foreign animal or vegetable origin. Research from many groups, including our own, has led to the identification, purification and characterization of numerous inhaled allergens from pollens and other plant and animal sources, as well as a variety of ingested and injected allergens [14, 17, 18]. In recent years, the cloning and sequencing of several different allergen complementary DNAs has led to a dramatic increase in our knowledge of their primary protein structures [19–30]. These data have been supplemented by amino acid sequencing, both total and partial (primarily N-terminal) [31–38]. In a few cases, including our recently completed nuclear magnetic resonance analyses of the *Amb t* V and *Amb a* V ragweed proteins [39, 40], the three-dimensional structures of allergenic molecules are known. The *Amb* V ragweed allergen homologues ($M_r = 4400–5000$) are comprised of single polypeptide chains of 40–45 amino acids, usually containing eight Cys residues which are all involved in disulphide bonds [23, 24, 31–33, 41]. We have recently cloned and sequenced *Amb a* V (short), *Amb t* V (giant) and *Amb p* V (western) ragweeds [23, 24, 42]. Interestingly, we found essentially no antigenic or allergenic cross-reactivity between *Amb a* V and *Amb t* V, although they share 49% amino acid sequence identity. We have also isolated and characterized two basically charged allergens, *Amb a* VI ($M_r = 11\,500$) [32] and *Amb a* VII [43].

Recently, some of the allergens have been shown to be homologous with other proteins and of known biological function. The major birch (*Betula verrucosa*) pollen allergen *Bet v* I and white-faced hornet venom allergen *Dol m* V have been found to be highly homologous to pathogenesis-related plant proteins [19, 25]. House-dust mite allergen *Der p* I has serine-protease activity [20]. Recently, a birch pollen profilin has been isolated and cloned and shown to be an allergen [29].

Role of HLA-D genes

The mechanism of the induction phase of Ia-restricted immune responsiveness to soluble antigens is now relatively well established, primarily from animal models [44–46]. Studies from several [47, 48] groups suggest that similar mechanisms are relevant in human responsiveness to soluble inhaled allergens. The peptide fragments generated from the degradation of allergens form the Ia−antigen complexes [49−52]. This complex subsequently interacts with a complementary TCR on a CD4$^+$ T-helper (T$_h$) cell to form an Ia−antigen−TCR complex (Fig. 16.1); this leads to cytokine production (including interleukin-4, IL-4) by the T$_h$ cells. IL-4 production by T$_{h2}$-like cells is required for B cells to differentiate into IgE-producing plasma cells and is therefore of particular relevance in atopic allergy [13, 53−55].

Analysis of responsiveness to well-defined pollen allergens has provided evidence that there is a striking association between the expression of HLA genes and atopic disease [56]. Work from our laboratory has focused on 'minor' allergens, like the *Amb* V and *Amb* VI homologues, toward which immune responsiveness tends to occur in an 'all-or-none fashion' and where, in population studies, a single (or two closely related) Ia molecule exhibits significant associations to serum IgE and IgG antibodies. We found that DR2/Dw2 is associated with IgE and IgG responsiveness to the *Amb* V allergens (Table 16.1) [57−60]. In subsequent studies, an association of the HLA-DR5 (DRw11) haplotype and the presence of *Amb a* VI specific IgE was observed [61]. In epidemiological studies, we found that HLA-DR3 is associated with *Lolium perenne* (rye grass) allergens, *Lol p* I, II and III [62, 63]. We also found that HLA-DR5 is associated with *Lol p* III. It has recently been indicated that the association of *Lol p* III to these two Ia molecules may be due to the conservation of amino acids in the amino terminal half of the domains (residues 9−11, EYSTS) of the β-chains of DR3 and DR5 [63−65].

No significant associations have been found between HLA-DR or DQ and responsiveness to certain allergens, particularly (but not exclusively) the more complex, relatively abundant allergens like *Amb a* I (M_r = 38 000). In such cases, different (or the same) agretopes may be recognized by several different Ia molecules, which would mask the HLA associations [17, 41]. For allergens of 'intermediate' complexity (M_r = 10 000−15 000), like *Lol p* II and III, it appears that there is an interaction between gene(s) regulating IgE production and HLA-linked *Ir* genes, such that HLA associations are found primarily in individuals possessing the 'low IgE' phenotype [12, 65]. In other cases (e.g. *Der f* II) there is evidence that HLA-DP molecules may be involved in allergen presentation [66]. Furthermore, Ia molecules produced by *trans*-complementation within an isotype (e.g. DQα−DQβ), or hybrid molecules (e.g. DQα−DPβ, *cis* or *trans*), may possibly be involved in specific immune recognition [67] and weak responsiveness to *Amb a* V (Marsh D *et al.* unpublished).

Role of T cells and studies on their epitopes

IgE responses are primarily initiated and regulated by CD4$^+$ T lymphocytes [47]. To understand the immunological properties of these T cells

Table 16.1 Significant associations of HLA with specific antibody responsiveness toward highly purified pollen allergens in atopic Caucasoid subjects

Systematic name	M_r	Major HLA association	Westinghouse subjects		Clinic patients		Overall P values*
			Positive	Negative	Positive	Negative	
Ambrosia artemisiifolia and *A. trifida* (short and giant ragweeds)							
Amb a V	5000	DR2/Dw2	9/9 (100%)	20/83 (24%)	27/29 (93%)	10/56 (18%)	$<10^{-9}$
Amb a VI	11500	DR5	11/13 (85%)	14/103 (14%)	6/15 (40%)	4/66 (6%)	$<10^{-6}$
Amb t V	4400	DR2/Dw2	3/4 (75%)	0/13 (0%)	3/3 (100%)	1/7 (14%)	$<10^{-3}$
Lolium perenne (perennial rye)							
Lol p I	27000	DR3	23/70 (33%)	9/65 (14%)	14/39 (36%)	2/28 (7%)	$<10^{-3}$
Lol p II	11000	DR3	11/28 (39%)	21/107 (20%)	9/19 (47%)	7/48 (15%)	10^{-3}
Lol p III	11000	DR3	13/30 (43%)	19/105 (18%)	13/23 (57%)	3/44 (7%)	$<10^{-5}$

* P values are given only for the most significant associations for analyses of IgE antibody data, except that IgG antibody data from immunized patients were used for Amb t V. No significant HLA-D associations were found for responsiveness to: Amb a I ($M_r = 37\,800$), Amb a III ($M_r = 12\,300$), Phl p V ($M_r = 27\,000$), Der f 1 ($M_r = 24\,000$) and Der f II ($M_r = 14\,500$) (Adapted from ref. 17 and unpublished).

and the physicochemical nature of the ternary complex formed between Ia, allergen and TCR, a number of T-cell clones specific for various allergens, such as ragweed, grass pollens, *Dermatophagoides* spp., cat allergens, honey bee venom, murine urinary protein, etc., were isolated from peripheral blood mononuclear cells (reviewed in ref. 47). Recently, using recombinant DNA and peptide synthesis approaches, a number of T-cell epitopes have been defined [47]. Using synthetic peptides (with Ala−Cys substitution) encompassing the entire *Amb a* V protein, it has been demonstrated that a 14-residue C-terminal peptide was able to block presentation of native *Amb a* V by the APC to the cloned T cells [60]. The information, however, on these epitopes is limited to date. More information will be needed to understand how these T cells enhance the switch to IgE antibody production, which is critical to allergic diseases.

The use of allergen-specific T-cell clones is important to investigate the contribution of individual HLA-D molecules in T-cell recognition at the molecular level. Using APCs containing the HLA-DR(α, β1 *1501) [or DR(α, β1 *1502), common in Orientals] molecules, it has been directly demonstrated that the responsiveness of *Amb a* V was restricted to these Ia molecules [59]. This has also been confirmed by using an anti-DR$\alpha\beta$1 monoclonal antibody (HU30), which blocked, in a dose-dependent manner, the cloned T-cell responses to *Amb a* V [59].

Role of T-cell-derived lymphokines

Lymphokines produced by certain CD4$^+$ T cells play a crucial role in IgE antibody production [16]. Mosmann and Coffman [68] originally defined two subsets of mouse CD4$^+$ Th cells: Th1 which produces IL-2, interferon (IFN)-γ and tumour necrosis factor (TNF)-β; and Th2, which produces IL-4, IL-5, IL-6 and IL-10. Subsequent studies have shown that atopic allergy is associated with the Th2 subset of CD4$^+$ cells. The development of B cells to IgE-secreting plasma cells is induced by IL-4 and suppressed by IFN-γ [69]. Analysis of lymphokine production profiles from atopic individuals showed a Th2-like secretion profile, whereas non-atopic individuals predominantly secrete IFN-γ, with little or no IL-4 [70, 71]. In addition, IL-4 has been defined as a 'switch factor' for IgE, which regulates transcription of the germ-line Cε gene [72, 73]. IL-4 also enhances the level of expression of FcεRII on lymphocytes and monocytes which, in turn, can further up-regulate IgE production [73]. Recent studies have shown that IL-4 is necessary, but not sufficient, for the induction of IgE synthesis [74]. When highly purified normal B cells are incubated with IL-4 and mixtures of T-cell-derived lymphokines, no IgE production is observed [75]. In both 'cognate' and 'non-cognate' interaction between B and T cells (i.e. with or without the involvement of class II molecules), a further costimulatory factor, apparently supplied by the activated T-cell membrane, is required for initial B-cell activation which leads to productive Cε transcripts and eventual IgE biosynthesis [72]. Recently, it has been shown that the stimulation of B cells with anti-CD40 monoclonal antibody and IL-4 induces large amounts of IgE antibody [76]. Therefore, interaction of CD40 with its ligand could be the costimulatory signal necessary for IgE synthesis in the presence of IL-4. Molecular cloning of the CD40 gene revealed that it is closely related to the receptors for nerve growth factor and TNF-α [77]. The natural ligand for CD40 is not known. It is also not known at which steps of the signal transduction pathways IL-4 and CD40 synergize for IgE production. Interestingly, IL-4 has been shown to up-regulate CD40 expression on B cells [78].

It has been indicated that multiple cytokines, derived from T cells or non-T cells, are able to modulate IL-4-dependent IgE synthesis [75]. IL-5 and IL-6 up-regulate IgE synthesis induced by IL-4 [76]. In contrast, IL-2, IL-1 and TNF-α had no effect [79].

Genetics of IgE regulation

Modern immunogenetic studies of allergic disease in humans were initiated by our group [80, 81] and by Levine *et al.* [82] following the crucial discoveries of MHC-linked *Ir* genes in animals [83, 84] and of IgE in humans [1]. The experiments of Levine, Vaz and others [85−88] showed that the ability of inbred mice to produce antibodies toward low doses of complex protein allergens is controlled by: (1) MHC-linked *Ir* genes determining specific antibody responses (of both the IgE and IgG classes); and (2) IgE-regulating gene(s) not linked to the MHC complex. These mouse studies showed that the segregation of specific *Ir* genes toward complex protein allergens could best be studied following immunogenically limiting low-dose immunization, with total allergen dosages about $10-100\,\mu g\,kg^{-1}$ [89, 90]. By contrast, seasonal dosages of inhaled pollen allergens usually total no more than $0.06-1\,\mu g$ (about $0.001-0.01\,\mu g\,kg^{-1}$) for adult humans [90]. We hypothesized that such ultralimiting allergen dosages, inhaled over a 6−8 week pollen season, would facilitate elucidation of the genetics of immune responsiveness in the highly polymorphic human population [89]. High total serum IgE levels are significantly associated with atopic rhinitis [1, 91] and with skin-test (ST) responsiveness to a panel of purified allergens [56]. Several twin studies have shown that log[total serum IgE] levels are largely determined by genetic factors [92]. Also, in a recent study, Blumenthal's group found that the pair-wise concordances for log[total IgE] for monozygotic twins (MZT) raised apart were similar to those for MZT raised together [93]. A recent large population study of Burrows *et al.* [94] demonstrated that high total IgE levels are associated with asthma, including in subjects who are ST⁻ to common inhalants. Our recent findings in adults are similar to those of Burrows *et al.*'s group. Both data sets strongly point to a greater role for IgE (and atopy) in asthma than many had assumed, and lend support to the effort to define genes critical for IgE regulation.

The evidence from several family studies of the genetics of total serum IgE levels points to the involvement of a major gene for IgE regulation that is not linked to HLA [95]. Different modes of inheritance for this postulated IgE-regulating gene have been suggested based on the distribution of total serum IgE levels in different families. Our initial study [56], and a subsequent study of Gerrard et al. [96], provided strong evidence for recessive inheritance of high IgE levels. Borecki et al. [97] showed that 'a single gene effect could influence both IgE production and liability to allergies'. However, further studies provided no clear support for any specific mode of inheritance [95]. These inconclusive results prompted our studies of 42 large Westinghouse families. We now conclude that there is a major gene that determines total IgE levels, but there is also significant 'polygenic' control. The strongest evidence supports the theory of recessive inheritance of high IgE, although codominant inheritance cannot be ruled out [98, 99].

Cookson et al. [100] suggest that a single, dominant atopy gene linked to the MS.51 genetic marker on chromosome 11q is necessary for the expression of atopy in 70–100% of atopics (LOD score of 5.6). In a related study, Lympany et al. [101] obtained a LOD ≈ 0.9, which does not confirm or definitively refute the Cookson hypothesis. Cookson et al. [100] have reported large Taq I restriction fragment length polymorphism fragments greater than 10 kb in several families, that were not found in studies by Krishnamoorthy R (unpublished) nor by Lympany et al. [101] and Roitman-Johnson et al. [102]. Using Cookson's phenotype (which combines ST positivity and/or 'high' total IgE levels), we have found at least four families out of 42 studied in detail that all have some ST^+ children, many with elevated total IgE; but in each case both parents are ST^- and have IgE levels less than 50 U ml^{-1} (120 ng ml^{-1}), well below Cookson's cut-point of 100 U ml^{-1} [103].

Concluding remarks

Modern technologies of molecular biology and cell biology have enabled us to clone a number of allergen genes and allergen-specific T cells. Assuming a continuous rapid rate of progress in the future, we should soon have enough material to ask some fundamental questions of immunology in humans, relating to: 1, the physicochemical nature of Ia–allergen–TCR interactions; 2, the TCR gene usage for allergic responses; and 3, the complex network of cytokines involved in allergic responsiveness. In addition, an understanding of Ia/T-cell epitopes and TCR gene usage may lead to vaccine design for efficient asthma and allergy management in the future.

No clear mode of inheritance of atopic disease is recognized. HLA-D genes contribute to atopy by regulating specific IgE responsiveness. The propensity of overall IgE production by an individual, however, is dependent on non-MHC-linked genes. Recent molecular genetic linkage studies indicated that the transmission of atopy was a dominant trait and a putative 'atopy gene' may be located on chromosome 11q. Other investigators, however, have been unable to confirm this finding. In any event, it is true that all individuals affected by atopic diseases have elevated levels of specific IgE. The genetic factors which control the overall IgE level have not been elucidated. It is obvious that a great deal of progress will be made in the near future to identify these genetic factors.

References

1 Ishizaka K, Ishizaka T. Human reaginic antibodies and immunoglobulin E. *J Allergy* 1968; 42: 330–63.

2 Unanue ER, Antigen-presenting function of the macrophage. *Annu Rev Immunol* 1984; 2: 395–428.

3 Berzofsky JA. The nature and role of antigen processing in T-cell activation. In: Cruse JM, Lewis RE, Jr, eds. *The Year in Immunology 1984–1985*. Basel: Karger S, 1985: 18–24.

4 Bjorkman PJ, Saper MA, Samraoui B, Bennett WS, Strominger JL, Wiley DC. Structure of the human class I histocompatibility antigen, HLA-A2. *Nature* 1987; 329: 506–12.

5 Bjorkman PJ, Saper MA, Samraoui B, Bennett WS, Strominger JL, Wiley DC. The foreign antigen binding site and T cell recognition regions of class I histocompatibility antigens. *Nature* 1987; 329: 512–18.

6 Babbitt BP, Allen PM, Matsueda G, Haber E, Unanue ER. Binding of immunogenic peptides to Ia histocompatibility molecules. *Nature* 1985; 317: 359–61.

7 Buus S, Colon S, Smith C, Freed JH, Miles C, Grey HM. Interaction of a 'processed' ovalbumin peptide and Ia molecules. *Proc Natl Acad Sci USA* 1986; 83: 3968–71.

8 Babbitt BP, Matsueda G, Haber E, Unanue ER, Allen PM. Antigenic competition at the level of peptide–Ia binding. *Proc Natl Acad Sci USA* 1986; 83: 4509–13.

9 Watts TH, Gaub HE, McConnell HM. T-cell mediated association of peptide antigen and major histocompatibility complex protein detected by energy transfer in an evanescent wave-field. *Nature* 1986; 320: 179–81.

10 Lapkoff CB, Goodfriend L. Isolation of a low molecular weight ragweed pollen allergen; Ra5. *Int Arch Allergy Appl Immunol* 1974; 46: 215–29.

11 Buus S, Sette A, Colon SM, Miles C, Grey H. The relation between MHC restriction and the capacity of Ia to bind immunogenic peptides. *Science* 1987; 235: 1353–8.

12 Willcox HNA, Marsh DG. Genetic regulation of antibody heterogeneity: its possible significance in human allergy. *Immunogenetics* 1978; 6: 209–25.

13 Romagnani S. Regulation and deregulation of human IgE synthesis. *Immunol Today* 1990; 11: 316–21.

14 Marsh DG, Norman PS. Antigens that cause atopic disease. In: Samter M, Talmage DW, Frank MM, Austin KS, Claman HN, eds. *Immunological Diseases*, 4th edn. Boston MA: Little, Brown and Co., 1988: 981–1008.

15 Marsh DG, Zwollo P, Huang SK, Ghosh B, Ansari AA. Molecular studies of

human response to allergens. *Cold Spring Harbor Symp Quant Biol* 1990; 54: 459−70.

16 Vercelli D, Geha RS. Regulation of IgE synthesis in humans: a tale of two signals. *J Allergy Clin Immunol* 1991; 88: 285−97.

17 Marsh DG. Immunogenetic and immunochemical factors determining immune responsiveness to allergens: studies in unrelated subjects. In: Marsh DG, Blumenthal MN, eds. *Genetic and Environmental Factors in Clinical Allergy.* Minneapolis, MN: University of Minnesota Press, 1990: 97−123.

18 Matthiesen F, Ipsen H, Løwenstein H. In: d'Amato G, ed. *Allergenic Pollens and Pollinosis in Europe.* Oxford: Blackwell Scientific Publications, 1991: 36.

19 Fang KSY, Vitale M, Fehlner P, King TP. cDNA cloning and primary structure of a white-face hornet venom allergen, antigen 5. *Proc Natl Acad Sci USA* 1988; 85: 895−9.

20 Chua KY, Stewart GA, Thomas WR *et al.* Sequence analysis of cDNA coding for a major house dust mite allergen, *Der p* I: homology with cysteine proteases. *J Exp Med* 1988; 167: 175−82.

21 Perez M, Ishioka GY, Walker LE, Chesnut R. cDNA cloning and immunological characterization of the rye grass allergen *Lol p* I. *J Biol Chem* 1990; 265: 16210−15.

22 Rafnar T, Griffith IJ, Kuo MC *et al.* Cloning of *Amb a* I (antigen E), the major allergen family of short ragweed pollen. *J Biol Chem* 1991; 266: 1229−36.

23 Ghosh B, Perry MP, Marsh DG. Cloning the cDNA encoding the *Amb t* V allergen from giant ragweed (*Ambrosia trifida*) pollen. *Gene* 1991; 101: 231−8.

24 Ghosh B, Marsh DG. Cloning cDNAs encoding *Amb* V allergens from ragweed (*Ambrosia*) pollens. *FASEB J* 1991; 5: A1662.

25 Breiteneder H, Pettenburger K, Bito A. *et al.* The gene coding for the major birch pollen allergen *Bet v* I, is highly homologous to a pea disease resistance response gene. *EMBO J* 1989; 8: 1935−8.

26 Silvanovich A, Astwood J, Zhang L *et al.* Nucleotide sequence analysis of three cDNAs coding for *Poa p* IX isoallergens of Kentucky bluegrass pollen. *J Biol Chem* 1991; 266: 1204−10.

27 Griffith IJ, Smith PM, Pollock J *et al.* Cloning and sequencing of *Lol p* I, the major allergenic protein of rye-grass pollen. *FEBS Lett* 1991; 279: 210−15.

28 Singh MB, Hough T, Theerakulpisut P *et al.* Isolation of cDNA encoding a newly identified major allergenic protein of rye-grass pollen: intracellular targeting to the amyloplast. *Proc Natl Acad Sci USA* 1991; 88: 1384−8.

29 Valenta R, Duchene M, Pettenburger K *et al.* Identification of profilin as a novel pollen allergen; IgE autoreactivity in sensitized individuals. *Science* 1991; 253: 557−60.

30 Morgenstein JP, Griffith IJ, Brauer AW *et al.* Amino acid sequence of a *Fel d* I, the major allergen of the domestic cat: protein sequence analysis and cDNA cloning. *Proc Natl Acad Sci USA* 1991; 88: 9690−4.

31 Mole LE, Goodfriend L, Lapkoff CB *et al.* The amino acid sequence of allergen Ra5. *Biochemistry* 1975; 14: 1216−20.

32 Roebber M, Hussain R, Klapper DG, Marsh DG. Isolation and properties of a new short ragweed pollen allergen, Ra6. *J Immunol* 1983; 131: 706−11.

33 Goodfriend L, Choudhury AM, Klapper DG *et al.* Ra5G, a homologue of Ra5 in giant ragweed pollen: isolation, HLA-DR-associated activity, and amino acid sequence. *Mol Immunol* 1985; 22: 899−906.

34 Roebber M, Klapper DG, Goodfriend L *et al.* Immunochemical and genetic studies of *Amb t* V (Ra5G), an Ra5 homologue from giant ragweed pollen. *J Immunol* 1985; 134: 3062−9.

35 Chapman MD, Aalberse RC, Brown MJ, Platts-Mills TAE. Monoclonal antibodies

to the major feline allergen *Fel d* I. II. Single step affinity purification of *Fel d* I, N-terminal sequence analysis, and development of a sensitive two-site immunoassay to assess *Fel d* I exposure. *J Immunol* 1988; 140: 812–18.

36 Ansari AA, Shenbagamurthi P, Marsh DG. Complete amino acid sequence of *Lolium perenne* (perennial rye grass) allergen, *Lol p* II. *J Biol Chem* 1989; 264: 11181–5.

37 Ansari AA, Shenbagamurthi P, Marsh DG. Complete primary structure of a *Lolium perenne* (perennial rye grass) allergen, *Lol p* III: comparison with known *Lol p* I and II sequences. *Biochemistry* 1989; 28: 8665–70.

38 Arruda LK, Platts-Mills TAE, Fox JW, *et al. Aspergillus fumigatus* allergen I, a major IgE-binding protein, is a member of the migogillin family of cytotoxins. *J Exp Med* 1990; 172: 1529–32.

39 Metzler WJ, Valentine K, Roebber M *et al.* Solution structures of ragweed allergen *Amb t* V. *Biochemistry* 1992; 31: 5117–27.

40 Metzler WJ, Valentine K, Roebber M *et al.* Proton resonance assignments and three-dimensional solution structure of the ragweed allergen *Amb a* V by nuclear magnetic resonance spectroscopy. *Biochemistry* 1992; 31: 8697–705.

41 Marsh DG. Defining human immune response fingerprints toward ultra-pure allergens: immunochemical and genetic aspects of responsiveness toward the *Amb* 5 (Ra5) homologues. Proceedings of the XII International Congress of Allergology and Clinical Immunology, Washington, DC, 1985. *Allergy Clin Immunol* 1986; 78 (Suppl.): 242-8.

42 Ghosh B, Perry MP, Rafnar T, Klapper DG, Marsh DG. *Amb p* V allergens from western ragweed (Ambrosia psilostachya) pollen. *J Allergy Clin Immunol* 1993; 91: 337.

43 Roebber M, Marsh DG. Isolation and characterization of allergen *Amb a* VII from short ragweed pollen. *J Allergy Clin Immunol* 1991; 87: 324.

44 Unanue ER, Allen PM. The basis for the immunoregulatory role of macrophages and other accessory cells. *Science* 1987; 236: 551–7.

45 Buus S, Sette A, Grey H. The interaction between protein derived immunogenic peptides and Ia. *Immunol Rev* 1987; 98: 115–41.

46 Guillet JG, Lai MZ, Briner TJ *et al.* Immunological self, nonself discrimination. *Science* 1987; 235: 865–70.

47 O'Hehir RE, Garman RD, Greenstein JL, Lamb JR. The specificity and regulation of T-cell responsiveness to allergens. *Annu Rev Immunol* 1991; 9: 67–95.

48 Gurka G, Ohman J, Rosenwasser LJ. Allergen-specific human T cell clones: derivation specificity, and activation requirements. *J Allergy Clin Immunol* 1990; 83: 945–54.

49 Macatonia SE, Knight SC, Edwards AJ *et al.* Localization of antigen on lymph node dendritic cells after exposure to the contact sensitizer fluorescein isothiocyanate. *J Exp Med* 1987; 166: 1654–67.

50 Kay AB. Mechanisms in allergic and chronic asthma which involve eosinophils, neutrophils, lymphocytes and other inflammatory cells. In: Kay AB, ed. *The Allergic Basis of Asthma*. London: Ballière Tindall, 1988: 1–14.

51 Bakke O, Dobberstein B. MHC class II-associated invariant chain contains a sorting signal for endosomal compartments. *Cell* 1990; 63: 707–16.

52 Lotteau V, Teyton L, Peleraux A *et al.* Intracellular transport of class II MHC molecules directed by invariant chain. *Nature* 1990; 348: 600–5.

53 Coffman RL, Ohara J, Bond MW *et al.* B cell stimulatory factor-1 enhances the IgE response of lipopolysaccharide-activated B cells. *J Immunol* 1986; 136: 4538–41.

54 Pene J, Rousset F, Briere F *et al.* IgE production by normal human B cells induced by alloreactive T cell clones is mediated by IL-4 and suppressed by

IFN-γ. *J Immunol* 1988; 141: 1218−24.

55 Vercelli D, Geha RS. Regulation of IgE synthesis in humans. *J Clin Immunol* 1989; 9: 75−83.

56 Marsh DG, Bias WB, Ishizaka K. Genetic control of basal serum immunoglobulin E level and its effect on specific reaginic sensitivity. *Proc Natl Acad Sci USA* 1974; 71: 3588−92.

57 Marsh DG, Hsu SH, Roebber M *et al*. HLA-Dw2: a genetic marker for human immune response to short ragweed pollen allergen Ra5. I. Response resulting primarily from natural antigenic exposure. *J Exp Med* 1982; 155: 1439−51.

58 Marsh DG, Hsu SH, Roebber M *et al*. HLA-Dw2: a genetic marker for human immune response to short ragweed pollen allergen Ra5. II. Response after ragweed immunotherapy. *J Exp Med* 1982; 155: 1452−63.

59 Huang SK, Zwollo P, Marsh DG. Class II MHC restriction of human T-cell responses to short ragweed allergen, *Amb a* V. *Eur J Immunol* 1991; 21: 1469−73.

60 Huang SK, Marsh DG. Human T-cell responses to ragweed allergens: *Amb* V homologues. *Immunology* 1991; 73: 363−5.

61 Marsh DG, Freidhoff LR, Ehrlich-Kautzky E *et al*. Immune responsiveness to *Ambrosia artemisiifolia* (short ragweed) pollen allergen *Amb a* VI (Ra6) is associated with HLA-DR5 in allergic humans. *Immunogenetics* 1987; 26: 230−6.

62 Freidhoff LR, Kautzky EE, Meyers DA, Ansari AA, Bias WB, Marsh DG. Association of HLA-DR3 with human immune response to *Lol p* I and *Lol p* II allergens in allergic subjects. *Tissue Antigens* 1988; 31: 211−19.

63 Ansari AA, Freidhoff LR, Meyers DA, Bias WB, Marsh DG. Human immune responsiveness to *Lolium perenne* grass pollen allergen *Lol p* III (Rye III) is associated with HLA-DR3 and DR5. *Hum Immunol* 1989; 25: 59−71.

64 Ansari AA, Freidhoff LR, Marsh DG. Molecular genetics of human immune response to *Lolium perenne* (rye) allergen, *Lol p* III. *Int Arch Allergy Appl Immunol* 1989; 88: 164−9.

65 Ansari AA, Shinomiya N, Zwollo P, Marsh DG. HLA-D gene studies in relation to immune responsiveness to a grass allergen, *Lol p* III. *Immunogenetics* 1991; 33: 24−32.

66 Eura M, Freidhoff LR, Ehrlich-Kautzky E *et al*. HLA-DPB polymorphism and IgE responsiveness to specific allergens. *11th International Histocompatibility Testing Workshop and Conference, Yokohama, Japan*, Abstr. no. PS-112-6, 1991: 235.

67 Charron D. Molecular basis of human leukocyte antigen class II disease associations. *Adv Immunol* 1990; 48: 107−59.

68 Mosmann TR, Coffman RL. Heterogeneity of cytokine patterns and functions of helper T-cells. *Adv Immunol* 1989; 46: 11.

69 Coffman RL, Seymour RW, Lebman DA *et al*. The role of helper T-cell products in mouse B cell differentiation and isotype regulation. *Immunol Rev* 1988; 102: 5−28.

70 Kapsenberg ML, Wierenga EA, Bos JD, Jansen HM. Functional subsets of allergen-reactive human CD4$^+$ T cells. *Immunol Today* 1991; 12: 392−5.

71 Parronchi P, Macchia D, Piccini MP *et al*. Allergen- and bacterial antigen-specific T-cell clones established from atopic donors show a different profile of cytokine production. *Proc Natl Acad Sci USA* 1991; 88: 4538−42.

72 Gauchat J, Lebman DA, Coffman RL *et al*. Structure and expression of germline ε transcripts in human B cells induced by interleukin 4 to switch to IgE production. *J Exp Med* 1990; 172: 463−73.

73 Paul WE. Interleukin-4: a prototypic immunoregulatory lymphokine. *Blood* 1991; 77: 1859−70.

74 Vercelli D, Jabara HH, Lauener RP, Geha RS. IL-4 inhibits the synthesis of IFN-γ

and induces the synthesis of IgE in human mixed lymphocyte cultures. *J Immunol* 1990; 144: 570−3.

75 Vercelli D, Jabara HH, Arai K *et al.* Endogenous interleukin 6 plays an obligatory role in interleukin 4-dependent human IgE synthesis. *Eur J Immunol* 1989; 19: 1419−24.

76 Jabara HH, Fu SM, Geha RS, Vercelli D. CD40 and IgE: Synergism between anti-CD40 monoclonal antibody and interleukin 4 in the induction of IgE synthesis by highly purified human B cells. *J Exp Med* 1990; 172: 1861−4.

77 Stamenkovic I, Clark EA, Seed B, A B-lymphocyte activation molecule related to the nerve growth factor receptor and induced by cytokines in carcinomas. *EMBO J* 1989; 8: 1403−10.

78 Clark EA, Shu GL, Luscher B *et al.* Activation of human B cells: comparison of the signal transduced by IL-4 to four different competence signals. *J Immunol* 1989; 143: 3873−80.

79 Pene J, Rousset F, Briere F *et al.* IgE production by normal human lymphocytes is induced by interleukin 4 and suppressed by interferons γ and α and prostaglandin E$_2$. *Proc Natl Acad Sci USA* 1988; 85: 6880−4.

80 Marsh DG, Bias WB, Hsu SH, Goodfriend L. Association of the HL-A7 cross-reacting group with a specific reaginic antibody response in allergic man. *Science* 1973; 179: 691−3.

81 Marsh DG, Bias WB, Hsu SH, Goodfriend L. Associations between major histo-compatibility (HL-A) antigens and specific reaginic antibody responses in allergic man. In: Goodfriend L, Sehon AH, Orange RP, eds. *Mechanisms in Allergy.* New York: Marcel Dekker Inc., 1973: 113−29.

82 Levine BB, Stember RH, Fotino M. Ragweed hay fever: genetic control and linkage to HLA haplotypes. *Science* 1972; 178: 1201.

83 McDevitt HO, Tyan ML. Genetic control of the antibody response in inbred mice: transfer of response by spleen cells and linkage to the major histocompati-bility (H-2) locus. *J Exp Med* 1968; 128: 1−11.

84 Benacerraf B, McDevitt HO. Histocompatibility-linked immune response genes. *Science* 1972; 175: 273−9.

85 Vaz NM, Levine BB. Immune responses of inbred mice to repeated low doses of antigen: relationship to histocompatibility (H-2) type. *Science* 1970; 168: 852−4.

86 Levine BB, Vaz NM. Two kinds of genetic control of reagin production in the mouse. *J Clin Invest* 1970; 49: 58a.

87 Watanabe N, Kojima S, Ovary Z. Suppression of IgE antibody production in SJL mice. I. Non-specific suppressor T cells. *J Exp Med* 1976; 143: 833−45.

88 Prouvost-Danon A, Mouton D, Abadie A *et al.* Genetic regulation of IgE and agglutinating antibody synthesis in lines of mice selected for high and low immune responsiveness. *Eur J Immunol* 1977; 7: 342−8.

89 Marsh DG. Allergens and the genetics of allergy. *Antigens* 1975; 3: 271−359.

90 Marsh DG, Meyers DA, Freidhoff LR *et al.* HLA-Dw2: a genetic marker for human immune response to short ragweed pollen allergen Ra5. II. Response after ragweed immunotherapy. *J Exp Med* 1982; 155: 1452−63.

91 Johansson SGO, Bennich HH, Berg T. The clinical significance of IgE. *Prog Clin Immunol* 1972; 1: 100−24.

92 Hanson B, McGue M, Roitman-Johnson B *et al.* Atopic disease and immuno-globulin E in twins reared apart and together. *Am J Hum Genet* 1991; 48: 873−9.

93 Blumenthal MN, Bonini S. Immunogenetics of specific immune responses to allergens in twins and families. In: Marsh DG, Blumenthal MN, eds. *Genetic and Environmental Factors in Clinical Allergy.* Minneapolis, MN: University of Minnesota Press, 1990: 132−9.

94 Burrows B, Martinez FD, Halonen M *et al.* Association of asthma with serum IgE

levels and skin-test reactivity to allergens. *N Engl J Med* 1989; 320: 271−7.

95 Meyers DA. Family analysis and genetic counseling for allergic diseases. In: Marsh DG, Blumenthal MN, eds. *Genetic and Environmental Factors in Clinical Allergy*. Minneapolis MN: University of Minnesota Press, 1990: 161−73.

96 Gerrard JW, Rao DC, Morton NE. A genetic study of immunoglobulin E. *Am J Hum Genet* 1978; 30: 46−58.

97 Borecki IB, Rao DC, Lalouel JM *et al*. Demonstration of a common major gene with pleiotropic effects on immunoglobulin E levels and allergy. *Genet Epidemiol* 1985; 2: 327−38.

98 Meyers DA, Beaty TH, Freidhoff LR, Marsh DG. Inheritance of total serum IgE (basal levels) in man. *Am J Hum Genet* 1987; 41: 51−62.

99 Meyers DA, Beaty TH, Colyer CR, Marsh DG. Genetics of total serum IgE levels: a regressive model approach to segregation analysis. *Genet Epidemiol* 1991; 8: 351−9.

100 Cookson WOCM, Sharp PA, Faux JA, Hopkin JM. Linkage between immuno-globulin E responses underlying asthma and rhinitis and chromosome 11q. *Lancet* 1989; i: 1292−5.

101 Lympany P, Welsh K, MacCochrane G *et al*. Genetic analysis using DNA poly-morphism of the linkage between chromosome 11q13 and atopy and bronchial hyperresponsiveness to methacholine. *J Allergy Clin Immunol* 1992; 89: 619−28.

102 Roitman-Johnson B, Rich S, Greenberg B *et al*. Genetics of atopy. *J Allergy Clin Immunol* 1992; 89: 267.

103 Marsh DG, Ghosh B, Rafnar T, Huang S-K. Molecular genetic studies of human immune responsiveness to ragweed pollen allergens. *Proceedings of the International Allergology and Clinical Immunology Meeting, Kyoto, 1991*; 130−137.

17 Interleukins in the pulmonary inflammatory response

GREGORY P. GEBA, RALPH J. ZITNIK
AND JACK A. ELIAS

Introduction

Historical overview

Erythema, swelling, heat and pain, the cardinal features of inflammation, were recognized as early as the year 30 BC by Celsus and redescribed between AD 130 and 200 by Galen [1]. Studies of these alterations have demonstrated a basic sequence of events that occurs in virtually all types of inflammatory response. This sequence includes:
1 vasodilation followed by transient vasoconstriction;
2 permeability alterations associated with the weepage of plasma proteins;
3 leucocyte margination to the vascular endothelium and subsequent migration into the interstitial space;
4 activation and proliferation of leucocytes at sites of injury; and
5 a fibroproliferative response characterized by dynamic alterations in fibroblast proliferation and matrix molecule production.
Studies in the twentieth century have added significantly to our appreciation of the complexity of the interactions that regulate these processes. In the 1920s Alexis Carrel demonstrated that leucocytes play an important role in wound healing. In 1966 J.R. David described 'migration inhibitory factor' (MIF) [2], the first non-antibody regulator of cellular function. As a result of these and subsequent studies it has become clear that the cell–cell interactions that are so important in inflammation and healing are mediated, to a great extent, by small cell-derived regulatory peptides called cytokines.

The description of MIF led students of biology to look for soluble factors that regulated other biological events. By the mid-1970s a wide variety of soluble bioactive factors had been described in a superficial fashion. In the late 1970s it became apparent that many of these activities were mediated by the same or similar molecules. In an attempt to remedy the linguistic nightmare that resulted, the Second International Lymphokine Workshop adopted a bioactivity-independent nomenclature for multifunctional cytokines. At this meeting the term interleukin (IL) was chosen for this group of regulators [2]. To date, 12 cytokines have been designated interleukins. For reasons that are not clear, however,

314

many other multifunctional cytokines are still referred to based on their original eponyms.

Mechanisms of cytokine function

The 'classic' cytokine is a glycosylated protein that is transiently produced by an appropriately stimulated effector cell and mediates its effects by binding to specific receptors on target tissues. It has autocrine effects when it modulates the phenotype of the cell that produced it, paracrine effects when it modulates the phenotype of nearby cells and endocrine effects when (like IL-6 induction of hepatic acute phase protein synthesis) it is produced at a site of injury and transported to a distant site where it mediates its effects [3]. In rare circumstances it has intracrine effects where it binds its receptor and mediates its effects before it gets out of the cell that produced it (Fig. 17.1). Recent studies have also demonstrated that cytokines such as platelet-derived growth factor (PDGF), IL-1, tumour necrosis factor (TNF) and transforming growth factor-α (TGF-α) may be cell-associated and/or exist as integral membrane proteins (Fig. 17.1). These molecules exert their effects via cell−cell contact and are important regulators of local inflammatory events. PDGF, basic fibroblast growth factor (bFGF) and TGF-β can also bind to extracellular matrix resulting in an exaggeration of their effects during times of matrix remodelling (Fig. 17.1).

Cytokine networking

With few exceptions, cytokines are multifunctional molecules. As a result they regulate a wide spectrum of immune and non-immune biological events, including inflammation, metabolism, cell growth and differentiation, morphogenesis, fibrogenesis and haemostasis. *In vitro* and *in vivo* studies have shown that the same cytokine can have different effects depending on its dose, the state of activation and/or maturation of the target cell and the presence of other cytokines in the local cellular microenvironment. An additional level of complexity has also been appreciated since cytokines frequently stimulate target tissues to produce bioactive cytokines. As a result, it is now clear that the biological effects of cytokines result from their direct effects on target tissues and their ability to interact with one another in regulating target cell function. Individual cytokines can be thought of as the letters in an alphabet or code that make up a complex cellular signalling language [2, 4]. The inflammatory and fibrotic responses can be viewed as complicated cascades or networks of interacting cytokines. The ultimate response of a cell to these networks is determined by the sum of the signals received at the cell membrane and modulated by the receptivity of the cell to these signals.

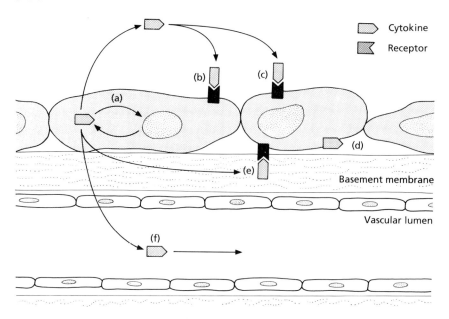

Fig. 17.1 Modes and sites of cytokine action. Cytokines are produced after appropriate stimulation. Their effects are intracrine (a) when they alter cell phenotype without being transported to the extracellular space. Once outside the cell they can have autocrine effects when they bind to receptors on the surface of the cell that produced the cytokine and regulate its function (b). They have paracrine effects when they bind to receptors on nearby cells (c) and endocrine effects when they enter the systemic circulation (f) and mediate their effects on distant target tissues. In addition to existing in a soluble form, some cytokines remain cell-associated (d) and some become incorporated into the extracellular matrix (e). In these locations cytokines are felt to play an important role in local cell–cell interactions and matrix remodelling, respectively.

Regulatory hierarchies

Many mediators of inflammatory and pathological processes have been elucidated over the past century. Some, such as histamine, serotonin, kinins, prostaglandins (PG), leukotrienes, neuropeptides and adrenergic and cholinergic neurotransmitters, have been well defined and their role in inflammation has received significant attention. In contrast, the cytokine network regulating inflammation is of more recent vintage. It is clear, however, that the regulatory effects of these mediators are not independent of one another. The regulatory effects of cytokines are part of a complex multifaceted apparatus that involves the nervous system, endocrine system and other regulators of the inflammatory response. Normal growth, repair and development are the result of the appropriate functioning and interaction of these regulatory processes. Dysregulation at any level, particularly dysregulated and/or abnormal cytokine production, is an important part of the pathogenesis of many human diseases (Fig. 17.2). Thus, the production of a cytokine can be part of a

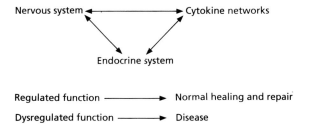

Fig. 17.2 Regulatory hierarchies. Schematic demonstration of the multiple interactions between the nervous system, endocrine system and cytokine networks. Regulated function and interaction of these processes contribute to normal healing and repair. Dysregulation at any site can contribute to disease pathogenesis.

beneficial physiological response or a dysregulated pathological response. It is only with the understanding that disease states can represent exaggerated normal responses that the role of a cytokine can be fully appreciated. In this light, the detection of a cytokine at a site of pathology, the ability of the cytokine to mimic a pathological response following local or systemic administration and the suppression of the pathological response by a specific cytokine antagonist can all be used as evidence that the cytokine plays a role in the pathogenesis of a specific disorder.

Inflammatory cytokines have been the topic of an extraordinary amount of recent investigative effort. As a result, the number of cytokines that have been described and our knowledge about each are increasing daily. It is beyond the scope of this chapter to cover all inflammatory cytokines described to date. Instead, we have provided a tabular overview of the interleukins and TNF (Table 17.1), described the scientific approach used to understand the biology of most cytokines and illustrated its application to IL-6. Lastly, there is an overview of the cytokine–cytokine interactions in the lung and their therapeutic implications. By necessity, many important cytokines, cytokine–cytokine interactions and cytokine–disease associations will not be mentioned or will be mentioned superficially.

Scientific approach to a cytokine

Early descriptions of most cytokines were superficial consisting of a description of a biological activity and a sketchy purification. To understand these molecules in greater depth, scientific approaches like the one outlined in Fig. 17.3 have been employed. Standard techniques of protein purification have been used to obtain information about the physical and chemical characteristics of specific cytokines and the complementary DNAs (cDNAs) that encode the cytokines have been isolated and sequenced to obtain their primary structures. Full-length cDNA clones in expression systems have been used to make recombinant cytokine

Table 17.1 Selected cytokines

Cytokine	Structure	Source	Chromosome	Receptor(s)	Major biological effects	References
IL-1	Two forms IL-1-α (often cell-associated) IL-1-β (often soluble regulator) 33 kD prohormones 17.5 kD mature cytokines Neither has signal peptide	Virtually all nucleated cells including monocytes, fibroblasts and endothelial cells	2	At least 2 types of high affinity receptors	Prototypic pleiotropic cytokine with wide ranging immune, inflammatory, metabolic, CNS and haematopoietic effects including fever induction, B- and T-lymphocyte stimulation, fibroblast activation and prostaglandin production, enhancement of leucocytes binding to vascular endothelium and the induction of a state of negative nitrogen balance	[1, 2, 118]
IL-1-ra	Secreted and intracellular forms 3rd member of IL-1 family	Monocytes Epithelial cells Alveolar macrophages Synovial cells	4	Binds both high affinity IL-1 receptors	Pure IL-1 receptor antagonist No bioactivity in own right	[67]
IL-2	19 kD glycoprotein	T lymphocytes	4	Multimeric IL-2 receptor complex with α- and β-chains	Induces T-cell proliferation Augments B-cell antibody production and proliferation Activates macrophages Induces natural killer cell proliferation and cytotoxic T-lymphocyte killing	[119, 120]

	Structure	Cell source		Receptor	Actions	Ref
IL-3	30–40 kD glycoprotein	T lymphocytes	5	IL-3 and GM-CSF receptors are multimeric structures with distinct α-subunits that compete for a common β-subunit	Stimulates granulocyte, macrophage, megakaryocyte, eosinophil, basophil and erythroid precursor proliferation and differentiation Stimulates mast cell proliferation	[121]
IL-4	140 amino acid glycoprotein	Th2 lymphocytes	5	140 kD structure 553 amino acid cytoplasmic domain	Stimulates B-cell proliferation Induces B-cell, IgE and IgG$_1$ production Stimulates Th2 lymphocyte proliferation Inhibits monocyte/endothelial cell cytokine production	[122]
IL-5	20 kD monomer 40–50 kD in biological fluids	Th2 lymphocytes	5	High affinity multimeric receptor complex Low affinity	Stimulates eosinophil proliferation Activates eosinophils Stimulates B-cell proliferation and immunoglobulin (Ig) production	[123]
IL-6	See text					
IL-7	25 kD glycoprotein	Bone marrow stromal cells Thymic epithelium T lymphocytes	NA	High and low affinity	Stimulates proliferation of pre-B cells Stimulates T-cell proliferation Induces macrophage cytokine production	[124, 125]
IL-8	79, 77 and 72 amino acid moieties between 8 and 10 kD	Alveolar macrophages Monocytes Fibroblasts Endothelial cells Epithelial cells Hepatocytes	4	High and low affinity	Chemotactic factor and activator of granulocytes	[85]

continued on p. 320

Table 17.1 *Continued*

Cytokine	Structure	Source	Chromosome	Receptor(s)	Major biological effects	References
IL-9	20–30 kD glycoprotein	T lymphocytes	5	NA	Prolongs T-cell survival Interacts with IL-3 and IL-4 to induce mast cell proliferation	[126, 127]
IL-10	18 kD polypeptide	Th2 lymphocytes	NA	NA	Inhibits Th1 lymphocyte production of LT, IFN-γ and IL-2. In so doing it inhibits Th1 cell function and decreases DTH-type responses Stimulates thymocyte proliferation Augments B-cell Ia expression Induces mast cell proliferation Inhibits monocyte cytokine production	[73, 74]
IL-11	23 kD	Stromal cells Fibroblasts	NA	NA	Stimulates plasmacytoma proliferation Supports macrophage progenitor proliferation Augments antibody production and IL-3-induced megakaryocyte formation	[128, 129]
IL-12	Heterodimer made up of 40 kD and 35 kD subunits	B lymphocytes	NA	NA	Synergizes with IL-2 in the generation of cytotoxic T lymphocytes and lymphokine-activated T cells Activates natural killer cells Stimulates IFN-γ production Augments antibody production and IL-3-induced megakaryocyte colony formation	[69, 130]
TNF	17.1 kD	Wide range of cells including: macrophage monocytes mast cells Th1 cells Th2 cells	6	2 types of cell-associated receptors Soluble receptor also described	Wide ranging biological effects Activates fibroblasts Activates endothelial cell integrin adhesion molecule expression Activates neutrophils Induces fever and acute phase protein synthesis Induces IL-1, IL-6, IL-8 and colony-stimulating factor production	[131,132]

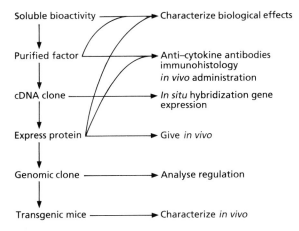

Fig. 17.3 Scientific approach to a cytokine. As noted in the left-hand column, many cytokines are initially identified as soluble bioactivities. They are subsequently purified, their primary structures obtained via cDNA cloning and their cDNA clones expressed to yield recombinant protein. Genomic clones are then isolated to provide structural detail about the genes that encode these cytokines and transgenic mice are produced which allow for a sophisticated understanding of the true *in vivo* role of these molecules. The biological effects of these cytokines can be studied in exquisite detail, taking advantage of cell supernatants, purified protein and recombinant protein. Monospecific neutralizing anti-cytokine antibodies can also be prepared using recombinant cytokine protein. They are extremely useful for tissue immunohistochemistry and can be given *in vivo*. The cDNA clones have been used to study the regulation of cytokine production *in vitro*. Techniques such as *in situ* hybridization also allow one to analyse the sites where cytokine mRNA is accumulating *in vivo*. The availability of large amounts of recombinant protein has allowed recombinant cytokines to be given *in vivo*. The structural information provided by the genomic clones has provided additional insight into the processes regulating cytokine gene transcription.

and recombinant or purified cytokine used to make anti-cytokine antibodies. The biological effects of these agents have been clarified using the highly purified or recombinant cytokines and monospecific anti-cytokine antibodies *in vivo* and *in vitro*. Antibodies against specific cytokines have also been used in tissue immunohistochemical studies to determine the sites of cytokine production in normal and diseased tissues. The cDNAs encoding these molecules have been used in Northern blot, slot blot and nuclear run-on assays to analyse the transcriptional and post-transcriptional processes that regulate cytokine production and in techniques such as *in situ* hybridization that identify the sites of cytokine messenger RNA (mRNA) accumulation *in vivo*. Genomic cloning has delineated the structure of the genes that encode these molecules. It has also provided cytokine promoters which have been analysed to dissect the elements that regulate cytokine gene transcription. Lastly, genomic and cDNA constructs can be introduced into cells at the earliest stage of foetal development resulting in the generation of transgenic animals.

Correlation between the phenotype of the animal and the over- and/or underexpression of a construct allows for a sophisticated analysis of the *in vivo* role of the protein.

Interleukin-6

Initial description and purification

Prior to its designation as a member of the interleukin family, IL-6 acquired a complex nomenclature which reflected its multiple biological effects: its weak antiviral activity resulted in its designation, interferon (IFN)-β_2 [5]; its ability to stimulate the proliferation of malignant B cells resulted in its designation, hybridoma–plasmacytoma growth factor [6]; its ability to induce B-cell differentiation and immunoglobulin (Ig) production resulted in its designation, B-cell differentiation factor [7]; its ability to induce IgG production by immortalized B-cell lines resulted in its designation, B-cell stimulation factor-2 [8]; its ability to induce hepatocyte production of acute phase proteins resulted in its designation, hepatocyte stimulating factor [9]; and its size resulted in the designation, 26 kD protein [10]. Purification of these proteins soon showed their similarity and multifunctional nature [9, 11]. Later cDNA cloning demonstrated their identity [12, 13] and resulted in the adoption of the term IL-6 for this molecule.

cDNA cloning

Characterization of cDNA clones encoding IL-6 has defined its primary structure and provided insight into the regulation of its production. The major transcription product of the IL-6 gene is a 1.3 kilobase (kb) mRNA with three transcription start sites, two poly-adenylation signals and AUUA sequences in its 3′ untranslated region similar to those in other rapidly degraded mRNAs [14, 15]. Its primary translation product is 212 amino acids in length and contains a 28 amino acid hydrophobic signal peptide, which is cleaved in the process of movement into the endoplasmic reticulum. This leaves a 184 amino acid peptide with a predicted molecular weight of approximately 21 kD [12]. This molecule undergoes extensive post-translational modification including N- and O-linked glycosylation, the formation of disulphide bridges and phosphorylation (Fig. 17.4) [14–17]. These modifications are, at least partially, tissue-specific, since endothelial cells preferentially produce a 45 kD form [18], monocytes preferentially produce a 24 kD species [16] and fibroblasts produce 23–25 and 28–30 kD IL-6 moieties [17, 19, 20].

Studies using bioassays, immunoassays (radioimmunoassays, enzyme-linked immunosorbent assays) and Northern blot analysis have demonstrated that IL-6 is produced by a wide variety of cells including mono-

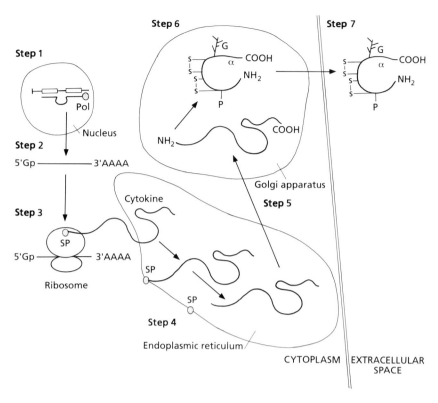

Fig. 17.4 Schematic version of the steps involved in the production of IL-6. The IL-6 gene is transcribed in the nucleus by an appropriate polymerase (Pol; step 1). In the cytoplasm it is appropriately processed including polyadenylation (step 2) and then undergoes translation by association with the multimeric ribosome (step 3). The completed translation product, including its signal peptide (SP), then enters the endoplasmic reticulum and the SP is cleaved before the IL-6 molecule is transported to the Golgi (step 5). In the Golgi post-translational modification occurs including phosphorylation (P), disulphide bridge formation (S—S) and glycosylation (G). The amino (NH_2) and carboxy (COOH) ends of the molecule also assume a position of proximity which is important for the bioactivity of the molecule. After appropriate post-translational modification, the IL-6 molecule is released into the extracellular space (step 7).

cytes, alveolar macrophages, fibroblasts, endothelial cells, mesangial cells, keratinocytes and B and T lymphocytes [16, 21, 22]. A wide variety of stimuli including IL-1, TNF, PDGF, TGF-β, DNA and RNA viruses, poly (I)-poly (C) and endotoxin, stimulate IL-6 production [19, 21–24]. TGF-β, retinoic acid, glucocorticoids and agents that increase cyclic adenosine monophosphate can inhibit IL-6 production under appropriate circumstances [22, 23, 25]. Interestingly, different cells produce IL-6 in response to different stimuli. For example, human lung fibroblasts produce large amounts of IL-6 in response to IL-1, modest amounts of IL-6 in response to TNF and little, if any, in response to endotoxin. In contrast, circulating blood monocytes and resident alveolar macrophages produce large amounts of IL-6 in response to endotoxin and minimal, if any, IL-6 in response to IL-1 or TNF [21].

By simultaneously assessing IL-6 protein production, mRNA accumulation and gene transcription (using nuclear run-on techniques), the transcriptional and post-transcriptional processes that stimulate and inhibit IL-6 production have been characterized. In virtually all cases, alterations in IL-6 protein production are associated with proportional alterations in IL-6 mRNA accumulation. Thus, pretranslational mechanisms appear to be most important in regulating IL-6 production. A number of studies have shown that alterations in IL-6 gene transcription and IL-6 mRNA degradation contribute to these pretranslational processes [19, 26].

Genomic cloning

The IL-6 gene has been localized to chromosome 7 [27]. Like the granulocyte−macrophage colony-stimulating factor (GM-CSF) gene it has five exons and four introns. To understand the processes regulating IL-6 transcription, the IL-6 promoter (obtained via genomic cloning) has been extensively analysed. These studies have shown that IL-6 transcription is regulated, to a significant degree, by nuclear proteins that bind to specific sequences (response elements) in the IL-6 promoter. At least three different stimulatory response elements have been described [28−30]. Interestingly, when steroids combine with the glucocorticoid nuclear receptor, the complex binds to the IL-6 promoter covering these stimulatory response elements and the TATA box, a regulatory sequence involved in gene transcription; this inhibits IL-6 transcription [25].

Characterization of biological effects of IL-6 using recombinant IL-6 and anti-IL-6 antibodies

Full-length IL-6 cDNA has been used in expression constructs to produce large amounts of recombinant IL-6 protein. The biological effects of recombinant IL-6 protein have been extensively investigated and neutralizing anti-IL-6 antibodies have been prepared. These studies have demonstrated that IL-6 has a diverse spectrum of biological activities and implicated IL-6 in the pathogenesis of a number of important diseases [22].

B-cell effects

IL-6 up-regulates IL-4-dependent IgE synthesis and mediates the terminal differentiation of B cells into immunoglobulin-producing cells [7, 8, 22, 31]. In the presence of IL-6, activated B cells are induced to produce IgG, IgM and IgA. IL-6 functions exclusively as a differentiation factor in normal B-cell development. It does not support the proliferation of normal B cells. In contrast, IL-6 is a potent growth factor for certain B-cell hybridoma and plasmacytoma lines [6].

T-cell effects

CD4[+] and CD8[+] thymocytes express IL-6 receptors and proliferate in response to IL-6. IL-6 also enhances the lectin-induced proliferation of peripheral blood T cells, interacts in a synergistic fashion with IL-1 in stimulating mouse thymocyte proliferation [20] and induces IL-2 receptor expression [32].

The acute phase response

The acute phase and febrile responses are part of the host's attempt to control and limit the tissue damage which occurs as a result of a wide variety of insults [9, 33]. IL-1, TNF and IL-6 are endogenous pyrogens [34]. IL-1, TNF, hepatocyte-stimulating factor III/leukaemia inhibiting factor and IL-6 [9, 33] regulate the acute phase response. IL-6, however, appears to be the most important. It induces hepatic uptake of amino acids and zinc, decreases gluconeogenesis, increases metallothionine production and regulates the production of acute phase proteins in a complex fashion. Gauldie et al. [3] showed that during an acute phase response IL-6 is not produced locally in the liver. Instead, IL-6 appears to be produced at the site of injury. It then travels in the circulation to the liver and stimulates hepatocytes in an endocrine manner.

Haematopoiesis

IL-6, alone or in combination with granulocyte colony-stimulating factor (G-CSF), GM-CSF, erythropoietin, IL-3 and/or IL-4, can modulate the proliferation and maturation of myeloid, erythroid and megakaryocytic lineage cells. When given to mice in vivo IL-6 stimulates pluripotent stem cell colony formation, enhances marrow transplant repopulation and accelerates total haematopoietic recovery after radiation [35]. IL-6 infusions also result in a pronounced reticulocytosis, bone marrow erythroid hyperplasia and thrombocytosis [36].

Endocrine effects

IL-6 stimulates adrenocorticotrophic hormone (ACTH) production [37]. It also stimulates the release of corticotrophin-releasing factor (CRF), pituitary cell secretion of luteinizing hormone, follicle stimulating hormone and prolactin, and adrenal cortical cells to produce corticosterone.

In vivo *effects*

In keeping with its impressive *in vitro* regulatory effects, IL-6 also appears to play an important role *in vivo* in a variety of infectious, inflammatory and malignant disorders [22].

Infectious disorders. Elevated levels of IL-6 have been found in patients with a wide variety of viral and bacterial infections [38−41]. Importantly, the levels of IL-6 in the serum of patients with meningococcal and other causes of sepsis [41] correlate with patient mortality. In keeping with these findings, exposure of normal human volunteers to intravenous endotoxin induces detectable levels of TNF followed 45 min to 1 h later by elevated serum IL-6 levels [42]. Many feel that IL-6 production in sepsis is a protective response. However, recent studies have implicated IL-6 in the pathogenesis of this disorder since anti-IL-6 antibodies markedly reduce the mortality of mice that received an otherwise lethal inoculum of bacteria [43]. IL-6 may also play a role in HIV-1 infection and HIV-1-related disorders since patients with HIV-1 infection have elevated levels of IL-6 in their serum, Kaposi's sarcoma cells produce IL-6 and proliferate in response to IL-6, and IL-6 directly up-regulates the production of HIV-1 in acutely, as well as chronically, infected monocytic cells [22, 44].

Inflammatory disorders. IL-6 levels are elevated in the serum within 7 h after incision in elective surgical procedures. The amount of IL-6 that is produced postoperatively correlates with the length as well as the complexity of the surgical procedure [45]. Elevated levels of IL-6 are also seen in patients with cutaneous burns, acute transplant rejection [46], insulin-dependent diabetes mellitus, Castleman's disease [22, 44], psoriasis [47], mesangio-proliferative glomerulonephritis [22, 44, 48] and Kawasaki's disease. The demonstration that keratinocytes from patients with psoriasis and mesangial cells from patients with mesangio-proliferative glomerulonephritis produce IL-6 and proliferate in response to IL-6 suggests that IL-6 is an autocrine and/or paracrine growth factor in these disorders [48−50]. IL-6 may be particularly important in arthritic disorders since the levels of synovial and circulating IL-6 are elevated in rheumatoid arthritis and elevated levels of IL-6 are also found in the synovial fluid of patients with septic arthritis, polymyalgia rheumatica, traumatic arthritis, gout, pseudogout, degenerative arthritis and ankylosing spondylitis [40, 51]. Patients with systemic lupus erythematosus (SLE) also have elevated serum levels of IL-6 [52].

Malignancy. Elevated levels of IL-6 have been noted in multiple myeloma, acute myeloblastic leukaemia (AML), Hodgkin's disease, non-Hodgkin's lymphomas, mycosis fungoides and a variety of solid tumours including hypernephromas and cardiac myxomas [22, 44, 53−55]. Myeloma and hypernephroma cells often proliferate in response to IL-6, suggesting that IL-6 plays a role as an autocrine or paracrine growth factor in these disorders [55].

Transgenic modelling

Transgenic technology allows recombinant DNA to be inserted into all of the cells of a living organism. Depending on the methods and construct employed, the *in vivo* effects of cytokine overproduction, cytokine under-production and cytokine production in an unusual location can be studied. Mice which overproduce IL-6 have been created by two separate means. Suematsu *et al.* produced a transgenic line in which the IL-6 gene was constitutively expressed under the control of the human immunoglobulin heavy chain enhancer. These animals experienced a massive plasmacytosis of lymphoid and non-lymphoid tissues and developed membranoproliferative glomerulonephritis [56]. IL-6 over-production was achieved in another model by infecting marrow stem cells with a retroviral IL-6 expression vector. These animals developed a condition resembling Castleman's disease, with anaemia, thrombocytosis, polyclonal hypergammaglobulinaemia and plasmacytoma formation [57]. Although the plasmacytomas observed in these animals are poly-clonal, repeatedly backcrossing transgenic animals with BALB/c mice resulted in the production of progeny with stable, monoclonal, trans-plantable plasmacytomas containing chromosomal translocations [22, 54].

Cytokine-producing cells in the lung

The normal lung has the ability to clear large quantities of inhaled particulates and antigens without developing an inflammatory response. However, acute and chronic inflammatory and fibrotic lung disorders are a common cause of morbidity and mortality. Cytokines and cytokine networking appear to play an important role in these very different responses. Before one can attempt to synthesize how cytokines contribute to these different responses, one must understand the cytokine profile of a number of important pulmonary effector cells.

Alveolar macrophages

The alveolar macrophage responds to many stimuli by producing a wide variety of cytokines that regulate pulmonary homeostasis. In response to stimuli such as endotoxin, it produces IL-1, TNF, IL-6, IL-8, TGF-β, PDGF-like peptides, TGF-α, insulin-like growth factor-1 (IGF-1), bFGF and IFN-γ [21, 58−66]. Interestingly, the capacity of the alveolar macrophage to produce these inflammatory cytokines differs significantly from its precursor cell, the circulating blood monocyte. On a per cell basis normal human alveolar macrophages stimulated with endotoxin elaborate significantly less soluble IL-1-β and significantly greater quantities of IL-6 and TNF than autologous blood monocytes [58, 59]. Alveolar macrophages also produce more IL-1 receptor antagonist (IL-1-ra) than blood monocytes [67]. The limited ability of the alveolar macrophage to elaborate IL-1-β appears to be due to a limitation in its ability to process the IL-1-β precursor [58]. The biological importance of the differences between monocytes and macrophages is not entirely clear. However, it is tempting to speculate that the decreased ability of the alveolar macrophage to produce soluble IL-1-β and its heightened ability to produce IL-1-ra are mechanisms that prevent routine loads of particulates from inducing pneumonia. As a result, mild or moderate insults might trigger either no, or only a mild, inflammatory response. In contrast, more severe insults would result in an influx of monocytes into the lung, as seen in sarcoidosis [68] and certain experimental models of pulmonary inflammation. This would lead to enhanced local production of IL-1 and heightened inflammation as a result of the direct effects of IL-1 and synergistic interactions between IL-1 and IL-6, TGF-β, IL-12 and TNF [19, 20, 23, 69].

Lymphocytes

In normal non-smoking subjects, less than 10% of lavage cells are lymphocytes and the majority are T cells. However, alterations in lymphocyte numbers are seen in smokers and in a number of lung diseases characterized by chronic inflammation [70]. In diseases such as sarcoidosis, increases in CD4$^+$ lymphocytes are noted histologically and by bronchoalveolar lavage [71]. In contrast, hypersensitivity pneumonitis, also a granulomatous disorder, is most commonly associated with a CD8$^+$ (suppressor cell) alveolitis [72]. In these disorders lymphocytes appear to be activated *in vivo*. For example, enhanced expression of the T-cell IL-2 receptor has been repeatedly noted upon in the study of T cells of patients with systemic sarcoidosis [71].

In vivo antibody/eosinophil mediated and delayed-type hypersensitivity reactions are often mutually exclusive [73, 74]. Recent advances in our understanding of CD4$^+$ (helper) lymphocytes have provided insight into the mechanisms that may be responsible for this exclusivity. Long-term mouse helper T-cell clones can be divided into two major classes based on the patterns of cytokines that they secrete in response to antigen or lectin stimulation. Th1 clones produce IL-2, IFN-γ and lymphotoxin, while Th2 clones secrete IL-4, IL-5, IL-6, P600 and IL-10. Both types of clones secrete IL-3, GM-CSF, TNF, preproenkephalin and several other inflammatory proteins (Fig. 17.5) [73]. As a result, these cells have very different functional profiles. Th1 cells preferentially induce

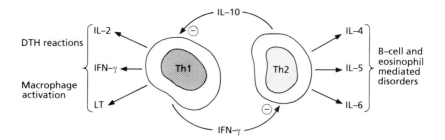

Fig. 17.5 Demonstration of the interactions between Th1 and Th2 lymphocytes. Stimulated Th1 lymphocytes produce IL-2, IFN-γ and lymphotoxin (LT). As a result, they play an important role in delayed-type hypersensitivity (DTH) reactions and macrophage activation. Stimulated Th2 cells produce IL-4, IL-5, IL-6 and IL-10. As a result, they play an important role in B-cell and eosinophil-mediated processes. The type of response that predominates appears to result from cross-talk between these two populations of cells. Th2-derived IL-10 inhibits Th1 cell cytokine production. Th1-derived IFN-γ inhibits Th2 cell proliferation.

delayed-type hypersensitivity reactions and Th2 cells provide help for B-cell antibody secretion (particularly for IgE responses) and eosinophil-mediated processes. The degree to which humoral, eosinophilic and delayed-type hypersensitivity reactions predominate may reflect the relative balance of IL-10, which inhibits Th1 cell cytokine production, and IFN-γ which inhibits Th1 cell proliferation (Fig. 17.5) [73, 74]. This may be particularly important in atopic asthma. In keeping with the importance of IgE and eosinophils in this disorder, bronchoalveolar lavage of these patients reveals an activated IL-3, IL-4, IL-5 and GM-CSF producing Th2-like T-cell population [75].

T-cells express heterodimeric membrane receptors for specific antigens. The characteristics of the two chains that make up these receptors allow T cells to be classified as α/β cells or γ/δ cells. The majority of $CD8^+$ and $CD4^+$ cells are $α/β^+$. Their cytokine profile has been reviewed above. γ/δ cells may be particularly important in the lung since they tend to assume a submucosal and mucosal location [76], appear in increased numbers during the resolution phase of influenza pneumonia [77] and may be increased in some patients with sarcoidosis [78]. Recent studies suggest that subsets of γ/δ T cells may have a unique cytokine profile characterized by the production of IL-2 and GM-CSF [79].

Fibroblasts

Most of the research on fibroblasts has focused on their production of structural and matrix proteins. However, it is becoming increasingly clear that fibroblasts are also important immune-effector cells at sites of inflammation. When appropriately stimulated, fibroblasts produce significant quantities of IL-6, IL-8, IL-1-α, colony stimulating factors, epidermal growth factor (EGF), IGF-1, stem cell growth factor, IL-11 and TGF-β [80]. IL-1 and TNF are major inducers of fibroblast IL-6, IL-1-α, IL-8 and IL-11 production. Importantly, incubating fibroblasts with IL-1 and TNF in combination results in a synergistic up-regulation of these cytokines [19, 81]. Stimulation with IL-1 and TNF in combination also causes fibroblasts to accumulate intracellular IL-1-β prohormone, but elaboration of biologically active extracellular IL-1-β protein does not occur [82]. Fibroblasts and alveolar macrophages are often capable of elaborating the same inflammatory cytokine. However, maximal production of these cytokines often occurs in response to different signals. Endotoxin is a potent stimulator of macrophage cytokine production while stimulating lung fibroblast cytokine production in a very modest fashion. In contrast, fibroblasts produce great quantities of inflammatory cytokines in response to IL-1 and TNF while monocytes respond to these cytokines minimally under most circumstances [21, 22, 80]. These findings suggest that alveolar macrophages produce inflammatory cytokines in a stimulus-specific fashion. In contrast, fibroblasts produce inflammatory cytokines in response to the IL-1 and/or TNF produced by macrophages responding to many different agents. This fibroblast response appears to be stimulus-independent and likely serves to augment pulmonary inflammation non-specifically.

Cytokine networks in the lung

Figure 17.6 is a simplified working model of the interactions of the interleukins and other selected cytokines in the regulation of lymphocyte and macrophage accumulation in the lung. The majority of alveolar macrophages in the lung are derived from circulating blood monocytes. They enter the lung along chemotactic gradients and have a limited capacity for self-replication [83]. Infectious agents and/or noxious stimuli reach the lung via the airways and stimulate resident alveolar macrophages to produce TNF, IL-6, IL-8, TGF-β and modest amounts of soluble IL-1-β. IL-8, in conjunction with IL-1, TNF and other neutrophil chemotactic agents, attracts neutrophils and initiates an acute inflammatory response. These and other inflammatory cytokines, in the presence of an appropriate antigen, an appropriate antigen-presenting cell and an appropriate major histocompatibility (MHC) antigen match, cause T-cell activation. Activated Th1 lymphocytes express high affinity IL-2 receptors and produce IL-2, IL-3 and IFN-γ. IL-2 acts in an autocrine fashion to stimulate T-cell proliferation and also serves to stimulate the growth of cytotoxic T lymphocytes (CTL) and natural killer (NK) cells. The IL-3 that is produced stimulates haematopoiesis and the IFN-γ that is produced activates local macrophages, stimulates CTL and NK cells and inhibits Th2 lymphocyte proliferation. The Th2 cells produce IL-3, IL-4, IL-5 and

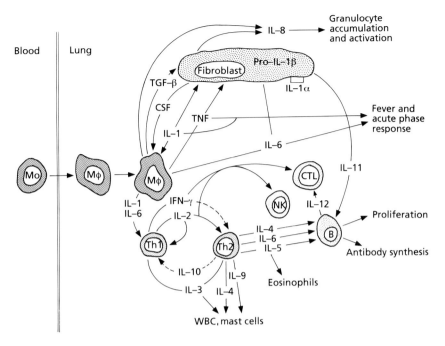

Fig. 17.6 Simplified schema of the major cytokine–cytokine interactions regulating macrophage and lymphocyte accumulation in the lung. B lymphocyte (B), Th1 helper T lymphocyte (Th1), Th2 helper T lymphocyte (Th2), natural killer lymphocyte (NK), cytotoxic T lymphocyte (CTL), monocytes (Mo) and macrophages (Mø). Solid lines indicate stimulation and broken lines indicate inhibition.

IL-6. IL-4 induces IgE production and in conjunction with IL-5 and IL-6 induces the proliferation and terminal differentiation of B cells into antibody-forming plasma cells. T cells also produce IL-9 which acts as a mast cell stimulator. Activated B cells are the likely source of IL-12 which stimulates CTL and lymphocyte-activated killer cell (LAK cell) proliferation. The IL-5 that is produced plays an important role in stimulating eosinophil growth and differentiation. The IL-1, TNF and IL-6 that are produced also gain access to the systemic circulation and stimulate hepatocyte production of acute phase proteins and induce fever. The degree to which B-cell and eosinophilic vs. delayed-type hypersensitivity reactions predominate probably depends on the balance between the production of IL-10 vs. IFN-γ.

The model as described above does not explain why some pulmonary insults result in transient inflammatory responses and others result in chronic pulmonary inflammation. Although the exact determinants of the severity and chronicity of inflammatory events are still a topic of investigation, a number of processes have been identified which, when initiated, can contribute to the development of chronic inflammation. First, the recruitment of blood monocytes in the lung would enhance local IL-1-β production. IL-1, via its direct effects and its ability to synergize with IL-6, TNF, TGF-β and IL-12 [19, 20, 23, 69], would augment a wide variety of pulmonary inflammatory responses. IL-1—IL-6 synergy would also further augment T-cell proliferation and T-cell activation [20]. Second, IL-1, TNF and TGF-β also have major effects on stromal cells. Individually and synergistically these cytokines induce the production of colony-stimulating factors, IL-6, IL-11, IL-1-α, the IL-1-β prohormone and IL-8 [19, 20, 23, 80—82, 84]. The colony-stimulating factors further enhance macrophage activation, IL-8 activates and recruits neutrophils [85] and IL-6 and IL-11 have major roles in the stimulation and proliferation of B cells and T cells [20, 32, 84]. As the result of this interaction, the stroma probably changes from a non-supportive environment to an environment that generates potent proinflammatory signals. This change may be a requirement for the development of a chronic pulmonary inflammatory response.

The fibrotic response in the normal lung can be stimulated for wound healing and lung anabolism and inhibited when healing is complete to prevent the development of pathological fibrosis. The degree to which basement membrane integrity is maintained and the extent of alveolar epithelial injury determine, to a great extent, whether normal or dysfunctional scarring occurs after pulmonary injury [86]. The role that cytokines play in regulating both normal and dysfunctional scarring has also been a topic of intense investigation. Platelet aggregation at sites of injury results in TGF-β, PDGF and EGF release. Macrophage activation results in IL-1, TNF, TGF-β, IFN-γ, PDGF, TGF-α and IGF-1 release. T-cell activation results in TGF-β, IFN-γ and lymphotoxin elaboration. Under appropriate circumstances, each cytokine has been shown to stimulate fibroblast proliferation and/or collagen production. Interestingly, IFN-γ and TNF individually can also inhibit fibroblast proliferation and collagen production [87, 88]. In addition, a number of laboratories have demonstrated that cytokines in combination tend to inhibit fibroblast function to a greater extent than they do individually. IL-1 and TNF in combination, IL-1 and TGF-β in combination and IFN-γ and TNF in combination all synergistically inhibit fibroblast function [89—91]. The complexity of the effects of cytokines and cytokine combinations on fibroblast function can clearly provide the stimulatory and inhibitory signals needed to regulate the fibrotic response appropriately. The complex interactions in this network also allow for a plausible hypothesis that explains the specialized pattern of centripetal scarring seen with granulomas and walled-off abscesses [92].

Therapeutic implications

Dysregulated cytokine production has been implicated in the pathogenesis of a large number of diseases (Table 17.2). Information of this sort has

Table 17.2 Selected cytokine—disease associations in pulmonary and critical-care medicine

Disease	Cytokine	References
Sepsis/endotoxaemia	Dysregulated/exaggerated IL-1, TNF, IL-6 and IL-8 production	[2, 41–43, 67, 118, 133, 134]
Sarcoidosis	Dysregulated/exaggerated IL-1-β, IL-2, TNF, G-CSF, GM-CSF, M-CSF, IFN-γ and IGF-1 production	[61, 62, 135–140]
Asthma	Dysregulated/exaggerated IL-3, IL-4, IL-5 and GM-CSF production	[75]
Idiopathic pulmonary fibrosis	Dysregulated/elevated IL-1, IL-8, PDGF, IGF-1 and TGF-β production	[61, 65, 141–144]

palpable clinical relevance since it leads to a vast number of new therapeutic options for patients with these disorders. Quite simply, once it is known that a cytokine is involved in a pathogenic process, its activity can be modified or the response of its target tissues modulated. As outlined in Table 17.3, cytokine activity can be modified by altering cytokine production, the administration of exogenous recombinant cytokine, gene implantation or interventions that block cytokine function. Target cell responses can be altered by modulating the expression of cytokine receptors, altering the function of the cytokine receptor or by killing the target cell using ligands coupled to specific toxins. Additional information about these approaches and clinically relevant examples of their utilization are detailed below.

Cytokine production can be blocked using drugs that block cytokine synthesis. Without knowing it, physicians may have been inhibiting cytokines for a long period of time, since it is now appreciated that a significant aspect of the immunosuppressive effects of corticosteroids and the immunomodulatory effects of retinoids result from their ability to regulate the production of IL-1 [93], TNF [94], IL-6 [25], TGF-β [95] and other cytokines. Cytokine production can also be regulated using antisense oligonucleotides. Antisense oligonucleotides are synthetic DNA molecules that correspond to the antisense (backwards) version of cytokine mRNA. They are transfected into cells using a variety of techniques. In these cells they bind to the mRNA that encodes the cytokine and prevent it from being translated into functional protein. *In vitro* studies suggest that this approach has significant potential. For example, IL-6 acts as an autocrine growth factor in plasma cell neoplasms since many myeloma and plasmacytoma cells constitutively produce IL-6 and proliferate in response to IL-6 [53–55]. Transfection with antisense IL-6 oligonucleotides decreases the proliferation and tumorigenicity of these cells causing them to take on a less malignant phenotype [55].

Table 17.3 Cytokine-based therapeutic options

Regulation of cytokine effector function

1 Regulation of cytokine production:
   (a) drugs;
   (b) antisense oligonucleotides.

2 Administration of recombinant cytokine.

3 Gene implantation.

4 Regulation of cytokine bioactivity:
   (a) drugs that bind cytokines;
   (b) anti-cytokine antibodies;
   (c) soluble cytokine receptors.

Regulation of target cell response

1 Block cytokine production:
   (a) drugs;
   (b) antisense oligonucleotides.

2 Block receptor function:
   (a) inhibit receptor signal transduction;
   (b) antireceptor antibodies;
   (c) non-functional cytokine ligand.

3 Kill target cell:
   (a) antireceptor antibodies coupled to toxin;
   (b) cytokine ligand coupled to toxin.

Techniques of modern molecular biology now allow large quantities of recombinant cytokine to be produced with relative ease. This has resulted in a rapid expansion of our knowledge of the therapeutic potential of these agents. When given systemically, G-CSF and GM-CSF appear to promote bone marrow recovery in patients that have received cancer chemotherapy and in those with aplastic anaemia [96, 97]. IL-2 has proven useful in salvage protocols of patients with metastatic malignancy [98, 99] and IL-3 may prove useful in patients with Diamond–Blackfan syndrome since it induces haematopoiesis when added to their bone marrow *in vitro* [100]. Cytokines may be particularly useful in the treatment of pulmonary disorders since administration via aerosol allows for lung-specific drug delivery and may minimize systemic side effects [101].

Gene implantation is an exciting area of medical technology in which genes encoding important molecules, including cytokines, can be introduced into various locations in the body. Studies of adenosine deaminase deficiency have shown that the adenosine deaminase gene can be transfected into a patient's leucocytes and that these cells produce functional adenosine deaminase protein [102]. Reinfusion of these leucocytes into the donor potentially can reverse the severe immunodeficiency associated with this disorder and is being pursued in clinical trials [102]. Recent studies have demonstrated that a catheter-directed process can be used to implant genes at specific arterial locations [103], intratracheal or intravascularly administered liposomes can selectively transfect functioning genes into the lung [104] and adenovirus vectors can transfect respiratory epithelium *in vivo* [105, 106]. This latter technique may be particularly useful in α_1-antitrypsin deficiency and cystic fibrosis, since adenovirus vectors have been used to transfer successfully the human α_1-antitrypsin and cystic fibrosis transmembrane conductance regulator genes *in vivo* [105, 106].

The biological activity of a cytokine can be modulated by drugs that inactivate the cytokine, by anti-cytokine antibodies that neutralize the cytokine and by soluble non-bioactive versions of cytokine receptors which bind the cytokine. There is an enlarging body of data supporting the utility of these last two approaches. Neutralizing antibodies against TNF [107] and IL-6 [43] increase survival in animal models of sepsis. Antibodies against TNF also suppress murine lupus erythematosus and ameliorate lung inflammation and fibrosis in models of bleomycin lung injury and silicosis [108–110]. Soluble forms of the TNF and IL-2 receptors occur naturally and soluble forms of the IL-1 and IL-4 receptors have been produced by genetic engineering [111, 112]. The soluble IL-1 receptor has been studied most extensively. When injected into mice it delays the rejection of grafted tissues [112]. This is felt to result from a competition for the cytokine between non-bioactive soluble receptors and bioactive cell-associated receptors. The therapeutic utility of mouse monoclonal antibodies against human cytokines is limited by the immunogenicity of the immunoglobulin molecule [113]. As a result, humanized mouse–human hybrids have been generated [113]. The naturally occurring and genetically engineered soluble cytokine receptors do not suffer from this limitation [111].

Drugs and antisense oligonucleotides can be used to modulate the expression of specific cytokine receptors and thereby regulate cytokine bioactivity. For example, the efficacy of retinoids in psoriasis may be related to their ability to inhibit IL-6 receptor expression [114]. Alternatively, the effect of a cytokine can be altered with: (a) drugs that specifically block the signal transduction processes employed by the cytokine receptor; (b) non-functional ligand analogues; and (c) antibodies that block the cytokine receptor. The IL-1 receptor antagonist (IL-1-ra) is a naturally occurring non-functional ligand analogue [67]. This member of the IL-1 family of proteins binds both type I and type II IL-1 receptors but does not transduce a signal. As a result, it blocks many of the effects of IL-1. Since it is a naturally occurring molecule it can be administered repeatedly without danger of sensitization. It has been shown to improve survival in animal models of sepsis [67] and decrease injury in animal models of immune complex colitis [115].

Antibodies against the IL-2 receptor also prevent the development of experimental diabetes mellitus [116] and transplant rejection [113].

A number of pathological processes are associated with the clonal expansion of inflammatory and/or malignant cells. If it is known that these cells express a specific cytokine receptor, they can be killed by treating them with anti-cytokine antibodies coupled to a specific toxin or the cytokine ligand coupled to a specific toxin [113]. The utility of this approach for malignancies that are perpetuated by autocrine growth factor production (such as IL-6 in multiple myeloma) is intuitively obvious [113]. Since this approach can provide cell-specific antigen-specific immunosuppression [117], it is also an exciting alternative to the non-specific immunosuppressives presently being employed clinically. This has been nicely demonstrated in transplantation where treatment with an IL-2-toxin conjugate reverses transplant rejection without altering the ability of the animal to respond appropriately to other stimuli [113].

Conclusions

Cytokine biology is a field in its infancy. The cytokine networks involved in various forms of inflammation and wound healing still need elucidation and their dysregulation in disease needs definition. In addition, our ability to differentiate between physiological and pathological cytokine production needs to be refined. However, there is little question that the interactions of cell biology, molecular biology and cytokine biology have opened up impressive new frontiers for medical therapeutics. As a result of this new knowledge, modern medicine will soon turn to the use of recombinant cytokines, anti-cytokine antibodies, soluble cytokine receptors, gene implantation, antisense oligonucleotides and other strategies to control inflammatory and fibrotic processes and thereby influence the outcome of human disease.

References

1 Dunn CJ. Cytokines as mediators of chronic inflammatory disease. In: Kimball ES, ed. *Cytokines and Inflammation*. Boca Raton, FL: CRC Press, Inc., 1991: 1–8.
2 Mizel SB. The interleukins. *FASEB J* 1989; 3: 2379–88.
3 Gauldie J, Northemann W, Fey GH. IL-6 functions as an exocrine hormone in inflammation. Hepatocytes undergoing acute phase responses require exogenous IL-6. *J Immunol* 1990; 144: 3804–08.
4 Sporn MB, Roberts AB. Peptide growth factors are multifunctional. *Nature* 1988; 332: 217–19.
5 Weissenbach J, Chernajovsky Y, Zeevi M *et al.* Two interferon mRNAs in human fibroblasts: *in vitro* translation and *Escherichia coli* cloning studies. *Proc Natl Acad Sci USA* 1980; 77: 7152–56.
6 Nordan R, Pumphrey J, Rudikoff S. Purification and NH_2 terminal amino acid sequence of a plasmacytoma growth factor derived from the murine macrophage cell line, P388D1. *J Immunol* 1987; 139: 813–17.

7 Hirano T, Teranishi T, Lin B *et al.* Human helper T-cell factor(s). IV. Demonstration of a human late-acting B cell differentiation factor acting on *Staphylococcus aureus* Cowan I-stimulated B cells. *J Immunol* 1984; 133: 798−802.

8 Teranishi T, Hirano T, Naomichi A *et al.* Human helper T cell factor(s) (ThF). II. Induction of IgG production in B lymphoblastoid cell lines and identification of T cell replacing factor (TRF)-like factor(s). *J Immunol* 1982; 128: 1903−8.

9 Gauldie J, Richards C, Harnish D *et al.* Interferon-β2/BSF-2 shares identity with monocyte-derived hepatocyte stimulating factor (HSF) and regulates the major acute phase protein response in liver cells. *Proc Natl Acad Sci USA* 1987; 85: 7251−5.

10 Content J, DeWit L, Pierard D *et al.* Secretory proteins induced in human fibroblasts under conditions used for the production of interferon beta. *Proc Natl Acad Sci USA* 1982; 79: 2768−72.

11 Poupart P, Vandenabeele P, Caypahs S *et al.* B cell growth modulating and differentiating activity of recombinant human 26-kD protein (BSF-2, HuIFN-β$_2$, HPGF). *EMBO J* 1987; 6: 1219−24.

12 Hirano T, Yasukawa K, Harada H *et al.* Complementary DNA for a novel human interleukin and (BSF-2) that induces B lymphocytes to produce immunoglobulin. *Nature* 1986; 324: 73−6.

13 Brakenhoff JP, deGroot ER, Evers R *et al.* Molecular cloning and expression of hybridoma growth factor in *Escherichia coli. J Immunol* 1987; 139: 4116−21.

14 Ray A, Sassone-Corsi P, Sehgal PB. A multiple cytokine- and second-messenger responsive element in the enhancer of the human IL-6 gene: similarities with c-*fos* gene regulation. *Mol Cell Biol* 1989; 9: 5537−47.

15 Yasukawa K, Hirano T, Watanabe Y *et al.* Structure and function of human B cell stimulatory factor-2 (BSF-2/IL-6) gene. *EMBO J* 1987; 6: 2939−45.

16 May LT, Ghrayeb J, Santhanam U *et al.* Synthesis and secretion of multiple forms of β$_2$-interferon/B-cell differentiation factor 2/hepatocyte-stimulating factor by human fibroblasts and monocytes. *J Biol Chem* 1988; 263: 7760−6.

17 Santhanam U, Ghrayeb J, Sehgal PB *et al.* Post-translational modifications of human interleukin-6. *Arch Biochem Biophys* 1989; 274: 161−70.

18 May LT, Torcia G, Cozzolino F *et al.* Interleukin-6 gene expression in human endothelial cells: RNA start sites, multiple IL-6 proteins, and inhibition of pro-liferation. *Biochem Biophys Res Commun* 1989; 159: 991−8.

19 Elias JA, Lentz V. IL-1 and tumor necrosis factor synergistically stimulate fibroblast IL-6 production and stabilize IL-6 messenger RNA. *J Immunol* 1990; 145: 161−6.

20 Elias JA, Trinchieri G, Beck JM *et al.* A synergistic interaction of IL-6 and IL-1 mediates the thymocyte-stimulating activity produced by recombinant IL-1-stimulated fibroblasts. *J Immunol* 1989; 142: 509−14.

21 Kotloff RM, Little J, Elias JA. Human alveolar macrophage and blood monocyte interleukin-6 production. *Am J Respir Cell Mol Biol* 190; 3: 497−505.

22 Zitnik R, Elias JA. Interleukin-6 in the lung. In: Kelly J. ed. Cytokines of the Lung. In *Lung Biology in Health and Disease*, Marcel Dekker, Inc., New York, NY. 1992: 229−80.

23 Elias JA, Lentz V, Cummings P. Transforming growth factor-β regulation of IL-6 production by unstimulated and IL-1 stimulated human fibroblasts. *J Immunol* 1991; 146: 3437−43.

24 Ray A, Tatter SB, May LT *et al.* Activation of human β$_2$-interferon/hepatocyte-stimulating factor/interleukin-6 promoter by cytokines, viruses, and second messenger agonists. *Proc Natl Acad Sci USA* 1988; 85: 6701−5.

25 Ray A, LaForge KS, Sehgal PB. On the mechanism for efficient repression of the interleukin-6 promoter by glucocorticoids: enhancer, TATA box, and RNA start site (Inr motif) occlusion. *Mol Cell Biol* 1990; 10: 5736−46.

26 Akashi M, Loussararian AH, Adelman DC *et al.* Role of lymphotoxin in expression of interleukin-6 in human fibroblasts. *J Clin Invest* 1990; 85: 121−9.

27 Bowcock AM, Kidd JR, Lathrop GM *et al.* The human 'interferon β2/hepatocyte stimulating factor/interleukin-6' gene: DNA polymorphism studies and localization to chromosome 7p21. *Genomics* 1988; 3: 8−16.

28 Ray A, Sassone-Corsi P, Sehgal PB. A multiple cytokine- and second messenger-responsive element in the enhancer of the human interleukin-6 gene: similarities with c-*fos* gene regulation. *Mol Cell Biol* 1989; 9: 5537−47.

29 Akira S, Isshiki H, Sugita T *et al.* A nuclear factor for IL-6 expression (NF-IL6) is a member of a C/EBP family. *EMBO J* 1990; 9: 1897.

30 Shimizu H, Mitomo K, Watanabe T *et al.* Involvement of a NF-kB-like transcription factor in the activation of the interleukin-6 gene by inflammatory lymphokines. *Mol Cell Biol* 1990; 10: 561−8.

31 Muraguchi A, Hirano T, Tang B *et al.* The essential role of B cell stimulatory factor 2 (BSF-2/IL-6) for the terminal differentiation of B cells. *J Exp Med* 1988; 167: 332−44.

32 Baroja ML, Ceuppens JL, VanDamme J *et al.* Cooperation between an anti-T cell (anti-CD28) monoclonal antibody and monocyte-produced IL-6 in the induction of T cell responsiveness to IL-2. *J Immunol* 1988; 141: 1502−7.

33 Baumann H, Richards C, Gauldie J. Interaction among hepatocyte stimulating factors, interleukin-1, and glucocorticoids for regulation of acute phase plasma proteins in human hepatoma (HepG2) cells. *J Immunol* 1987; 139: 4122−8.

34 LeMay L, Vander A, Kluger MJ. Role of interleukin-6 in fever in rats. *Am J Physiol* 1990; 258: R798−803.

35 Patchen ML, MacVittie TJ, Williams JL *et al.* Administration of interleukin-6 stimulates multilineage hematopoiesis and accelerates recovery from radiation-induced hematopoietic depression. *Blood* 1991; 77: 472−80.

36 Ulich TR, del Castillo J, Guo K. *In vivo* hematologic effects of recombinant interleukin-6 on hematopoiesis and circulating numbers of RBCs and WBCs. *Blood* 1989; 73: 108.

37 Naitoh Y, Fukata J, Tominga T *et al.* Interleukin-6 stimulates the secretion of adrenocorticotrophic hormone in conscious, freely moving rats. *Biochem Biophys Res Commun* 1988; 155: 1459−63.

38 Frei K, Leist TP, Meager A *et al.* Production of B cell stimulatory factor-2 and interferon-γ in the central nervous system during viral meningitis and encephalitis. Evaluation in a murine model of infection and in patients. *J Exp Med* 1988; 168: 449−53.

39 Kern P, Hemmer J, VanDamme J *et al.* Elevated tumor necrosis factor alpha and interleukin-6 serum levels as markers for complicated *Plasmodium falciparum* malaria. *Am J Med* 1989; 87: 139−43.

40 Bharwaj N, Santhanam U, Lau L *et al.* IL-6/IFN-β2 in synovial effusions of patients with rheumatoid arthritis and other inflammatory arthritides. *J Immunol* 1989; 143: 2153−9.

41 Waage A, Brantzaeg P, Halstensen A *et al.* The complex pattern of cytokines in serum from patients with meningiococcal septic shock. *J Exp Med* 1989; 169: 333−8.

42 VanDeventer SJH, Buller HR, ten Cate JW *et al.* Experimental endotoxemia in humans: analysis of cytokine release and coagulation, fibrinolytic, and complement pathways. *Blood* 1990; 76: 2520−6.

43 Starnes HF, Pearce MK, Tewari A *et al.* Anti-IL-6 monoclonal antibodies protect against lethal *Escherichia coli* infection and lethal tumor necrosis factor alpha challenge in mice. *J Immunol* 1990; 145: 4185−91.

44 Hirano T, Akira S, Taga T, Kishimoto T. Biological and clinical aspects of

interleukin-6. *Immunol Today* 1990; 11: 443−9.

45 Nishimoto N, Yoshizaki K, Tagoh H *et al.* Elevation of serum interleukin 6 prior to acute phase proteins on inflammation by surgical operation. *Clin Immunol Immunopathol* 1989; 50: 399−401.

46 Van Oers MHJ, Van Der Heyden A, Aarden LA. Interleukin-6 (IL-6) in serum and urine of renal transplant recipients. *Clin Exp Immunol* 1988; 71: 314−9.

47 Grossman RM, Kreuger J, Yourish D *et al.* Interleukin-6 is expressed at high levels in psoriatic skin and stimulates proliferation of cultured human keratinocytes. *Proc Natl Acad Sci USA* 1989; 86: 6367−71.

48 Horii Y, Muraguchi A, Iwano M *et al.* Involvement of IL-6 in mesangial proliferative glomerulonephritis. *J Immunol* 1989; 143: 3949−55.

49 Ruef C, Budde K, Lacy J *et al.* Interleukin 6 is an autocrine growth factor for mesangial cells. *Kidney Int* 1990; 38: 249−57.

50 Zoja C, Wang JM, Bettoni S *et al.* Interleukin-1-β and tumor necrosis factor-α induce gene expression and production of leukocyte chemotactic factors, colony stimulating factors, and interleukin-6 in human mesangial cells. *Am J Pathol* 1991; 138: 991−1003.

51 Waage A, Kaufmann C, Espevik T *et al.* Interleukin-6 in synovial fluid from patients with arthritis. *Clin Immunol Immunopathol* 1989; 50: 394−8.

52 Linker-Israeli M, Deans RJ, Wallace DJ *et al.* Elevated levels of endogenous IL-6 in systemic lupus erythematosus. A putative role in pathogenesis. *J Immunol* 1991; 147: 117−123.

53 Vink A, Coulie P, Warnier G *et al.* Mouse plasmacytoma growth *in vivo*: enhancement by interleukin-6 (IL-6) and inhibition by antibodies directed against IL-6 or its receptor. *J Exp Med* 1990; 172: 997−1000.

54 Hirano T. Interleukin-6 (IL-6) and its receptor: Their role in plasma cell neoplasias. *Int J Cell Cloning* 1991; 9: 166−84.

55 Levy Y, Tsapis A, Brouet J-C. Interleukin-6 antisense oligonucleotides inhibit the growth of human myeloma cell lines. *J Clin Invest* 1991; 88: 696−9.

56 Suematsu ST, Matsuda K, Aozasa N *et al.* IgG1 plasmacytosis in interleukin-6 transgenic mice. *Proc Natl Acad Sci USA* 1989; 86: 7547−51.

57 Brandt SJ, Bodine DM, Dunbar CE *et al.* Dysregulated interleukin 6 expression produces a syndrome resembling Castleman's disease in mice. *J Clin Invest* 1990; 86: 592−9.

58 Wewers MD, Herzyk DJ. Alveolar macrophages differ from blood monocytes in human IL-1-β release. Quantitation by enzyme-linked immunoassay. *J Immunol* 1989; 143: 1635−41.

59 Rich EA, Panuska JR, Wallis RS *et al.* Dyscoordinate expression of tumor necrosis factor-alpha by human blood monocytes and alveolar macrophages. *Am Rev Respir Dis* 1989; 139: 1010−6.

60 Rankin JA, Sylvester I, Smith S *et al.* Macrophages cultured *in vitro* release leukotriene B$_4$ and neutrophil attractant/activation protein (interleukin 8) sequentially in response to stimulation with lipopolysaccharide and zymosan. *J Clin Invest* 1990; 86: 1556−64.

61 Rom WN, Basset P, Fells GA *et al.* Alveolar macrophages release an insulin-like growth factor 1-type molecule. *J Clin Invest* 1988; 82: 1685−93.

62 Robinson BW, McLemore TL, Crystal RG. γ-Interferon is spontaneously released by alveolar macrophages and lung T lymphocytes in patients with pulmonary sarcoidosis. *J Clin Invest* 1985; 75: 1488−95.

63 Rappolee DA, Mark D, Banda MJ *et al.* Wound macrophages express TGF-α and other growth factors *in vivo*: analysis by mRNA phenotyping. *Science* 1988; 241: 708−12.

64 Assoian RK, Fleurdelys BE, Stevenson HC *et al.* Expression and secretion of type

B transforming growth factor by activated human macrophages. *Proc Natl Acad Sci USA* 1987; 84: 6020–4.

65 Nagaoka I, Trapnell BC, Crystal RG. Upregulation of platelet-derived growth factor-α and -β gene expression in alveolar macrophages of individuals with idiopathic pulmonary fibrosis. *J Clin Invest* 1990; 85: 2023–7.

66 Nathan C, Sporn M. Cytokines in context. *J Cell Biol* 1991; 113: 981–6.

67 Arend WP. Interleukin-1 receptor antagonist. A new member of the interleukin 1 family. *J Clin Invest* 1991; 88: 1445–51.

68 Hance AJ, Douches S, Winchester RJ *et al*. Characterization of mononuclear phagocyte subpopulations in the human lung using monoclonal antibodies: changes in alveolar macrophage phenotype associated with pulmonary sarcoidosis. *J Immunol* 1985; 134: 284–92.

69 Gubler U, Chua AO, Schoenhaut DS *et al*. Coexpression of two distinct genes is required to generate secreted bioactive cytotoxic lymphocyte maturation factor. *Proc Natl Acad Sci USA* 1991; 88: 4143–7.

70 The BAL Cooperative Group Steering Committee. Bronchoalveolar lavage constituents in healthy individuals, idiopathic pulmonary fibrosis, and selected comparison groups. *Am Rev Respir Dis* 1990; 141: S169–202.

71 Campbell DA, Poulter LW, Dubois RM. Immunocompetent cells in bronchoalveolar lavage reflect the cell populations in transbronchial biopsies in pulmonary sarcoidosis. *Am Rev Respir Dis* 1985; 132: 1300–06.

72 Trentin L, Migone N, Zambello R *et al*. Mechanisms accounting for lymphocytic alveolitis in hypersensitivity pneumonitis. *J Immunol* 1990; 145: 2147–54.

73 Street NE, Mosmann TR. Functional diversity of T lymphocytes due to secretion of different cytokine patterns. *FASEB J* 1991; 5: 171–7.

74 Fiorentino DF, Bond MW, Mosmann TR. Two types of mouse T helper cells. IV. Th2 clones secrete a factor that inhibits cytokine production by Th1 clones. *J Exp Med* 1989; 170: 2081–95.

75 Robinson DS, Hamid Q, Ying S *et al*. Predominant T_{H2}-like bronchoalveolar T-lymphocyte population in atopic asthma. *N Engl J Med* 1992; 326: 298–304.

76 Augustin A, Kubo RT, Sim G-K. Resident pulmonary lymphocytes expressing the γ/δ T-cell receptor. *Nature* 1989; 340: 239–41.

77 Carding SR, Allan W, Kyes S *et al*. Late dominance of the inflammatory process in murine influenza by γ/δ T cells. *J Exp Med* 1990; 172: 1225–31.

78 Balbi B, Moller DR, Kirby M *et al*. Increased numbers of T lymphocytes with γ/δ positive antigen receptors in a subgroup of individuals with pulmonary sarcoidosis. *J Clin Invest* 1990; 85: 1353–61.

79 Morita CT, Verna S, Aparicio P *et al*. Functionally distinct subsets of human γ/δ T cells. *Eur J Immunol* 1991; 21: 2999–3007.

80 Elias JA, Zitnik R, Ray P. Fibroblast immune-effector function. In: Phipps R, ed. *Pulmonary Fibroblast Heterogeneity*. Boca Raton, FL CRC Press 1992: 295–322.

81 Elias JA, Reynolds MM. Interleukin-1 and tumor necrosis factor synergistically stimulate fibroblast interleukin-1-α production. *Am J Respir Cell Biol* 1990; 3: 13–20.

82 Elias JA, Reynolds MM, Kern JA. Fibroblast interleukin-1-β: Synergistic stimulation by recombinant IL-1 and tumor necrosis factor and post-transcriptional regulation. *Proc Natl Acad Sci USA* 1989; 86: 6171–5.

83 Van Oud Alblas B, Van Der Linden-Schrever B, Van Furth R. Origin and kinetics of pulmonary macrophages during an inflammatory reaction induced by intraalveolar administration of aerosolized heat killed BCG. *Am Rev Respir Dis* 1983; 128: 276–81.

84 Paul SR, Bennett F, Calvetti JA *et al*. Molecular cloning of a cDNA encoding interleukin-11, a stromal cell-derived lymphopoietic and hematopoietic cytokine. *Proc Natl Acad Sci USA* 1990; 87: 7512–6.

85 Baggiolini M, Walz A, Kunkel SL. Neutrophil-activating peptide-1/interleukin-8, a novel cytokine that activates neutrophils. *J Clin Invest* 1989; 84: 1045—9.

86 Crouch E. Pathobiology of pulmonary fibrosis. *Am J Physiol* 1990; 259: L159—84.

87 Solis-Herruzo JA, Brenner DA, Chojkier M. Tumor necrosis factor α inhibits collagen gene transcription and collagen synthesis in cultured human fibroblasts. *J Biol Chem* 1988; 263: 5841—5.

88 Czaja MJ, Weiner FR, Eghbali M *et al*. Differential effects of γ-interferon on collagen and fibronectin gene expression. *J Biol Chem* 1987; 262: 13348—51.

89 Elias JA, Freundlich B, Adams SL *et al*. Regulation of human lung fibroblast collagen production by recombinant interleukin-1, tumor necrosis factor, and interferon-γ. *Ann N Y Acad Sci* 1990; 580: 233—44.

90 Heino J, Heinonen T. Interleukin-1-β prevents the stimulatory effect of transforming growth factor-β on collagen gene expression in human skin fibroblasts. *Biochem J* 1990; 271: 827—30.

91 Kahari V-M, Chen YQ, Su MW *et al*. Tumor necrosis factor-α and interferon-γ suppress the activation of human Type I collagen gene expression by transforming growth factor-β1. *J Clin Invest* 1990; 86: 1489—95.

92 Elias JA, Freundlich B, Kern JA *et al*. Cytokine networks in the regulation of inflammation and fibrosis in the lung. *Chest* 1990; 97: 1439—45.

93 Kern JA, Lamb RJ, Reed JC *et al*. Dexamethasone inhibition of interleukin-1-β production by human monocytes. *J Clin Invest* 1988; 81: 237—44.

94 North RJ, Havell EA. Glucocorticoid-mediated inhibition of endotoxin-induced intratumor necrosis factor production and tumor hemorrhagic necrosis and regression. *J Exp Med* 1989; 170: 703—10.

95 Glick AB, Flanders KC, Danielpour D *et al*. Retinoic acid induces transforming growth factor-β2 in cultured keratinocytes and mouse epidermis. *Cell Regul* 1989; 1: 87—97.

96 Vadjan-Raj S, Buescher S, LeMaistre A *et al*. Stimulation of hematopoiesis in patients with bone marrow failure and in patients with malignancy by recombinant human granulocyte—macrophage colony-stimulating factor. *Blood* 1988; 72: 134—41.

97 Kojima S, Fukuda M, Miyajima Y *et al*. Treatment of aplastic anemia in children with recombinant human granulocyte colony-stimulating factor. *Blood* 1991; 77: 937—41.

98 Rosenberg SA, Packard BS, Aebersold PM *et al*. Use of tumor infiltrating lymphocytes and IL-2 in the immunotherapy of patients with metastatic melanoma. A preliminary report. *N Engl J Med* 1989; 319: 1676—80.

99 Rodolfo M, Sulvey C, Bassi C *et al*. Adoptive immunotherapy of mouse carcinoma with recombinant interleukin-2 alone or combined with lymphokine activated killer cells or tumor immune lymphocytes: survival benefit of adjuvant, postsurgical treatments in comparison with experimental metastasis model. *Cancer Immunol Immunother* 1990; 31: 28—36.

100 Halperin DS, Estrov Z, Freedman MH. Diamond—Blackfan anemia: promotion of marrow hematopoiesis *in vitro* by the use of recombinant IL-3. *Blood* 1989; 73: 1168—74.

101 Jaffe HA, Buhl R, Mastrangeli A *et al*. Organ specific cytokine therapy. Local activation of mononuclear phagocytes by delivery of an aerosol of recombinant interferon-γ to the human lung. *J Clin Invest* 1991; 88: 297—302.

102 Culver K, Cornetta K, Morgan R *et al*. Lymphocytes as cellular vehicles for gene therapy in mouse and man. *Proc Natl Acad Sci USA* 1991; 88: 3155—9.

103 Nabel EG, Plautz G, Nabel GJ. Site-specific gene expression *in vivo* by direct gene transfer into the arterial wall. *Science* 1990; 249: 1285—8.

104 Brigham KL, Meyrick B, Christman B *et al*. Rapid communication: *in vivo*

transfection of murine lungs with a functioning prokaryotic gene using a liposome vehicle. *Am J Med Sci* 1989; 298: 278−81.

105 Rosenfeld MA, Siegfried W, Yoshimura K *et al*. Adenovirus-mediated transfer of a recombinant α1-antitrypsin gene to the lung epithelium *in vivo*. *Science* 1991; 252: 431.

106 Rosenfeld MA, Yoshimura K, Trapnell BC *et al*. *In vivo* transfer of the human cystic fibrosis transmembrane conductance regulator gene to the airway epithelium. *Cell* 1992; 68: 143−55.

107 Opal SM, Cross AS, Sadoff JC *et al*. Efficacy of antilipopolysaccharide and anti-tumor necrosis factor monoclonal antibodies in a neutropenic rat model of pseudomonas sepsis. *J Clin Invest* 1991; 88: 885−90.

108 Deguchi Y, Kishimoto S. Tumor necrosis factor/cachectin plays a key role in autoimmune pulmonary inflammation in lupus-prone mice. *Clin Exp Immunol* 1991; 85: 392.

109 Piguet PF, Collart MA, Grau GE *et al*. Tumor necrosis factor/cachectin plays a key role in bleomycin-induced pneumopathy and fibrosis. *J Exp Med* 1989; 170: 655−63.

110 Piguet PF, Collart MA, Grau GE *et al*. Requirement of tumor necrosis factor for development of silica-induced pulmonary fibrosis. *Nature* 1990; 344: 245−7.

111 Durum SK, Mealy K. Hilton Head revisited — cytokine explosion of the 80s takes shape for the 90s. *Immunol Today* 1990; 11: 103−6.

112 Fanslow WC, Sims JE, Sassenfeld H *et al*. Regulation of alloreactivity *in vivo* by a soluble form of the interleukin-1 receptor. *Science* 1990; 248: 739−42.

113 Waldmann TA, Grant A, Tendler C *et al*. Lymphokine receptor-directed therapy: a model of immune intervention. *J Clin Immunol* 1990; 10: 19S−28S.

114 Sidell N, Taga T, Hirano T *et al*. Retinoic acid-induced growth inhibition of a human myeloma cell line via down-regulation of IL-6 receptors. *J Immunol* 1991; 146: 3809−14.

115 Cominelli F, Nast CC, Clark BD *et al*. Interleukin-1 (IL-1) gene expression, synthesis, and effect of specific IL-1 receptor blockade in rabbit immune complex colitis. *J Clin Invest* 1990; 86: 972−80.

116 Gaulton GN, Markmann JE. Regulation of lymphocyte growth by antagonists of interleukin-2 or its cellular receptor. *Immunol Res* 1988; 7: 113−35.

117 Bastos MG, Pankewycz O, Rubin-Kelley VE *et al*. Concomitant administration of hapten and IL-2 toxin results in specific depletion of antigen-activated T cell clones. *J Immunol* 1990; 145: 353−9.

118 Dinarello CA, Savage N. Interleukin-1 and its receptor. *Crit Rev Immunol* 1989; 9: 1−20.

119 Smith KA. Interleukin-2: inception, impact and implications. *Science* 1988; 240: 1169−76.

120 Hatakeyama M, Tangiguchi T. Interleukin-2. In: Sporn MB, Roberts AB, eds. *Peptide Growth Factors and Their Receptors I*. New York: Springer-Verlag, 1990: 523.

121 Ihle JN. Interleukin-3. In: Sporn MB, Roberts AB eds. *Peptide Growth Factors and Their Receptors I*. New York: Springer-Verlag, 1990: 541.

122 Paul WE. Interleukin-4: a prototypic immunoregulatory lymphokine. *Blood* 1991; 77: 1859−70.

123 Honjo T, Takatsu K. Interleukin-5. In: Sporn MB, Roberts AB, eds. *Peptide Growth Factors and Their Receptors I*. New York: Springer-Verlag, 1990: 609.

124 Henney CS. Interleukin-7: effects on early events in lymphopoiesis. *Immunol Today* 1989; 10: 170−3.

125 Alderson MR, Tough TW, Ziegler SF *et al*. Interleukin-7 induces cytokine secretion and tumoricidal activity by human peripheral blood monocytes. *J Exp Med* 1991; 173: 923−30.

126 Hultner L, Druez C, Moeller J *et al.* Mast cell growth enhancing activity (MEA) is structurally related and functionally identical to the novel mouse T cell growth factor P40 (interleukin-9). *Eur J Immunol* 1990; 20: 1413−6.

127 Donahue RE, Yang Y-C, Clark SC. Human P40 T cell growth factor (interleukin-9) supports erythroid colony formation. *Blood* 1990; 75: 2271−5.

128 Musashi M, Yang Y-C, Paul SR *et al.* Direct and synergistic effects of interleukin-11 on murine hemopoiesis in culture. *Proc Natl Acad Sci USA* 1991; 88: 765−9.

129 Bruno E, Briddell RA, Cooper RJ *et al.* Effects of recombinant interleukin-11 on human megakaryocyte progenitor cells. *Exp Hematol* 1991; 19: 378−81.

130 Gately MK, Desai BB, Wolitzky AG *et al.* Regulation of human lymphocyte proliferation by a heterodimeric cytokine, IL-12 (cytotoxic lymphocyte maturation factor). *J Immunol* 1991; 147: 874−82.

131 Beutler B, Cerami A. The biology of cachectin/TNF, a primary mediator of the host response. *Annu Rev Immunol* 1989; 7: 625−55.

132 Rosenblum MG, Donato NJ. Tumor necrosis factor α: multifaceted peptide hormone. *Crit Rev Immunol* 1989; 9: 21−44.

133 Tracey KJ, Lowry SF, Cerami A. Cachectin/TNF-α in septic shock and septic adult respiratory distress syndrome. *Am Rev Respir Dis* 1988; 138: 1377−9.

134 Martich GD, Danner RL, Ceska M, Suffredini AF. Detection of interleukin-8 and tumor necrosis factor in normal humans after intravenous endotoxin: the effect of antiinflammatory agents. *J Exp Med* 1991; 173: 1021−41.

135 Hunninghake GW. Release of interleukin-1 by alveolar macrophages of patients with active pulmonary sarcoidosis. *Am Rev Respir Dis* 1984; 129: 569−72.

136 Bachwich PR, Lynch JP, Larrick J *et al.* Tumor necrosis factor production by human sarcoid alveolar macrophages. *Am J Pathol* 1986; 125: 421−5.

137 Tazi A, Nioche S, Chastre J *et al.* Spontaneous release of granulocyte colony-stimulating factor (G-CSF) by alveolar macrophages in the course of bacterial pneumonia and sarcoidosis: endotoxin-dependent and endotoxin-independent G-CSF release by cells recovered by bronchoalveolar lavage. *Am J Respir Cell Mol Biol* 1991; 4: 140−7.

138 Itoh A, Yamaguchi E, Kuzumaki N *et al.* Expression of granulocyte−macrophage colony-stimulating factor mRNA by inflammatory cells in the sarcoid lung. *Am J Respir Cell Mol Biol* 1990; 3: 245−9.

139 Kreipe H, Radzun HJ, Heidorn K *et al.* Proliferation, macrophage colony-stimulating factor, and macrophage colony-stimulating factor-receptor expression of alveolar macrophages in active sarcoidosis. *Lab Invest* 1990; 62: 697−703.

140 Hancock WW, Muller WA, Cotran RS. Interleukin 2 receptors are expressed by alveolar macrophages during pulmonary sarcoidosis and are inducible by lymphokine treatment of normal human lung macrophages, blood monocytes, and monocyte cell lines. *J Immunol* 1987; 138: 185−191.

141 Eden E, Turino GM. Interleukin-1 production from human alveolar macrophages in lung disease. *J Clin Immunol* 1986; 6: 326−33.

142 Carre PC, Mortenson RL, King TE *et al.* Increased expression of the interleukin-8 gene by alveolar macrophages in idiopathic pulmonary fibrosis, a potential mechanism for the recruitment and activation of neutrophils in lung fibrosis. *J Clin Invest* 1991; 88: 1802−10.

143 Martinet Y, Rom WN *et al.* Exaggerated spontaneous release of platelet-derived growth factor by alveolar macrophages from patients with idiopathic pulmonary fibrosis. *N Engl J Med* 1987; 1317: 202−9.

144 Khalil N, O'Connor RN, Unruh HW *et al.* Increased production and immuno-histochemical localization of transforming growth factor-β in idiopathic pulmonary fibrosis. *Am J Respir Cell Mol Biol* 1991; 5: 155−62.

18 Gene therapy

ROBERT A. STOCKLEY

Introduction

As our basic understanding of the processes of gene control and their implications for cell replication, protein production and the control of tissue damage and repair increases, the potential for interfering at several stages with molecular biological technology will also advance. Indeed, many examples have been cited in the preceding chapters where the potential of molecular biological methods is already being explored, and in some cases used, to influence disease states.

For instance, lung tumours have been associated with overexpression of the *myc* oncogenes [1]. The product of this gene is a known growth factor and its uncontrolled production has been implicated in many human tumours. Why this oncogene escapes normal regulatory control is largely unknown, but in some tumours the messenger RNA (mRNA) produced is abnormal and can contain extra sequences derived from the introns [2] as shown in Fig. 18.1. This provides a novel potential approach to therapy. The introduction of oligonucleotides into replicating cells can inactivate appropriate complementary species of mRNA. In the case of the abnormal *myc* oncogene transcript a probe can be developed that is specific for the abnormal mRNA. Introduction of this probe will inactivate the abnormal mRNA but not hybridize with any normal *myc* mRNA, which should be under cellular control and hence not mitogenic (Fig. 18.1).

Alternative methodologies may also exist to deal with malignant disease. One such approach was mentioned in Chapter 1, where a chimeric protein had been produced through molecular biological methods consisting of the diphtheria toxin coupled to a binding region for the interleukin-2 receptor. This enables a cytotoxic protein to be targeted to cells which only express the relevant receptor. The approach has been used successfully in haematological malignancy [3], but may have a potential role in lung tumours if introduced via the airways and/or intravenously.

Clearly, the benefits of such an approach would be enormous in lung malignancy, which is one of the major forms of solid tumour and where overall prognosis is poor. However, at the moment our understanding of oncogene expression and the role of anti-oncogenes and other controlling factors of cell replication is relatively patchy.

344

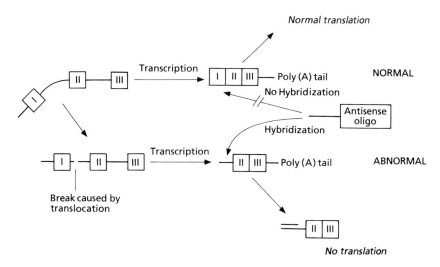

Fig. 18.1 Use of specific antisense oligonucleotide to inactivate abnormal mRNA produced by translocation of exon 1 and exon/intron splice region. From McManaway ME, Neckers LM, Loke SL *et al. Lancet*, 1990; 335: 808–11.

On the other hand, knowledge about gene deficiency states and their relationship to respiratory disease is more advanced. Furthermore, it seems conceptually easier to replace or supplement a deficient gene and its product than to control overexpression of a normal cellular control system. For this reason technological developments have advanced more rapidly and generated more interest in the field of gene replacement.

α_1-Antitrypsin deficiency and cystic fibrosis (associated with deficient membrane expression of the cystic fibrosis transmembrane conducting regulator) are the most common inherited diseases of white people (approximately 1 in 2000 live births for each). Both are associated with significant morbidity and mortality primarily as a result of progressive destructive lung disease. The genetic defects responsible for these diseases are becoming well defined and there is a great deal of activity directed towards the possibility of gene therapy.

α_1-Antitrypsin deficiency

A variety of genetic defects have been identified leading to α_1-antitrypsin deficiency. These include rare defects, such as gene deletion [4], point mutations leading to premature termination of transcription [5] and the production of unstable mRNA [6]. However, by far the most common severe deficiency state is the Z allele characterized by a point mutation resulting in a change of the amino acid at position 342 from glutamic acid to lysine [7]. Although this does not affect gene transcription [8], or translation [9], the defect results in polymerization of the protein and its retention at the rough endoplasmic reticulum [10]. The net result is greatly decreased secretion of the protein resulting in plasma and lung deficiency. It is believed that low to absent levels of α_1-antitrypsin in the lung are related to unopposed tissue damage by enzymes normally controlled by the α_1-antitrypsin [11].

Thus, in theory, if the lung can be altered to produce sufficient of its own α_1-antitrypsin it should be able to protect itself from the destructive effects of the enzymes normally controlled by the inhibitor.

Cystic fibrosis

This disease is characterized by abnormalities of the cystic fibrosis trans-membrane conductive regulator (CFTR) gene on chromosome 7. The common mutation (70% of cases) is the deletion of the codon for phenylalanine at position 508 [12]. The disease is associated with a defect in the function of the cellular chloride channel [13] and replacement of the gene *in vitro* 'normalizes' the defective channel [14]. Although it is possible that CFTR plays a critical role in intracellular protein processing [15], it is generally believed that the defective chloride channel results in abnormal mucus production in the airways. This in turn results in mucus retention, bacterial colonization, an associated inflammatory response and epithelial damage.

If this hypothesis is true the introduction of the normal CFTR gene into the airways should correct the chloride defect and return mucus production to normal, thereby breaking the chain of events.

Gene delivery

For effective gene delivery a system has to be devised to introduce the required sequence into an appropriate cell so that it can generate its product. At present several potential delivery systems are being studied although it is likely that more will be devised.

Two physical means of delivery have shown promise. First, the transfer of plasmid DNA in liposomes. This method has the advantages of the use of highly purified, well-characterized DNA and stable integration of DNA into the cells is not required. However, gene expression is only transient and it is necessary to repeat therapy frequently.

Second, the DNA can be bound to a ligand which is recognized by specific receptors on the target cell. For instance, complexing of DNA with transferrin results in DNA transfer to target cells that express the transferrin receptor [16]. Again the agent is highly purified and more prolonged expression can be obtained. Recent studies *in vivo* with Nagase analbuminaemic rats have shown that the albumin gene can be transferred to cells if attached to an asialoglycoprotein, which binds to and is internalized by its respective hepatocyte receptor. If in addition cell replication occurs, gene expression can be prolonged for several weeks [17].

The alternative to these physical means has been the development of viral vectors to deliver the genes by 'infecting' the target cell. At present most work has been carried out with either retroviruses or, more recently, adenovirus vectors.

Retroviral vectors

Retroviruses used as vectors are those in which all viral genes have been removed or altered so that 'infection' of the cell does not result in the production of viral proteins and hence viral replication. However, in order to generate sufficient viruses for gene transfer, initial replication is carried out in a retrovirus packaging cell, which does produce the viral proteins but does not have the ability to replicate. Thus if the DNA form of the retrovirus vector is introduced into these cells they produce virions that carry vector RNA and can infect target cells but will not thereafter replicate and spread.

The vector RNA codes for reverse transcriptase and the relevant gene product, together with relevant transcription control elements. Once inside the cell the released RNA makes reverse transcriptase and thereby converts itself into DNA, which becomes incorporated as a functional gene in the cellular genome. This process is shown diagrammatically in Fig. 18.2.

This approach has been shown to introduce the α_1-antitrypsin gene into animal cells *in vitro* resulting in secretion of the protein [18]. Furthermore, when these cells are implanted into the peritoneal cavity of experimental animals the protein can be detected in the plasma and lung [18]. In a similar way the normal CFTR gene can be transferred into human cell lines or epithelial cells derived from cystic fibrosis patients and will correct the abnormal chloride channel [14, 19].

The whole process of gene transfer using retroviruses is termed **transduction** to differentiate it from the normal infective process leading to viral replication, cell death and viral spread. The process is highly efficient in replicating cells and the integration of the genes into the cellular genome is precise and stable. However, there are several major disadvantages especially if the target is the human lung epithelium. First, the retrovirus vectors are unable to 'infect' non-replicating cells [20], which form the majority in the airways. Second, it is difficult to be sure of the characterization of the preparations because they are made by cultured cells. Retrovirus vectors are complex mixtures of protein and nucleic acids and may become contaminated with replication competent retroviruses that may be present in the packaging cells. In addition, cellular RNA species may be included in the virion and, since they cannot be removed, they may become incorporated in the target cell

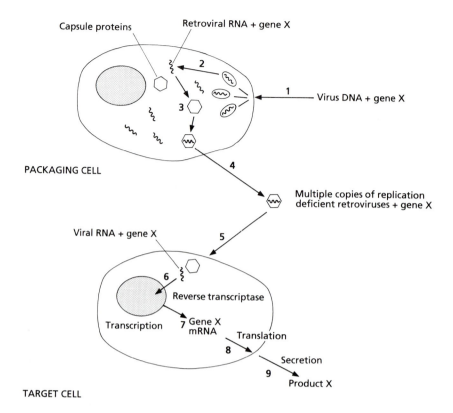

Fig. 18.2 Diagrammatic representation of methodology required for gene delivery using retroviruses. Step 1 — introduction of virus DNA into packaging cell; step 2 — generation of viral RNA; step 3 — packaging of viral RNA with capsule proteins produced by packaging cell; step 4 — harvesting; step 5 — 'infection' of target cell; step 6 — transfer of virus DNA to cell genome; step 7 — transcription of target gene; step 8 — translation of target gene; step 9 — secretion of product.

genome [21]. The implications of this complication have to be determined.

Another major potential hazard is the possibility of mutagenesis as a result of activation of an oncogene by insertion of the new gene. This problem may remain theoretical as retroviral activation of cellular onco-genes in experimental animals only occurs with spreading infection of replication competent viruses. Nevertheless, there is concern that replication defective viruses may revert to replication competent viruses, perhaps during packaging by recombination with other viral sequences in the packaging cells. Only extensive *in vivo* experimentation will deter-mine the long-term safety of the retroviral vectors.

Adenovirus vectors

More recently adenoviruses have been used as an alternative vector. These viruses have several advantages over retroviruses: first, they can carry large segments of DNA up to 36 kilobase pairs; second, they can be obtained in very high titre; and third, they can infect non-replicating cells. This latter property makes adenoviruses an attractive vector for gene delivery to the epithelial cells in the lung. In addition, recombination is rare, there are no known human malignancies associated with adenovirus infections and vaccines have been given safely.

The adenovirus vector is constructed by removal of the E3 region (to permit encapsulation of the recombinant sequence containing the exogenous gene), and part of the E1a coding sequence (to impair viral replication). The exogenous gene expression cassette consists of the gene to be delivered and the adenovirus major late promoter as well as a polyadenylation signal (see Fig. 18.3).

Using this type of vector the α_1-antitrypsin gene has been delivered into the lungs of experimental animals. The viral DNA undergoes illegitimate recombination with the epithelial cell genome and the α_1-antitrypsin gene is expressed. The isolated epithelial cells secreted α_1-antitrypsin *in vitro* and the protein can be detected in bronchial lining fluid for at least 7 days [22].

A similar study with CFTR has shown successful gene transfer *in vivo* and expression of the gene has been detected even after several weeks. Furthermore, the protein was present immunologically at least 2 weeks after transduction [23].

These early results seem encouraging. However, several problems remain. The vectors still contain many of the adenovirus genes that code for antigenic proteins and since the vector only infects non-replicating cells the 'treatment' will have to be repeated on a regular basis as old cells die and are replaced. It is likely that activation of the pulmonary immune system will render the vector ineffective due to prevention of cell infection and clearance of the virus. Furthermore, the gene may not

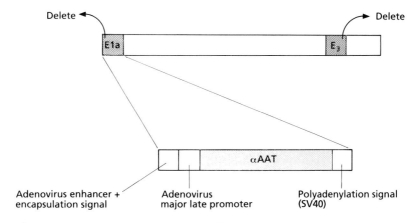

Fig. 18.3 Diagrammatic representation of construction of adenovirus DNA containing α_1-antitrypsin together with relevant controlling sequences and polyadenylation signal.

reach and be expressed in the appropriate cells or its product may not be delivered to the appropriate site. For instance, if CFTR deficiency is responsible for abnormal mucus production the gene must reach the glandular cells responsible for mucus production. In addition, delivery of the α_1-antitrypsin gene will be ineffective unless the protein is secreted into the lung interstitium where connective tissue damage by proteolytic enzymes results in the development of emphysema. Furthermore, once the diseases are established even effective gene expression may not alter disease progression. Thus, it may be more appropriate to commence therapy prior to the onset of disease, although both cystic fibrosis [24] and α_1-antitrypsin deficiency [25] show widely variable lung manifestations and hence therapy may be unnecessary for many patients.

Conclusions

The technology involved and the elegance of experiments in gene therapy are impressive and offer great potential for prevention and correction of many progressive diseases. However, at present gene replacement would only be applicable to a small minority of patients with lung disease. Targets other than those discussed above include lung fibrosis in subjects with deficient expression of the superoxide dismutase gene [26], and emphysema in subjects with cutis laxa resulting in deficient expression of the elastin gene [27]. Thus progress will depend upon overcoming problems of safety (preliminary studies of CF gene replacement have resulted in one case of severe pneumonitis that may reflect viral load), activation of immunity, frequency of administration, reaching the desired target cell and cost benefit. Nevertheless, medical science is renowned for its ingenuity and tenacity and progress will undoubtedly continue.

References

1 Nau MM, Brooks BJ, Battey J et al. L-*myc*, a new *myc*-related gene amplified and expressed in human small cell lung cancer. *Nature* 1985; 318: 69–73.
2 McManaway ME, Neckers LM, Loke SL et al. Tumor-specific inhibition of lymphoma growth by an antisense oligodeoxynucleotide. *Lancet* 1990; 335: 808–11.
3 Lemaistre CF, Rosenblum MG, Reuben JM et al. Therapeutic effects of genetically engineered toxin (DAB$_{486}$ IL-2) in patients with chronic lymphatic leukaemia. *Lancet* 1991; 337: 1124–5.
4 Takahashi H, Crystal RG. α_1Antitrypsin Null$_{isola\ de\ procida}$: a novel subclass of $\alpha_1$antitrypsin deficiency alleles caused by deletion of all $\alpha_1$antitrypsin coding of exons. *Am J Hum Genet* 1990; 47: 403–13.
5 Satoh K, Nukiwa T, Brantly M et al. Emphysema associated with complete absence of $\alpha_1$antitrypsin in serum and the homozygous inheritance of a stop codon in an $\alpha_1$antitrypsin coding exon. *Am J Hum Genet* 1988; 42: 77–83.
6 Garver RI, Mornex J-F, Nukiwa T et al. Alpha1-antitrypsin deficiency and emphy-

sema caused by homozygous inheritance of non-expressing alpha1-antitrypsin genes. *N Engl J Med* 1986; 314: 762−6.

7 Kidd VJ, Golbus MS, Wallace RB, Itakura K, Woo SLC. Prenatal diagnosis of alpha-1-antitrypsin deficiency by direct analysis of the mutation site in the gene. *N Engl J Med* 1984; 310: 639−42.

8 Mornex JF, Chytil-Weir A, Martinet Y *et al*. Expression of the alpha1-antitrypsin gene in mononuclear phagocytes of normal and alpha1-antitrypsin deficient individuals. *J Clin Invest* 1986; 77: 1952−61.

9 Verbanac KM, Heath EC. Biosynthesis processing and secretion of M and Z variant human alpha-1-antitrypsin. *J Biol Chem* 1986; 261: 9979−89.

10 Lomas DA, Evans DLC, Finch JT, Carrell RW. The mechanism of Z $\alpha_1$antitrypsin accumulation in liver. *Nature* 1992; 357: 605−7.

11 Stockley RA. Alpha-1-antitrypsin and the pathogenesis of emphysema. *Lung* 1987; 165: 61−77.

12 Kierem B, Rommens JM, Buchanan JA *et al*. Identification of the cystic fibrosis gene: genetic analysis. *Science* 1989; 245: 1073−80.

13 Widdicombe JH, Welsh MJ, Finkebeiner WE. Cystic fibrosis decreases the apical membrane chloride permeability of monolayers cultured from cells of tracheal epithelium. *Proc Natl Acad Sci USA* 1985; 82: 6167−71.

14 Rich DP, Anderson MP, Gregory RJ *et al*. Expression of cystic fibrosis transmembrane conductance regulator corrects defective chloride channel regulation in cystic fibrosis airway epithelial cells. *Nature* 1990; 347: 358−63.

15 Barasch J, Kiss B, Prince A *et al*. Defective acidification of intracellular organelles in cystic fibrosis. *Nature* 1991; 352: 70−3.

16 Curiel DT, Agarwal S, Romer MU *et al*. Gene transfer to respiratory epithelial cells via the receptor-mediated endocytosis pathway. *Am J Respir Cell Mol Biol* 1992; 6: 247−52.

17 Wu GY, Wilson JM, Shalaby F *et al*. Receptor-mediated gene delivery *in vivo*. Partial correction of genetic analbuminemia in Nagase rats. *J Biol Chem* 1991; 266: 14338−42.

18 Garver RI, Chytil A, Courtney M, Crystal RG. Clonal gene therapy: transplanted mouse fibroblast clones express human α_1-antitrypsin gene *in vivo*. *Science* 1987; 237: 762−4.

19 Drumm ML, Pope HA, Cliff WH *et al*. Correction of the cystic fibrosis defect *in vitro* by retro-virus mediated gene transfer. *Cell* 1990; 62: 1227−33.

20 Miller DG, Adam MA, Miller AD. Gene transfer by retrovirus vectors occurs only in cells that are actively replicating at the time of infection. *Mol Cell Biol* 1990; 10: 4239−42.

21 Miller AD. Retrovirus packaging cells. *Hum Gene Ther* 1990; 1: 5−14.

22 Rosenfeld MA, Siegfried W, Yoshimura K *et al*. Adenovirus-mediated transfer of a recombinant $\alpha_1$antitrypsin gene to the lung epithelium *in vivo*. *Science* 1991; 252: 431−4.

23 Rosenfeld MA, Yoshimura K, Trapnell BC *et al*. *In vivo* transfer of the human cystic fibrosis transmembrane conductance regulator gene to the airway epithelium. *Cell* 1992; 68: 143−55.

24 Kierem E, Corey M, Kerem B-S *et al*. The relationship between genotype and phenotype in cystic fibrosis − analysis of the most common mutation (ΔF_{508}). *N Engl J Med* 1990; 323: 1517−22.

25 Silverman EK, Pierce JA, Province MA, Rao DC, Campbell EJ. Variability of pulmonary function in $\alpha_1$antitrypsin deficiency: clinical correlates. *Ann Intern Med* 1989; 111: 982−91.

26 Ackerman AD, Fackler JC, Tuck-Miller CM *et al*. Partial monosomy 21, diminished activity of superoxide dismutase and pulmonary oxygen toxicity. *N Engl J Med*

1988; 318: 1666–9.

27 Olsen DR, Fazio MJ, Shambon AT, Rosenbloom J, Uitto J. Cutix laxa: reduced elastin gene expression in skin fibroblast cultures as determined by hybridization with a homologous cDNA and an Exon 1-specific oligonucleotide. *J Biol Chem* 1988; 263: 6465–7.

Index

Note: Page numbers in *italic* refer to figures; those in **bold** refer to tables